James Jackson Putnam and Psychoanalysis

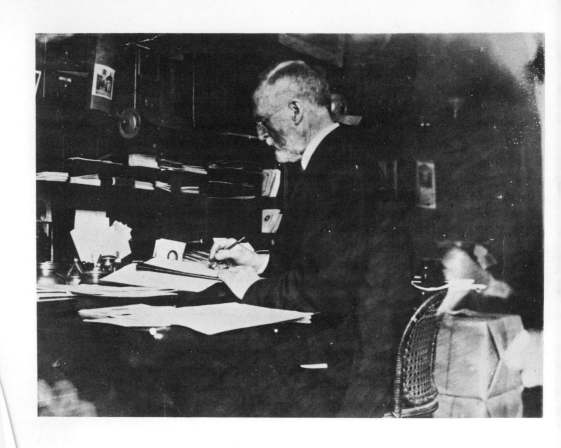

James Jackson Putnam and Psychoanalysis

Letters between Putnam and Sigmund Freud,
Ernest Jones, William James, Sandor Ferenczi,
and Morton Prince, 1877–1917

Edited with an introductory essay by Nathan G. Hale, Jr.

Translations of German texts by Judith Bernays Heller

Harvard University Press   Cambridge, Massachusetts   1971

ⓒf   A Commonwealth Fund Book

This volume is published as part of a long-standing
cooperative program between the
Harvard University Press and the Commonwealth Fund,
a philanthropic foundation,
to encourage the publication of significant
scholarly books in medicine and health.

Acknowledgments

This volume owes a heavy debt to the generosity of many people. Marian C. Putnam provided knowledge, suggestions, and patience that were inestimably helpful. Judith Bernays Heller, Professor Freud's niece, gave without stint of her invaluable knowledge of her uncle and of the early years of psychoanalysis, in addition to translating the German texts. Particular thanks are due to the late Ernst Freud, as well as to the Freud family, the London Institute of Psycho-Analysis, the Francis A. Countway Library of Medicine, Boston, Mrs. Ernest Jones, Michael Balint, Kurt Eissler and the Freud Archives, and Mrs. Morton Peabody Prince. Edmund Brill provided a Putnam letter that Ernest Jones had given to his father, A. A. Brill. Charles Moorfield Storey made available Putnam letters to his father. Thanks are due Robert Granville Hall, Eunice Winters, and Beatrice Crossman. The Clark University Library, the William Henry Welch Library of the Johns Hopkins University, and the Houghton Library of Harvard University kindly gave permission to quote from manuscripts in their possession. Ann Orlov, of the Harvard University Press, encouraged the project through a protracted period of preparation. Elizabeth Riklin, Alphonse Maeder, H. Walser, Gay Wilson Allen, Dorothy Ross supplied important data. Drs. Norman Reider, Henry Viets, and John Abbott provided information about neurology and psychoanalysis. John Clendenning and Frank Oppenheim, S.J., gave invaluable information about Josiah Royce, and the late Jacob Loewenberg read Putnam's letters to Freud, for their possible relation to Royce's philosophy. Richard Wolfe, Rare Books Librarian, and the staff of the Francis A. Countway Library of Medicine were tireless in facilitating the editorial work. Ann Bradsher, Katherine Olschki, Helga Kraft, and Helga Moldenhauer assisted with texts and editing. Ann Bradsher, Henry Farnham May, Samuel Haber, Anne Sherrill, and Drs. Norman Reider and John Abbott read the Introduction. The manuscript was typed by Marjorie E. Sprague, Ellen Wolfe, and Phyllis Fidiam.

Nathan G. Hale, Jr.

Berkeley, California
Autumn 1970

A Note on Texts

The printed text reproduces the writer's final, corrected version. This is especially important in the case of Putnam, who often crossed out and interpolated, a rarity for Freud, Jones, and Ferenczi. Whatever the occasional interest of Putnam's changes, their retention would have resulted in a text burdensome for the reader. About one-third of Putnam's letters were typewritten, probably by a secretary; letters of the other correspondents were handwritten. Original spellings and abbreviations have been preserved with this exception: ampersands or their equivalent have been transcribed as "and." Freud wrote two letters to Putnam, those of January 22, 1911, and January 26, 1916, in Roman script, the rest in Gothic. The following letters were transcribed by the Freud Archives: May 14, 1911; November 5, 1911; Christmas, 1911; March 28, 1912; June 25, 1912; July 18, 1912; August 20, 1912; November 28, 1912; December 3, 1912; January 1, 1913; January 21, 1913; March 11, 1913; November 13, 1913; March 30, 1914; May 17, 1914; June 19, 1914. The other Freud letters and all the Ferenczi letters were transcribed by Judith Bernays Heller, who retained the original spellings. Originals of the Freud-Putnam letters are in the Freud Archives, Library of Congress. The holographs of Putnam's letters to Jones are in the Jones Papers in the London Institute of Psycho-Analysis. The original of the letter of Putnam to Jones, February 24, 1911, is in the Brill Archives, Library of Congress. Unless otherwise noted, originals of all other letters and documents are in the Putnam Papers, the Francis A. Countway Library of Medicine, Boston.

Shortened Forms and Abbreviations

Ad Psa   James Jackson Putnam, *Addresses on Psycho-Analysis* (London, Vienna, New York: The International Psycho-Analytical Press, 1921).

PPsa   Ernest Jones, *Papers on Psycho-Analysis* (London: Baillière Tindall and Cox, 1913; New York: William Wood and Co., 1913). Revised editions were issued by both publishers in 1918, 1924, 1938, 1948.

SE   *The Standard Edition of the Complete Psychological Works of Sigmund Freud*, trans. from the German under the general editorship of James Strachey, in collaboration with Anna Freud, with the assistance of Alix Strachey and Alan Tyson, and with Angela Richards as editorial assistant, vols. I–XXIII (London: The Hogarth Press and the Institute of Psycho-Analysis, 1953–1966).

Jahrbuch   *Jahrbuch für psychoanalytische und psychopathologische Forschungen* [Yearbook for Psychoanalytic and Psychopathological Research].

Zentralblatt   *Zentralblatt für Psychoanalyse. Medizinische Monatschrift für Seelenkunde* [Journal for Psychoanalysis. Medical Monthly for Psychology].

Zeitschrift   *Internationale Zeitschrift für ärztliche Psychoanalyse* [International Journal for Medical Psychoanalysis]. With volume 6, "ärztliche" was dropped from the title.

Ψ The Greek letter psi occasionally was used by the correspondents to stand for the first element of psychoanalysis.

Contents

Foreword

BY MARIAN C. PUTNAM

In Freud's essay "On the History of the Psychoanalytic Movement," he wrote of my father: "The esteem he enjoyed throughout America on account of his high moral character and unflinching love of truth was of great service to psycho-analysis and protected it against the denunciations which in all probability would otherwise have overwhelmed it." *

Like Freud, my father was educated in the classical tradition and was a tremendous worker. A poor sleeper, he did most of his reading and writing between three and seven or eight in the morning, when he began to see patients at home or took his daily exercise, running at a dogtrot along the Charles River to the Massachusetts General Hospital, where he had early established an outpatient clinic for nervous diseases, or he went to the Harvard Medical School to teach.

His practice was an active one, and no mealtime went by that he was not called to the telephone at least two or three times. His offices were on the first floor of our house, and as children we were expected to pass through the hallway quickly and without noise. We were admonished never to disclose the identity of a patient we might have seen entering the house, and we were forbidden to use the word "nervous," an invidious term which my father believed described neither his patients nor their problems.

His family and close friends knew him as a charming, gentle, overconscientious person — though by no means without humor — slow to anger, public-spirited, thoughtfully purposeful in his every undertaking, whether personal or professional. Even while gardening or sailing on summer weekends with his family in Cotuit on Cape Cod, or mountain climbing, reading, and con-

* "Zur Geschichte der psychoanalytischen Bewegung," *Jahrbuch der Psychoanalyse,* 6 (1914), 228; SE, XIV, 31.

versing in his beloved Adirondacks for the vacation month of September, he was constantly thinking about problems philosophical, social, or artistic. He loved the beauty and mysteries of nature, describing them eloquently in innumerable letters. He loved music, took part in group singing, and encouraged his children to play some instrument or sing German lieder while he accompanied them on the piano. When I, the least expressive of the family, was the soloist, he used to urge me, "Make them cry!" He was keenly interested in his children's development, eager that they should live up to the highest principles and work and learn as avidly as he himself had done. While I was studying German, he wrote to me exclusively in that language.

My father was thirty-eight when he married Marian Cabot, eleven years his junior, with whom he had already shared years of work in the Associated Charities of Boston. They often had met with a small group of his cousins and friends to read poetry and discuss philosophy; but above all they had been companions at the "Shanty" in the Adirondack Mountains for two or three weeks each summer.

In contrast to my father, who was the youngest of four in a reserved household, my mother came from a large affectionate family of eight brothers and sisters and many cousins who lived within walking distance of each other. Her diary before her marriage showed that she visited some close relative — grandmother, aunt, married sister or close friend — practically every day of her life. If she were separated from them, she kept in constant touch by letter; and after her marriage she and my father wrote to each other every day that they were apart. She was a conservative, practical person, who maintained a well-ordered, hospitable household for her busy husband, their five children, and my father's oldest sister. My mother was greatly beloved by her children's friends, who came frequently to the house. My father valued her intelligent common sense, occasionally coming upstairs from his office to seek her advice about some patient's family problems. She was sympathetic with all his interests, and loved to listen to his philosophic discussions with William James and others.

Nothing, however, in my father's background or hers prepared her for his interest in psychoanalysis. When he accepted the validity of this new science, she reacted with tragic bitterness, feeling that he had been mistakenly lured into a false path which would ruin his professional standing. His practice indeed did fall off, for her view was shared by many of his colleagues. Nevertheless when in 1920 she was asked to send his psychoanalytic manuscripts and reprints to form the first volume published by the International Psychoanalytical Press, she not only complied but contributed financially to the publication.

I have little recollection of his early interest in psychoanalysis, except that occasionally a few strange men assembled in my father's library. They were not invited upstairs to join the family, nor were their discussions reported to us by my father.

Unfortunately I had to undergo an appendectomy in Boston just before the memorable visit of Drs. Freud, Jung, and Ferenczi to our camp in the Adirondacks. I know only that Mrs. Henry Bowditch, herself a German, had decked out the camp in German emblems in their honor, only to find that they were respectively Austrian, Swiss, and Hungarian.

From this time on there was no turning back for my father. Already he had begun to verify some of the conclusions of psychoanalysis. His personal acquaintance with Freud confirmed his commitment. Open-mindedness and love of truth were qualities many had admired in him. No one was too simple or too young to receive a serious hearing from him. New ideas and new light on old ideas were his meat and drink. But open-mindedness did not preclude steadfastness, a quality illustrated by the following letter to me, which was jotted down one sleepless night while we were all in Paris a month or two before the 1911 Psychoanalytic Congress in Weimar:

1911

Midnight reflections for what they are worth —

Dear Molly

I woke up at midnight (an hour and a half or more ago) with the beginnings of 40 things going through my mind, part of them suggested by what you said, part by a letter of Cousin Fanny Morse's, part by the general tendency to think over my paper forever and ever, part by too much café au Pré Catelain, and after vainly trying other means of getting rid of them I am now trying this means, which is at least a pleasant one.

You said, with good reason, that London and Paris make Boston seem tiny, but it is true for more reasons than that of size.

Travelling as we do it is hard to get hold of the real life and inner history of the places we see, but if we could get this it would outway all the rest in richness and significance. Real history, whether of individuals or nations, means the series of efforts through which men have, half blindly, tried to find freedom and express love. Read, for example, Victor Hugo's Les Misèrables and take even the accounts he gives (unless I greatly err) of the "gamins" of Paris, homeless boys who used to eat what they could get and sleep under the arches of the bridges, but who, nevertheless, had a real spirit of freedom and courage. Then take Jean himself, who carried the same spirit a stage further.

Then consider the extraordinary courage the resentful poor have shown, the great if terrible Revolution and the many barricades, so bravely defended. Then consider what a change has come over the whole people and how the spirit of the Hugenots has prevailed gradually more and more, even permeating the Government, which has become a Government of the people. Then think of the many good institutions of reform, such as those that Aunt Bessie came over to hear and talk about, years ago.

The only fault that I have to find with Cousin Fanny Morse is that which at heart she believes. I am sure that what I said is true, — namely, that history, at bottom, is an account of the efforts of men to find freedom and show love — yet she is sometimes impatient with the particular efforts of particular men, to bring about these results. She is too much governed by the fact that such men are often distasteful to her, either personally or in their methods, or that they show too little respect for the *good* things and beautiful things of the past. Of course I admit that but I feel strongly that one can't stay on both sides of the fence, and for my part I throw in my lot with the radicals and the reformers.

Or rather, I will say this: I shall try to keep free from any general promises or general conclusions except where some important issue is at stake, but I shall try, above all, to see that I do not let personal comfort and prejudice stand in the way of *the people's* progress. So, *on the whole,* I feel much more than formerly inclined to go in for socialistic movements and to see the good side of the men who are devoting themselves to such schemes. For similar reasons I have given up taking wine, simply because its use is a curse to the people as a whole and there is a *practical chance* to create a sentiment against it. The most important movements in history have been and will be the (unpicturesque) *people's movements* and the history of the King-fellars is of little significance except as seen against the background of the history of *the people* and as bearing on the people's life.

Institutions, and the evidences of the *struggles of the people;* those are what we really want to see — whether at Versailles or Chartres.

Now I must go to bed.

JJP

James Jackson Putnam and Psychoanalysis

Introduction

Putnam's Role in the Psychoanalytic Movement

At sixty-three, an age when most people resist innovation, James Jackson Putnam took up the cause of psychoanalysis. One of America's most distinguished specialists in nervous diseases, a pillar of the professional life of Boston, he seemed an unlikely acquisition for the beleaguered young psychoanalytic movement. After 1905 when Freud's theories became more widely known in Europe and America they were vigorously denounced as mystical and pornographic. Putnam's reputation for unimpeachable integrity and scientific acumen played a crucial role in the American reception of psychoanalysis. Although he saw himself as neither unusually courageous nor given to controversy, he secured a hearing for Freud's views among the nation's neurologists, and his prestige greatly facilitated the organization of the American Psychoanalytic Association. Putnam's conversion is all the more surprising because in 1906 he had published the first clinical test of psychoanalysis in an English-speaking country and had concluded that Freud's claims were stimulating but exaggerated.

Two personal encounters altered Putnam's attitude. In December 1908, he met Ernest Jones, a brash twenty-nine-year-old demonstrator in psychiatry at the University of Toronto who was visiting Boston to present Freud's views. The following September he met Freud, who had traveled to Worcester, Massachusetts, to receive his first academic honor at tiny, unorthodox Clark University. Putnam held long and earnest discussions with both men.

The correspondence that followed these meetings illuminates the emergence of psychoanalysis in the United States with unusual sweep and clarity. These letters shed unexpected light on the personalities of the psychoanalytic pioneers who revealed themselves to each other with special frankness. They discussed not only their patients' symptoms, dreams, and parapraxes but their own. They described their anger and discouragement, as well as their sense of discovery and achievement. Sometimes they wrote hastily and impulsively, late at night or in the early morning hours, on trains, in hotels, or in the country. Candor and haste give many of these letters an unusual freshness and immediacy.

Like Ernest Jones in Toronto, Putnam at first tried out Freud's techniques alone, without the support of colleagues who shared his commitment. This isolation forced him to rely on correspondence to resolve problems of theory and method he encountered in his practice. His letters record the apprenticeship of a distinguished physician in a new historic profession. Freud presented psychoanalysis to his American friend as an open and experimental system: it was far from complete, and there was ample room for new contributions. Putnam's long experience in the treatment of nervous diseases enabled him to relate Freud's discoveries cogently to earlier developments in neurology and psychotherapy. However, Putnam's interests transcended technical details.

For seven years Putnam discussed with Freud problems of ethics and the nature of man. Putnam's American optimism, nourished in his youth on Emerson and the Unitarians, clashed with Freud's increasing disillusionment. Freud saw himself as a God forsaken "incredulous Jew." [1] Putnam cherished a universe with "love and hope in it from the start." [2] From the standpoint of a native American philosophical idealism, Putnam criticized what he believed to be the reductionist elements in Freud's position. He anticipated many of the questions later pursued by psychoanalytic ego psychologists as well as by psychotherapists outside the movement.

Putnam's stubborn insistence on moral and philosophical idealism was among the influences that led Freud to take up the study of religion and of conscience. The exchange deeply affected them both.

"You convince me," Freud wrote, "that I have not lived and worked in vain, for men such as you will see to it that the ideas I have arrived at in so much pain and anguish will not be lost to

[1] Freud to Putnam, August 18, 1910.
[2] Putnam to William James, June 25, 1910.

humanity. What more could one desire." [3] "Your visit," Putnam
insisted, "was a more significant event to me than you can easily
imagine, for it helped to change radically the whole course of my
life and thought." [4]

These letters also illuminate the transformation of psychoanalysis into an organized social movement, a development in which
Putnam played an important, if initially reluctant role. Because
the psychoanalysts needed his support and because they admired
him, they responded carefully to his questions and attempted to
meet his objections.

Freud himself, eager to preserve the integrity of his theories and
techniques, took the initiative in organizing the movement in
Europe and America.[5] He insisted on the foundation of the American Psychoanalytic Association, and these letters provide some of
the first information available about its organization. The growth
of the movement was accompanied by personal disputes and bitter
doctrinal schisms. Hoping that Putnam would not desert the
cause, Freud candidly described his reactions to these melancholy,
yet seemingly inevitable developments.

The first psychoanalysts were self-chosen and zealous advocates,
and they had a clear sense of their historic roles in an important
new movement. As a result they saved much of their correspondence. These letters are all that has survived in the possession of
the Freud, Jones, and Putnam families.[6]

Background and Encounters, 1846–1909

Putnam's New England character, which he himself regarded
with mixed feelings, provided the basis for his commitment and
his usefulness to the psychoanalytic movement. His "history," he
informed Ernest Jones, was responsible for much that was "mischievous," preventing him, for example, from writing frankly
about childhood sexuality for a lay audience.[7] Yet Putnam's tra-

[3] Freud to Putnam, September 29, 1910.
[4] Putnam to Freud, September 11, 1912.
[5] Freud to Putnam, June 16, 1910; Jones to Putnam, August 14, 1910.
[6] A single perfunctory note from Jung to Putnam about the impending Weimar
Congress has been omitted.
[7] Putnam to Jones, July 21, 1915.

dition had nourished in him a passion for professional innovation and for beleaguered causes. He was able to open doors and influence appointments not only because of his post at Harvard and his scientific attainments but because of his reputation for uncompromising idealism. In 1909, the jurist and reformer Moorfield Storey, a friend from Boston Latin School and Harvard College, was moved to write to him: "We New Englanders are an inexpressive race, and find it hard to say what we really think to each other, but it is now more than fifty years since we met and once in half a century one may be forgiven for breaking through the ice of silence. Let me therefore say to you what I have often said of you. That in all these fifty years I have no memory of you that is not delightful, and that I have never known a more absolutely unselfish, pure hearted and high minded man." [8]

Putnam absorbed a moral strenuousness and a judicious radicalism that were as much a part of his New England tradition as the "ice of silence." He was graduated from Harvard in 1866 at the age of 20. His college essays, set pieces on conventional topics, displayed many of the values, personal traits, and professional aims that marked his subsequent life. Writing in the shadow of the Civil War, Putnam urged a timely adherence to principles: large conflicts could be prevented by uncompromising early stands. Raised a Unitarian, he rejected Original Sin, yet accepted the reality of evil, the necessity of moral struggle, and the Judgment of God. A man's life was weighed by his improvement of himself and his contribution to progress, defined as the "good of the community" and the "discovery of truth." [9] Putnam's vision of progress also linked scientific knowledge and unpopular truth.

Mankind was pulled forward by a great man, "more original and more energetic than his contemporaries," who grasped a truth "far ahead of what the world is prepared to receive and then the world comes gradually from scorn and denial, to acknowledge the supremacy of the discovery and the greatness of the discoverer." [10] All the "great truths which now appear to us self-evident," were started by a minority and consequently "we should be careful how

[8] Moorfield Storey to Putnam, December 26, 1909.
[9] "Whether the Untrained Impulses of the Human Mind Incline More to Good or Evil?" [undated]; "A Death-bed's a Detector of the Heart," November 11, 1863; [Bad Examples, undated, untitled].
[10] [The Establishment of Truth, undated, untitled].

we reject a doctrine because its supporters may be few." [11] Putnam's exemplars were religious and scientific — Johannes Kepler, the astronomer, or William Ellery Channing, the Unitarian divine. Their causes required the "marvelous fanaticism," the "pure and unselfish devotion" of a Saint Francis.[12] A few years later, in a letter to Storey, Putnam argued that only those who could withstand temptation and the severest moral tests were truly virtuous.[13]

Probably from childhood, Putnam's own character had been carefully scrutinized. He was born into New England's professional aristocracy, socially secure, if not always well-to-do. His brother, Charles, two years older than he, was tireless and outgoing. His father, an early specialist in obstetrics and women's diseases, was unassuming and unobtrusive. His mother, according to family tradition, was somewhat nervous. Her father and his namesake, James Jackson, had been a founder of the Massachusetts General Hospital and acknowledged head of the medical profession in Boston. His grandfather's key and seal were given to Putnam while he was in medical school by a family friend over whom Dr. Jackson had watched during a long illness. "On the seal," she wrote, "I had engraved the arms and beautiful motto of his family which so many of them have nobly justified — uprightness and honor being their ideal of true happiness . . . May it [serve] . . . to keep his love, and holy, spotless example ever before you, so that you may live to be truly worthy of the name you bear." [14]

Putnam's mother anxiously admonished him: "Pray don't over-walk this hot weather, but do all to make yourself all right for good honest study next year." [15] She cautioned: "Some good society must not be entirely neglected, yet you are surely right in guarding carefully *any wasted* time." [16]

Not only virtue, hard work, and unpopular truth, but specialized professional knowledge contributed to progress. At Harvard Putnam expressed contempt for the polite classical education of

---

[11] "The Reasons for Free Speech," no. 10 [undated].

[12] "St. Francis," June 15, [no.] 20.

[13] Putnam to Storey, February 13, 1867, in possession of Charles Moorfield Storey.

[14] Aunt Anna [Cabot Lowell] to Putnam, October 21, 1867. "Dr. James Jackson," *Boston Medical and Surgical Journal,* 77 (September 5, 1867), 106–109, and "Charles G. Putnam, M.D.," *ibid.,* 92 (February 11, 1875), 163–165.

[15] Elizabeth Cabot Putnam to Putnam, Sunday noon [1864].

[16] Unsigned, undated, in the handwriting of Elizabeth Cabot Putnam.

young men of his social class. Instead of the "dead dogmas of Greece and Rome," it was better to study the "living ideas of the nineteenth century." His ideal was the German student who might spend a lifetime studying the "fly's wing or some other microscopic subject," or the man who devoted himself "directly or indirectly to one branch of industry or one trait of task or intellect." [17] This was a highly significant ideal in a young American when the scientific professions, including the medical specialties, were as yet largely unorganized.

Neurology, which was not at that time fully established in America, became Putnam's first important unpopular cause. Because of their increasingly detailed knowledge of the brain and nervous system, neurologists claimed to treat a wide variety of illnesses, ranging from insanity and brain tumors to headaches and hysteria. They thus aroused the ire of general practitioners and of alienists who specialized in the care of the insane. Putnam's interest in this new field probably was stimulated by Charles E. Brown-Séquard, a pioneer French-American scientist, who taught physiology and pathology at Harvard Medical School. There Putnam made a life-long friend of his fellow medical student William James and completed the three years' course in 1869. His inaugural dissertation, "A Report of Some Experiments on the Reflex Contraction of Blood Vessels," based on observations by Brown-Séquard, was published in the *Boston Medical and Surgical Journal*.[18] In 1869 he was House Pupil at the Massachusetts General Hospital.

In May of 1870 Putnam left for two years in Europe to study electrotherapeutics and neurology. His brother, who also had graduated from Harvard Medical School, already was abroad studying pediatrics. That year the first successful experiments using electrical stimulation to determine localization of brain functions were published. During the next two decades the first modern knowledge of the minute anatomy and physiology of the brain was consolidated, an achievement brilliantly summarized in William James's *Principles of Psychology*. At first some neurologists fervently believed that within the foreseeable future the operations of the brain and nervous system would be completely known and

---

[17] "On Education," Forensic I, October 6, 1865.
[18] "A Report of Some Experiments on the Reflex Contractions of Blood Vessels," *Boston Medical and Surgical Journal*, 82 (June 23, 1870), 469–472.

all nervous and mental diseases would be assigned to specific physiological causes. The zeal for physiological theorizing outran exact knowledge, and the enthusiasm of the classical, materialistic neurologists often blinded them to their own assumptions. A few of these require brief summary because all the first psychotherapists from Morton Prince to Putnam and Freud had to resolve the problems this approach created.

Neurologists devoted their primary systematic attention to the physical aspects of the brain and nervous system. Instead of focusing on psychological processes, neurologists concentrated on anatomy and pathology, sometimes in ways that were as speculative as metaphysics, a fact that later became apparent to James, to Freud, and to Putnam, if not to many neurologists. The brain was the "organ of mind," and every psychological state corresponded to a definite condition of the brain and nervous system. Complex functions of mind and brain could be analyzed into simple elements. Borrowing from faculty psychology, many neurologists assumed that mental states could be reduced to combinations of sensations and memory images. Analogously, the brain was made up of overlapping centers, each controlling a different elemental function, such as vision or speech. Inhibition and intellect were controlled by the frontal lobes of the cortex. Aphasia or disturbances of speech, caused by lesions of the brain, seemed to provide a model that bridged cerebral and psychological processes.

Nervous and mental illness, whenever possible, were ascribed to localized lesions, definite injuries to tissue. The primary model for psychiatric illness was syphilitic insanity, in which postmortem examinations revealed tangible, diffuse morbid processes.[19] Nervous and mental diseases occurred chiefly in those with defective heredity.

Many neurologists thought of the brain and the mind as closed parallel systems. A few, such as Morton Prince, began to attack this view because it seemed to preclude the influence of the mind on the body. Others, Freud among them, felt that parallelism allowed them to construct a purely psychological system of causes, without attempting to explore their correlation with physical

[19] For a transitional view that still retained much of the classical outlook, see Bernard Sachs, "Advances in Neurology and Their Relation to Psychiatry," *Proceedings of the American Medico-Psychological Association*, 4 (1897), 132–149.

processes. But these departures did not become influential until the 1890's.

Putnam studied in Europe with the major contributors to the new neurological knowledge — Theodore Meynert at the University of Vienna, John Hughlings Jackson in London, Jean Martin Charcot in Paris. All three profoundly influenced Freud a decade later.

Putnam's first European trip opened in May of 1870 like the traditional Grand Tour. He visited Warwick Castle, and galleries in Holland and Belgium, where Van Dyck pleased and Reubens disgusted, except for his portraits and religious paintings. Putnam traveled down the Rhine past Cologne, whose cathedral tower he hoped one day to see completed.

During the summer of 1870, he studied physiology and microscopy in Leipzig, his first taste of German research, which he described for his cousin and confidante, Miss Frances R. Morse, also a close friend of William James. "My professor of microscopy devotes his whole time to teaching and studying that science for almost no pay and we have a fine laboratory, I believe at the expense of the King of Saxony." He wrote to his father contrasting the German emphasis on "pure science" and the "discovery of as many physiological facts as possible, whether apparently important or not" with the scientific ignorance of such eminent Boston physicians as Oliver Wendell Holmes.[20]

That winter in Vienna, he worked on the anatomy of the brain with Meynert, and volunteered to complete a translation of Meynert's "On the Brain of Mammals," which was published in the United States in 1872.[21] Putnam was impressed by Meynert's lectures on Mental Diseases during which he "touched on the Mechanism of Thought in a very masterly and scientific manner." Meynert's pathology of the brain was based on 800 specimens which he had weighed and examined himself although it was rumored that Frau Meynert had sliced the best specimens herself. Putnam also

[20] Putnam to Frances Morse [1870]; Putnam to Charles Gideon Putnam, Leipzig, July 11, 1870. Franz Schweigger-Seidel (1834–1871) was professor of histology and Carl Ludwig (1816–1895), of physiology in the University of Leipzig.

[21] Putnam to Elizabeth Cabot Putnam, Vienna, September 9, 1871, and October 12, [1871]. The translation appeared in Professor S. Stricker, *A Manual of Histology* (New York: William Wood, 1872), pp. 650–766; Putnam to his sister Annie [Putnam], Vienna, October 27, 1871.

studied electrotherapeutics with Moritz Benedikt, whom he judged to be a "random harum-scarum empiric." Putnam resolved to avoid becoming a mere "electropath," a "battery-doctor" who mechanically specialized in a newfashioned treatment rather than in a profound knowledge of disease and diagnosis.[22]

The next winter was passed in Berlin with his Harvard classmate, the physician Edward Emerson, fourth son of Ralph Waldo Emerson. They lived in "two scraps of rooms" into which the sun never shone and where they were visited by the white-haired American Ambassador, George Bancroft, who had known Dr. Jackson. Putnam studied at the medical school and its hospital, the Charité, which had a famous section devoted to nervous diseases. He followed the lectures of the great Rudolph Virchow, who taught pathology, "really systematically." [23] On the way home, he listened briefly in Paris to the great neurologist Jean Martin Charcot and saw the famous physiologist Claude Bernard, a "fine looking old man in a velvet cap and fur-trimmed coat." [24] By 1872 Putnam had mastered German, wrote tolerable French, and had absorbed the most up-to-date knowledge of the brain and nervous system. He was impressed by the specialized outpatient departments of the European hospitals, where "several men may be teaching the same subject *every day* without interfering with each other," and he hoped to introduce a similar system at home.[25] Above all, he had absorbed the German insistence on careful laboratory techniques and demonstrable somatic causes.

On his return to Boston in the spring of 1872, he found his brother already specializing in pediatrics and becoming a leader in the city's charitable and social work. Putnam himself, according to tradition, set up a neurological laboratory in his own home. He collaborated with William James and Henry Pickering Bowditch in experiments on the localization of brain functions. Throughout his life he made important contributions to organic neurology — studies of adult poliomyelitis, paraesthesia of the

[22] Putnam to Elizabeth Cabot Putnam, Berlin, February 2, 1872; Putnam to Elizabeth Cabot Putnam, Vienna, March 27, 1871; Putnam to Lillie [?], Vienna, September 21, 1871.

[23] Putnam to Elizabeth Cabot Putnam, Berlin, November 24, 1871; Putnam to Elizabeth Cabot Putnam, Berlin, March 4, 1872.

[24] Putnam to Elizabeth Cabot Putnam, Paris, April 23, 1872.

[25] Putnam to Elizabeth Cabot Putnam, Vienna, December 13, 1870.

hands, system diseases of the spinal cord, brain tumors. In 1874 Putnam became a founder of the American Neurological Association and in 1888 served as president.[26]

Putnam's successive changes of title reflect the growing recognition of neurology as a distinct specialty. In 1872 he was appointed "Electrician" at the Massachusetts General Hospital, in charge of its "magnetic and electric apparatus"; a year later this became "Physician to Out-Patients with Diseases of the Nervous System." He worked in a small room on a small budget, treating patients, many of them immigrants, whose troubles ranged from paresis to hysteria. In 1873 he became Lecturer on the Application of Electricity in Nervous Diseases at Harvard Medical School. In 1874 his title was changed to Instructor in Diseases of the Nervous System and in 1893 he became Harvard's first full professor of that subject.

In 1874, braving the scorn of plumbers, Putnam began painstaking research on lead and arsenic that involved him in problems of industrial medicine and community health. He concluded that lead water pipes and the manufacture of rubber articles caused far more lead poisoning than had been suspected. He also established that arsenic poisoning from wallpaper and cloth was common and called for legislative protection against this "widespread public danger." [27]

Putnam's next unpopular cause was the medical education of women. In 1879 he vainly urged the Harvard Medical School to admit them. The University of Zurich, he argued, already had been successfully training women in medicine, and there was a growing demand for their services. Such women were not, as the *Boston Medical and Surgical Journal* alleged, "nihilists," "advanced thinkers," or "representatives of some ephemeral sect." Women, as well as men, should benefit from the new program of four years' study demanded by the Harvard Medical School. Let us "not fall into the fallacy of maintaining that the standard in-

---

[26] William Hammond to Putnam, November 18, 1874; "Charles Pickering Putnam," *Boston Medical and Surgical Journal,* 170 (May 7, 1914), 741–742. For suggestions of a complex sibling relationship, see Putnam to Freud, September 30, 1911; Freud to Putnam, October 5, 1911; Jones to Putnam, October 31, 1911.

[27] "On Chronic Arsenic Poisoning, Especially from Wallpaper, Based on the Analysis of Twenty-five Cases in Which Arsenic was found in the Urine," *Boston Medical and Surgical Journal,* 120 (March 7, 1889), 235.

sisted on by Harvard, with so much labor, is applicable to men alone, the second best being good enough for women," he wrote.[28]

For the first ten years of his career Putnam sarcastically denounced mental therapeutics and theories of functional neurosis because they seemed unscientific.[29] Then he underwent a gradual but complete change of heart. By the mid 1890's he was experimenting with hypnosis and psychotherapy, which at the time were almost as suspect as the medical education of women. No clear distinctions then were drawn between the medical psychology of dreams and hypnosis or psychic research in thought transference and the soul's survival of bodily death. William James, Morton Prince, and, to a very limited extent, Putnam, were interested in both.[30] Many physicians, especially those outside Boston, associated mental treatment not only with spook hunting but with practitioners of Christian Science and the New Thought. These "irregulars" were stealing patients from neurologists and treating them so successfully that mental therapeutics could be dismissed no longer.[31] In Boston competition grew so brisk that segments of the medical establishment attempted to outlaw the practitioners, a proposal ardently fought by James on grounds that their therapeutic experiments were invaluable.

As a result of this unorthodox competition, Putnam and a small circle in Boston between 1890 and 1909 developed the most sophisticated and scientific psychotherapy in the English-speaking world. The Boston "school" was notable for the informal cooperation of psychologists, philosophers, neurologists, and psychiatrists. Among them were William James, Josiah Royce, and Hugo Münsterberg from Harvard, Putnam and Prince, and Edward Cowles, who directed the McLean Asylum, for generations the

[28] "Women at Zurich," *Boston Medical and Surgical Journal,* 101 (October 16, 1879), 567.

[29] "Neuralgia," in William Pepper, ed., *A System of Practical Medicine by American Authors* (Philadelphia: Lea Bros., 1886), V, 1221; see Putnam's remarks on the paper by the American neurologist George M. Beard (1839–1883), "The Influence of the Mind in the Causation and Cure of Disease — The Potency of Definite Expectation," *Journal of Nervous and Mental Disease,* 3 (July 1876), 433.

[30] All three, as well as Royce, were members of the American Society for Psychical Research. See *Proceedings of the American Society for Psychical Research,* 1 (1885–1889), 52, 572, and *Journal of the American Society for Psychical Research,* 1 (June 1907), 349.

[31] Putnam, "Remarks on the Psychical Treatment of Neurasthenia," *Boston Medical and Surgical Journal,* 132 (May 23, 1895), 505.

refuge of Boston's mentally ill "best people." James and Putnam also were in close touch with Adolf Meyer who visited from Worcester, where from 1896 to 1902 he was clinical director of the Insane Hospital and taught at Clark University.[32]

Although the Boston circle was aware of Freud's psychological work almost from its inception, he contributed little to their methods of mental treatment or their theories of the subconscious. These were based on their own original work and on the remarkable discoveries of the French psychopathologists, chiefly Charcot, Hippolyte Bernheim, and Pierre Janet. As late as 1906 Putnam interpreted Freud much as William James had first described him — as a valuable gloss on Janet.[33]

Beginning in the 1880's, it had become clear to Putnam that many symptoms he had once considered to be entirely physiological were in fact psychological in origin. From careful studies of the traumatic neuroses of working-class patients, he concluded, as had Charcot and others, that many conditions attributed to physical injury were in fact hysterical. They were also involuntary, and sometimes serious and lasting. This was an unpopular stand, because many neurologists argued that such symptoms must be deliberately simulated by patients who wanted compensation.[34]

Two other major contributions reinforced Putnam's increasingly psychological interpretation of the neuroses. Pierre Janet demonstrated that shock and strain could alter the memory so that certain

[32] See Putnam to Adolf Meyer, March 5, [1899], May 9, 1899, August 3, 1899, February 21, [1902]; William James to Adolf Meyer, February 2, 1899, November 28, 1901, September 22, 1909, in the Meyer Papers, the William H. Welch Medical Library, the Johns Hopkins University.

[33] See W.J. [William James], "Ueber den psychischen Mechanismus hysterischer Phänomene. J. Breuer und S. Freud. (Mendel's Neurol. Centralbl., 1893, pp. 4, 43)" [On the Psychical Mechanism of Hysterical Phenomena. J. Breuer and S. Freud.], *Psychological Review*, 1 (March 1894), 199. Putnam was probably acquainted with Freud's neurological work and had seen J. Mitchell Clarke's review, "Dr. Joseph Breuer and Dr. Sigmund Freud, *Studien über Hysterie*" [Studies on Hysteria], Leipzig and Vienna: F. Deuticke, 1895, which appeared in *Brain*, 19 (1896), 401–414, and F. W. H. Myers, "The Mechanism of Hysteria," *Proceedings of the Society for Psychical Research* (London), 9 (1893–1894), 12–14.

[34] "Recent Investigations into the Pathology of So-Called Concussion of the Spine," *Boston Medical and Surgical Journal*, 109 (September 6, 1883), 217–220; "Typical Hysterical Symptoms in Man Due to Injury and Their Medico-Legal Significance." Read at the tenth annual meeting of the American Neurological Association, June 18, 1884, *Journal of Nervous and Mental Disease*, 11 (July 1884), 496–501; "On the Etiology and Pathogenesis of the Post-Traumatic Psychoses and Neuroses," *Journal of Nervous and Mental Disease*, 25 (November 1898), 769–799.

ideas, usually intensely painful, became "dissociated" or "split off" from ordinary awareness. Yet, these fixed ideas remained active and could cause hallucinations, paralyses, vomiting, confusion, anesthesia, and so forth. Building on Janet, Morton Prince argued that many neurotic symptoms resulted from the association of a mental state with a physical process. Repetition and habit turned these associated conditions into autonomous mechanisms. For example, the sight of roses, real or artificial, could set off hay fever.[35]

The habit pattern, the fixed idea, the traumatic shock functioned outside the personal consciousness or the direct control of the will, presumably in that portion of the mind that carried out a command months after it had been given to a hypnotized subject or that woke the nurse with clocklike regularity. These active mental processes, dissociated from awareness, were termed subconscious. Prince called them "co-conscious" states, and Putnam, the "sub-personal consciousness." Some Boston psychologists, notably Münsterberg, argued that they were purely neural processes and involved no consciousness at all. This issue still was unresolved in 1909.[36]

Putnam developed his psychotherapy from these observations. He defined health as a moving equilibrium of conscious and subconscious, of mental and bodily processes. This coordination gave a person a consistent sense of character and the ability to act efficiently in the present. In nervous disorders, this harmony was broken, and subconscious processes dominated the personality. The therapist's task was to heal these dissociations, which, as Janet and others had demonstrated, sometimes went back to childhood.[37] By the skillful "analysis" of memory, with or without hypnosis, the "morbid chain" that led back to the original cause was discovered and assimilated. Putnam placed increasing emphasis on the analysis of memory. But he retained another method. The patient was en-

[35] "Association Neuroses: A Study of the Pathology of Hysterical Joint Affections, Neurasthenia and Allied Forms of Neuro-Mimesis, *Journal of Nervous and Mental Disease,* 18 (May 1891), 256–282, "Habit Neuroses as True Functional Diseases," *Boston Medical and Surgical Journal,* 139 (December 15, 1898), 589–592.

[36] Prince, Hugo Münsterberg et al., "A Symposium on the Subconscious," *Journal of Abnormal Psychology,* 2 (1907–1908), 22–43, 58–80, published as *Subconscious Phenomena* (Boston: Richard G. Badger, 1910); Putnam, "Not the Disease Only, but Also the Man," Shattuck Lecture (1899), Massachusetts Medical Society, *Medical Communications,* 18 (1899–1901), 64.

[37] "A Consideration of Mental Therapeutics as Employed by Special Students of the Subject," *Boston Medical and Surgical Journal,* 151 (August 18, 1904), 181.

couraged to reconceptualize his view of himself and to change his character. If a neurasthenic, he was taught not to "act out" his fears or his nervous weakness, but gradually to demonstrate his capacities and courage. As William James had shown, it was useful deliberately to adopt an attitude of hope and confidence.

A stringent critique of classical neurology accompanied the new therapy. Morton Prince, who believed in the interaction of mind and body, attacked Hughlings Jackson's theory of psycho-physical parallelism in 1885. Putnam by 1899 was denouncing heredity as the medical equivalent of false doctrines of "original sin" and "predestination." William James was insisting that men and women possessed reserves of energy they seldom utilized, thus refuting the traditional nineteenth-century wisdom that each person possessed a limited "bank account" of nervous energy, and that this could be rapidly exhausted in those who inherited a tainted constitution. The more rigid theories of brain localization and of aphasia were being discarded in the 1890's and early 1900's. Putnam insisted by 1906 that consciousness was the ultimate reality, and that a knowledge of cerebral action could only supplement what could be learned from speech and gesture.[38]

The psychotherapists prided themselves on their detailed "analytic" case histories that described the patient's whole life and on their painstaking treatment, which in some cases lasted three years or more. Putnam argued that training in psychology was as important for physicians as physics or chemistry. The new psychotherapy had become as demanding as surgery and required equally careful preparation, an analogy Freud was also fond of drawing.

Between 1904 and 1907 psychotherapy won growing but limited acceptance. It was being tried chiefly at university connected hospitals and clinics in Boston, New York, and Baltimore, and physicians across the country began experimenting with it. In 1904 Pierre Janet, the most noted of the foreign psychopathologists, lectured at the Lowell Institute in Boston and in 1906 at Harvard and

[38] "The Bearing of Philosophy on Psychiatry, with Special Reference to the Treatment of Psychasthenia," *British Medical Journal* (October 20, 1906), pp. 1021–1023, and "Not the Disease Only, but Also the Man," p. 72; Prince, *The Nature of Mind and Human Automatism* (Philadelphia: J. B. Lippincott, 1885), and "American Neurology of the Past, Neurology of the Future," *Journal of Nervous and Mental Disease,* 42 (June 1915), 445–454.

other medical schools.[39] In two respects, Janet was less optimistic than the Bostonians. Like most French physicians, he regarded nervous disorders as the result of a weakened constitution, the final product of inherited degeneracy. He often relied on suggestion and on cautious regimes that restricted his patients' activities, so as to avoid the taxing tasks, the excitements, the occasions for decision that contributed to their nervous disorders.

Studies of sexuality and oblique criticism of the prevailing reticence were an important aspect of the new psychopathology. If New Englanders often carried prudery to extremes, as William James argued, they also were among America's first students of sexuality. Morton Prince, in the 1890's, had argued that sadism and homosexuality resulted not from inherited degeneracy, then the common view, but from patterns of habit and association that had roots deep in the individual's past.[40] Josiah Royce, who was thoroughly familiar with Krafft-Ebing, informed his physician friends in Boston that disturbances in "self-consciousness," or the "self-image" as it might now be called, frequently occurred in connection with sexual problems.[41] At Clark University, G. Stanley Hall for years had encouraged studies of sexuality.

Putnam was consulted, as were other neurologists, by patients with a wide range of sexual problems. In 1874, for example, a young man from a small New England town had asked to be "fitted for marriage" because he believed his "generative powers" had been almost entirely destroyed by masturbation.[42] In treating sexual neurasthenia, a syndrome that included impotence and morbid fears, Putnam counseled: where "self-restraint is needed its difficulties and possibilities should be clearly pointed out, with a view to the stimulation of the will and the counteraction of morbid self-reproach. It should be recognized that sexual intercourse is not the main object of marriage . . . On the other hand, an unnatural struggle for extreme abstinence is not good for the

[39] Janet's Harvard lectures were dedicated to Putnam and published as *The Major Symptoms of Hysteria* (New York: The Macmillan Co., 1907).

[40] "Sexual Perversion or Vice? A Pathological and Therapeutic Inquiry," *Journal of Nervous and Mental Disease*, 25 (April 1898), 237–256, and "A Case of Ideational Sadism," *Boston Medical and Surgical Journal*, 135 (August 20, 1896), 194–197.

[41] "Some Observations on the Anomalies of Self-Consciousness," in *Studies of Good and Evil* (New York: D. Appleton and Co., 1898), p. 190.

[42] Letter to Putnam, November 9, 1874.

neurasthenic patient, and the physician can often bring material aid to the patient in arriving at a wise conclusion as to detail." [43]

The informal contacts of the Boston circle reinforced Putnam's growing interest in psychoanalysis and in Freud's sexual theories between 1904 and 1907. On the periphery of the Boston group, G. Stanley Hall published his monumental *Adolescence* in 1904, which stressed Freud's findings about the importance of sexual traumas in the neuroses. That year Boris Sidis, a brilliant, prickly psychopathologist, moved to Boston from New York, and in 1905 recommended Freud's *Traumdeutung* and *Zur Psychopathologie des Altagslebens* to James, his former teacher.[44] Adolf Meyer, with whom Putnam corresponded, soon found Freud's sexual theories valuable because of the light they shed on the sexual disturbances that often were observed in psychotic patients. At the New York Psychiatric Institute, which he directed, Meyer acquainted his staff with Carl Jung's association tests and his application of Freud's theories to dementia praecox. The Institute became the most important early center for the dissemination of psychoanalysis.

By 1909 no single school or method of psychotherapy dominated American medicine. Hypnosis was declining in prestige, and more emphasis was being placed on "analysis," persuasion, and explanation. From many independent sources came studies of childhood, sexuality, dreams, and the subconscious. In 1906 Morton Prince founded the *Journal of Abnormal Psychology*, the first devoted exclusively to psychotherapy in English, and Putnam was one of the editors. But Prince deliberately refrained from creating a "school," lest the hostility of the medical profession be increased.

Many conservative physicians were alarmed by the growing enthusiasm for psychotherapy. A distinguished New York neurologist told his colleagues in 1908 that he did not worry "over the influence of mind over body," because he had been "very much busier . . . trying to find out what are the physical conditions that give rise to mental disturbance." [45]

---

[43] "Neurasthenia," in Alfred Lee Loomis, M.D., and William Gilman Thompson, M.D., eds., *A System of Practical Medicine by American Authors* (New York: Lea Bros., 1898), IV, 595.

[44] Boris Sidis to William James, October 9, 1905, the James Papers, the Houghton Library, Harvard University, by permission of the Harvard College Library.

[45] Remarks of Bernard Sachs in Discussion of S. Weir Mitchell, "Rest Treatment

A highly comprising lay popularity had set in. An adaptation of Morton Prince's study of the multiple personalities of Sally Beauchamp played to capacity audiences on Broadway. Magazines gave unprecedented publicity in 1908 and 1909 to the Emmanuel Movement, originating in Boston, which encouraged the clergy to treat nervous disorders by scientific psychotherapy. Putnam, who had been a sponsor, withdrew his support because medical supervision was inadequate.[46]

Of all the methods of psychotherapy, psychoanalysis was the most controversial, the most elaborate, time-consuming, and relentlessly psychological. A campaign against it was opened by conservative Philadelphia neurologists in 1908 at the American Neurological Association, and Putnam himself announced his disbelief in psychoanalysis, although he declared it was a "distinct contribution." [47]

Two years before, in 1906, he had published a lengthy evaluation in the first issue of the *Journal of Abnormal Psychology*. Putnam then interpreted psychoanalytic therapy in the tradition of Janet, as the cathartic confession of traumatic memories, an approach Freud had given up years before. According to Putnam, Freud placed his hand on the patient's forehead, urged him to relax and to search his memory, as a "housekeeper dusts the remotest corners of her rooms, in order to bring to life anything and everything, no matter how disagreeable, how offensively sexual, which may be related to the condition which is at stake, or may even come into the mind, without at first seeming to have any relationship to this condition." [48]

Putnam objected that when he tried this method with hysterical patients at the Massachusetts General Hospital, a detailed confession of traumatic sexual experiences often failed to cure. Or the memories were accessible without psychoanalysis. His theoretical

---

in Relation to Psychotherapy," *Journal of Nervous and Mental Disease*, 35 (December 1908), 784.

[46] Putnam to the Reverend Elwood Worcester, May 27, 1907, and September 12, 1908; Putnam, "The Service to the Nervous Invalid of the Physician and the Minister," *Harvard Theological Review*, 2 (April 1909), 235–250.

[47] Discussion of S. Weir Mitchell, "Rest Treatment in Relation to Psychotherapy," pp. 781–782.

[48] "Recent Experiences in the Study and Treatment of Hysteria at the Massachusetts General Hospital; with Remarks on Freud's Method of Treatment by 'Psycho-Analysis,' " *Journal of Abnormal Psychology*, 1 (April 1906), 30.

disagreement was more important. Memories were not tangible and intact, like dents in a piece of brass or books in a library. Rather, the mind was fluid; every current impression modified all past ones, much as a new planet would modify the operations of a solar system. A symptom might outlive its original significance and take on an entirely different meaning. Psychoanalysis did not discharge a past affect but substituted a "new mental state" for an earlier one. It was better to foster "healthy," "rational" associations than to dwell on the repugnant details of noxious memories. Freud's therapy was difficult and often unnecessary.

Although Putnam reserved judgment about Freud's sexual theories, his description of them missed their significance. He ignored childhood sexuality and the Oedipus complex, although listing the major works in which they were described. Freud had come to insist on the role of repressed tendencies to sexual inversion in the neuroses, with keenness and "amazing fullness of detail." Long insistent on the psychotherapist's need for a broad, philosophical culture, Putnam also praised Freud's "fluent style, abundance of illustration . . . evidence of wide reading, general cultivation and imaginative ability." [49] Thus by 1906 Putnam had tested his own version of Freud's psychoanalysis from a detached, yet sympathetic viewpoint, but was by no means convinced of its merits.

In December 1908 he met Ernest Jones who visited Morton Prince's splendid house on Beacon Street to discuss psychoanalysis with the Boston circle. Only Putnam seemed seriously interested in learning more about Freud's theories.

Putnam, Jones recalled, behaved "with a deference quite absurd in the circumstances, and then, with his characteristic frankness, said he was disappointed in my appearance since he had expected to meet a tall man with a gray beard." [50]

On the surface, Jones might not have seemed qualified to dispel Putnam's doubts. He was a brilliant neurologist, but endowed with an "omnipotence complex" and a caustic tongue. The son of a Welsh colliery clerk who became a mining engineer, Jones attended University College, Cardiff, and had been trained at Uni-

[49] "Recent Experiences in the Study and Treatment of Hysteria at the Massachusetts General Hospital," p. 27.
[50] *Free Associations* (New York: Basic Books, 1959), p. 189.

versity Hospital in London. Recently he had been dismissed from the staff of a London hospital for attempting to discover, in accordance with Freud's theories, a sexual basis for the hysterical paralysis of a ten-year-old girl.

He had taken a position as demonstrator in psychiatry at the University of Toronto, at the bottom of the academic ladder. But he had impressive letters of recommendation from William Osler, a friend of Putnam, and from several London neurologists.[51] Already Jones had written more than twenty papers and had an unusual gift for clear, orderly argument. He was intense, decisive, and energetic, a driving perfectionist. He was plagued by rheumatoid arthritis.

As an adolescent Jones had suffered intensely from a sense of guilt. He had been preoccupied with religion, philosophy, and the salvation of his soul, which he came to interpret as "atonement" with the father. In London he had listened to the Fabian socialists H. G. Wells, Bernard Shaw, and Sidney Webb. He regarded himself as an idealist committed to the reform of society. He had an acute sense of conflict, of Saint Paul's war of the members against the law of the mind. Jones's idealism, his intransigent advocacy, and his sensitivity to inner conflict may have appealed to Putnam.

Jones's own growing understanding of psychoanalysis had been fostered by recent contacts with Jung and Freud. In 1905 Jones had begun experimenting with psychoanalysis, improving his German in order to learn more about it. In 1907 he visited Jung, then assistant director at the Burghölzli Clinic in Zurich. There Jones met A. A. Brill, a young American psychiatrist, who had worked with Adolf Meyer at the Psychiatric Institute of the New York State Hospitals on Ward's Island.

For Jones and Brill, as for Jung and most of the first psychoanalysts, their relationship with Freud was decisive. At the first Psychoanalytic Congress in Salzburg in 1908 they heard Freud present the famous rat man case for four hours. Freud became for Brill a father figure who reconciled him to his Jewish heritage. To Jones,

[51] Cyril Greenland, "Ernest Jones in Toronto 1908–1913, a Fragment of Biography," *Canadian Psychiatric Association Journal*, 6 (June 1961), 132–139, and *ibid.*, 11 (December 1966), 512–519.

Freud, for all his brilliance, seemed vulnerable, a man Jones wished to protect, and later he saw himself as the "bonny fighter" for Freud that Huxley had been for Darwin.

In the spring of 1908 the two young physicians visited Vienna, dined with Freud, and attended Wednesday night meetings of Freud's circle. Brill asked for and received the rights to translate Freud's work into English. He returned to New York, a struggling young physician determined to take up the practice of psychoanalysis. Jones moved to Toronto, a city he quickly came to detest because of its "puritanism" and "provinciality." He devoted his energies to mastering psychoanalytic theory and technique, presenting it to others in trenchant, lucid essays and addresses.

As a result of his conversations with Jones, Putnam reconsidered the two major hypotheses he had ignored or doubted — the importance of childhood sexuality and the persisting effects of early experiences. Putnam's new enthusiasm was exhibited in a paper to the American Therapeutic Congress in New Haven in May 1909. It was the first meeting of this organization of general physicians to be devoted exclusively to psychotherapy. All the current methods — hypnotism, suggestion, re-education — had their advocates. The Boston group attended in force, and Ernest Jones came down from Toronto to open the "campaign for psychoanalysis." He said little of Freud's sexual theories, explaining psychoanalysis as a new method of psychotherapy as painstaking and radical as surgery. In an address on character formation Putnam, in passing, observed that Freud had discovered how "mental twists and habits" formed in childhood could persist into adult life in forms "strangely altered and concealed." [52] With the knowledge that could be obtained through psychoanalysis, traits that previously had seemed beyond control could be altered. Putnam cautioned that Freud's methods still required further evaluation, but that the more he learned about them the more he was convinced of their significance. His new appreciation of the importance of early experience had been confirmed by a former patient, Miss Susan Blow, a leader of the American kindergarten movement to whom he had sent the New Haven paper. She wrote back that she

[52] "The Relation of Character Formation to Psychotherapy," in Morton Prince, ed., *Psychotherapeutics* (Boston: Richard G. Badger, 1909), pp. 166–186.

had suffered tortures in childhood from repressions and conceal-
ments, and that her childhood fears had been worsened by her
family's blue Presbyterianism.[53]

Putnam next defended the sexual inquiries of psychoanalysis in
a stinging letter to the *Boston Medical and Surgical Journal* written on June 10, 1909. The *Journal* had condemned a German
essay on psychoanalysis without bothering to summarize or publish
it. The most startling new element in Putnam's protest was this:
the "eternal, the fierce yet often needless conflict between natural
instincts and an artificial social organization striving blindly and
often cruelly for the mastery." This conflict caused an "immense
variety of neuroses and psychoses" and more "unadulterated misery
than cancer or tuberculosis or perhaps than both combined." [54]

Although Putnam had begun to try psychoanalysis with his patients, he was not yet fully committed. Three years later, he recalled that when he first read an article of Freud's on the sexual
origin of the neuroses he had put the paper down in disgust. Was
Freud honest or merely an eccentric notoriety seeker, he had
wondered? [55] As with others, so with Putnam, his encounter with
Freud was crucial.

After 1905 as Freud emerged from what he called his "splendid
isolation," he met increasing opposition. He long had hoped that
others would test his findings and add to them by the new techniques he had devised. Until then, however, psychoanalysis had
remained the nearly exclusive possession of himself and his circle
of personal followers in Vienna — talented, but sometimes obscure young men not all of them physicians and none professors
of medicine. In 1904 Freud learned that Eugen Bleuler, professor
of psychiatry at the University of Zurich, and his assistant Carl
Jung had been working with psychoanalysis for some years. Having for many reasons felt isolated from university and medical life
in Vienna, Freud hoped that psychoanalysis might become a
recognized part of scientific and medical discipline, at least outside
his native city. Yet in 1908 and 1909, the prospects were not brilliant. Bleuler, for all his friendliness, remained ambivalent. Freud

---

[53] Blow to Putnam, June 10, 1909.
[54] Putnam to editor, *Boston Medical and Surgical Journal,* 161 (July 1, 1909), 37.
[55] "On Freud's Psycho-Analytic Method and Its Evolution," *Boston Medical and Surgical Journal,* 166 (January 25, 1912), 121; Ad Psa, 121.

wrote to his young disciple Karl Abraham, a former physician at the Burghölzli, that Bleuler's defection was "imminent" and Bleuler's relations with Jung "strained to the breaking point." [56] The major German authorities in neurology and psychiatry regularly were denouncing psychoanalysis.

Then, quite unexpectedly came the possibility of establishing psychoanalysis in the new world. In December, the month Ernest Jones first visited Boston, Freud received an invitation from G. Stanley Hall to lecture at the Twentieth Anniversary Celebration of Clark University.[57] Freud refused at first because he could not sacrifice three weeks' earnings in July to make the trip before his customary vacation in August or September. However, the date for the celebration was changed, the fee was raised from $400 to $750, and an honorary degree was included. Freud wrote again to Abraham, March 9, 1909: "And now for the big news. I have accepted the repeated invitation of Clark University, Worcester, Mass., near Boston, to give a series of lectures there in the week beginning September 6th . . . I am very curious about what will happen there and about the outcome of these lectures. The trip may certainly be mentioned, it is as sure as anything human can be. Perhaps it will annoy some people in Berlin as well as in Vienna. That cannot do any harm." [58]

Hall hoped the celebration would attract a "select audience of the best American professors and students of psychology and psychiatry," he had informed Freud. On April 13, 1909, Hall wrote again: "We have given out no notices as yet; nevertheless, in some way the news of your coming has reached a number of people in this country who have been profoundly interested in your work and have written us expressing their pleasure and their desire to hear whatever you may have to say to us.

"Janet, who has visited this country and given a similar course of public lectures, has had a profound influence in turning the attention of our leading and especially our younger students of

---

[56] Letter of September 29, 1908, in *A Psycho-Analytic Dialogue: The Letters of Sigmund Freud and Karl Abraham, 1907–1926,* edited by Hilda C. Abraham and Ernst L. Freud, translated by Bernard Marsh and Hilda C. Abraham (New York: Basic Books, 1965), pp. 51–52.

[57] Hall to Freud, December 15, 1908, Clark University Papers.

[58] In *A Psycho-Analytic Dialogue,* p. 75.

abnormal psychology from the exclusively somatic and neurological to a more psychological basis. We believe that a concise statement of your own results and point of view would now be exceedingly opportune, and perhaps in some sense mark an epoch in the history of these studies in this country." [59]

When Freud came to Worcester in September, Putnam and William James made an effort to hear him. They were part of an audience that included many present and future leaders of American intellectual life, the anthropologist Franz Boas, Adolf Meyer, and Hall himself, with James, the founder of American academic psychology. On September 12, the *Worcester Telegram* reported: "Conference Brings Savants together: Long-Haired Type Hard to Discover: Men with Bulging Brains have Time for Occasional Smiles."

Impressed by Freud's comprehensive and skillful presentation, and by his personality and brilliance, Putnam invited him and his colleagues Carl Jung and Sandor Ferenczi to his camp at Keene Valley in the Adirondacks. There, around the fire, they continued their discussions. Putnam wrote to Ernest Jones that the visit was on the whole satisfactory. "They were curiously unlike most of the other persons gathered here, but I believe they found the experience an interesting one." [60]

Freud, ill with a mild attack of appendicitis, sent his family this wry description on September 16:

"It was four weeks ago today that I set out. This will probably be the last letter that arrives before I do. Of all the things that I have experienced in America, this is by far the most amazing. Imagine a camp in a forest wilderness situated somewhat like the mountain pasture on the Loser where the inn is. Stones, moss, groups of trees, uneven ground which, on three sides, runs into thickly wooded hills. On this land, a group of roughly hewn small log cabins, each one, as we discover, with a name. One of them is called the Stoop and is the parlor, where there is a library, a piano, writing desks and cardtables. Another the "Hall of Knights" with amusing old objects, has a fireplace in the center and benches along the walls, like a peasant dining room; the others are living quarters. Ours with only three rooms is called Chatterbox. Everything is left very rough and primitive but it comes off. Mixing bowls serve as wash bowls, china mugs for glasses, etc. But

[59] Hall to Freud, letter, Clark University Papers.
[60] Letter of November 22, 1909.

naturally nothing is lacking and is supplied in one form or another. We have discovered that there are special books on camping in which instruction is given about all this primitive equipment.

"Our reception at half past two consisted of an invitation to take a walk up the nearest mountain, where we had an opportunity of becoming acquainted with the utter wildness of such an American landscape. We took trails and came down slopes to which even my horns and hoofs were not equal.

"Fortunately it is raining today. There are many squirrels and porcupines in these woods; the latter are invisible so far. Even black bears are said to be seen in winter.

"We had supper in the company of the ladies. One of the hostesses, a lady from Leipzig, is extremely affected. The unmarried sister of Dr. Putnam, a well-preserved lady of middle age, accompanied on the piano a young girl who sang English songs, and then Jung sang German songs.

"The Putnam family understands German, has often been to Germany and also to Vienna. Ferenczi and I were taught an amusing board game by two young girls. Amazing! This morning I sorely missed a barber for all I can do is comb my hair. Fortunately there is the greatest informality in dress, or at least so it seems. Breakfast was very original and plentiful. In short, there will be much to tell you about.

"We shall start on the last lap of our journey, the day after tomorrow, going to New York, perhaps on the Hudson River. We expect to arrive in New York on the evening of the 18th. My love to all of you. Only 14 days more!

Pa." [61]

Before Freud left, Putnam mentioned that he would write an article about psychoanalysis, possibly to lay at rest the rumors that surrounded it. Putnam had satisfied his New England conscience as to the integrity of Freud and his disciples. He soon wrote to Freud that he would incline to accept his views "much the more" for having had the pleasure of making his acquaintance.[62]

In Prince's *Journal,* Putnam characterized psychoanalysis in terms similar to those he had used in his Harvard college essays nearly five decades before. Personal virtue, technical innovation, an unpopular cause — all these early enthusiasms were now applied to psychoanalysis. It offered new truths too little appreciated, advanced by a small band of courageous men, who were not merely zealous but also "kindly, unassuming, tolerant, earnest and sincere." [63]

[61] Letter from Putnam Camp, September 16, 1909.
[62] Letter of November 17, 1909.
[63] "Personal Impressions of Sigmund Freud and His Work, with Special Reference

The Psychoanalytic Movement, 1909–1918

In his first letter to Freud, Putnam observed that although he could not confirm all Freud's conclusions, there was so much that he could verify he was in no mood for hostile criticism.[64] Putnam's commitment to psychoanalysis involved a complex blending of emotional and scientific processes. First had come a new willingness to judge psychoanalysis based on his personal encounters with Jones and Freud. Then Putnam deepened his theoretical and practical knowledge. By April of 1910, six months after their correspondence began, Freud's "views" had become "the cause." [65] An outward sign of this common bond was the Greek letter psi which Freud and Putnam occasionally used to stand for the first three letters of psychoanalysis.[66] In May 1910 Putnam publicly proclaimed his new convictions and directly confronted the hostility that had accompanied the growth of psychoanalysis almost from its inception. This experience led him to defend Freud all the more vigorously. Finally, the status of psychoanalysis as a distinctive specialty was confirmed by the founding of professional organizations and a journal, acts which further deepened commitment and inflamed opposition.

Ernest Jones seemed to sense Putnam's need to champion unpopular truths. Soon after the Clark Conference he asked Putnam to "strike a blow" at materialism by speaking on the psychoanalytic treatment of the neuroses at a meeting of the Canadian Medical Association the following spring. "The tender plant of psychoanalysis in America," [67] Jones warned, was in danger of being crushed by those who, unlike Putnam, were too blind to appreciate new truths. Putnam replied within three days that he not only accepted the invitation but was writing two papers "on Freud matters" for Prince's *Journal*.[68] Putnam marshalled all his energies, his prestige, and his eloquence on behalf of psychoanalysis. His contribution

---

to His Recent Lectures at Clark University" (part 2), *Journal of Abnormal Psychology*, 4 (February–March 1910), 379; Ad Psa, 30.

[64] Letter of November 17, 1909.

[65] Putnam to Freud, April 14, 1910.

[66] Now a common abbreviation in psychology, the Greek letter "psi" does not appear in letters of G. Stanley Hall.

[67] Letter of November 19, 1909.

[68] Letter of November 22, 1909.

lay, not in new clinical or theoretical knowledge, as he himself realized, but in skillfully presenting the "cause" to neurologists and physicians. It was Putnam who chiefly secured for Freud's views a serious public hearing. He spoke in May 1910 before the American Neurological Association in Washington, in November of 1911 to the Harvey Society of New York, in June of 1914 before the Section on Nervous and Mental Diseases of the American Medcial Association. It was nearly four years after Putnam's first paper that William Alanson White, superintendent of the Government Hospital for the Insane in Washington, D.C., addressed the nation's psychiatrists periphrastically on the subject of psychoanalysis.[69] Although Putnam became emeritus in 1912 he lectured on psychoanalysis at Harvard Medical School from 1913 through 1915, and probably secured the appointment of a psychoanalytic psychologist to the staff of the Massachusetts General Hospital in 1911.[70]

Putnam's commitment was accompanied by a sustained burst of productivity, as if confirming the faith of his friend William James in the hidden energies of men. Like many psychoanalytic pioneers, Putnam always had been hard-working, prolific in contributions to his field. From 1909 until his death in 1918 he published twenty-two papers on psychoanalysis, and still others on organic neurology. He assisted in a translation, wrote reviews and memorials and a book for laymen. His work on behalf of psychoanalysis, he later wrote, provided more "intense and engrossing labor" than any previous task. It also involved "much readjustment — sometimes far from pleasant but very satisfactory in its results." [71] He became somewhat isolated from his Boston colleagues and attended fewer meetings of the Boston Society of Neurology and Psychiatry, where his criticism of other methods of treatment provoked opposition.[72] His practice diminished.[73]

---

[69] "The Genetic Concept in Psychiatry," *American Journal of Insanity*, 70 (October 1913), 441–446.

[70] *Announcements of the Medical School of Harvard University* (1912–1913), p. 50; *ibid.* (1914–1915), p. 64. Louville Eugene Emerson, who held a doctorate in psychology from Harvard and became a member of the American Psychoanalytic Association, was appointed in 1911 to the Psychoneurological Department; see *Sixth Annual Report of the Social Service Department, Massachusetts General Hospital*, p. 18, and *Massachusetts General Hospital, Ward G. Records*, vol. IV (September 21, 1911), p. 130.

[71] "The Present Status of Psychoanalysis," *Boston Medical and Surgical Journal*, 170 (June 11, 1914), 897; Ad Psa, 254.

[72] Putnam spoke on "Studies in Psychoanalysis" on December 15, 1910. See Putnam to Jones, January 5, 1911; Minutes of the Boston Society of Neurology and

Ernest Jones also poured out a stream of articles, many of which became part of the psychoanalytic canon — the Hamlet essay, studies of sublimation and education, a lucid exposition of Freud's theory of dreams, a psychoanalytic critique of hypnosis and suggestion. Many physicians and psychologists believed he was the clearest expositor of Freud's theories writing in English. He was also a tireless organizer. "You are certainly the most energetic, precise and prompt and efficient individual I have ever met," Putnam wrote in 1910.[74] Not merely energy and belief account for this degree of activity. Freud provided models that opened up for systematic investigation aspects of behavior that before had been largely ignored.

Although Putnam's richly detailed papers on psychoanalysis have received less attention than Jones's, they lucidly connect psychoanalysis with the whole past of psychotherapy. Putnam carefully read everything Freud, Jung, and the other psychoanalysts had written, especially the *Three Contributions to a Theory of Sexuality* which he had not understood before. He applied this new knowledge to his patients and to himself and experienced a growing sense of illumination. Between the spring of 1909 and May 1910, Putnam tested the new method on about twenty patients suffering from anxiety-neurosis, hysteria, neurasthenia, fears, impulsions, impotence, stammering.[75] He informed Freud that he was obtaining deeper insights into his patients than ever before.[76] By June 1910, Putnam had reassessed completely his own professional outlook: "I could almost point to the moments when I first learned clearly what was meant by the conversion of desire to fear; the relationship of death and pain to the sexual instinct; the significance of parents for the mental development of the child; the tendency of the neuropathic patient unconsciously to seek ever new objects of desire, etc." [77] Putnam stressed the uniqueness of Freud's

Psychiatry, the Francis A. Countway Library of Medicine, Boston. For the derisive comments of one member, see J. W. Courtney, "The Views of Plato and Freud on the Etiology and Treatment of Hysteria: A Comparison and Critical Study," *Boston Medical and Surgical Journal,* 168 (May 1, 1913), 649–652.

[73] Putnam to Jones, May 12, 1915.

[74] Putnam to Jones, October 14, 1910.

[75] "Personal Experience with Freud's Psychoanalytic Method." Read before the American Neurological Association, May 3, 1910. *Journal of Nervous and Mental Disease,* 37 (November 1910), 657; Ad Psa, 31.

[76] Letter of November 17, 1909.

[77] "Personal Experience with Freud's Psychoanalytic Method," p. 673; Ad Psa, 51.

achievement: the unprecedented depth of his penetration of the unconscious, his discovery of the meaning of dreams, the searching and merciless thoroughness of his therapy.

Psychoanalysis held out hope for obsessions, doubts, and compulsions that even the "keen and able Janet" regarded as relatively hopeless. Instead of the theoretical fluidity of mind and the therapy of substitution, Putnam now stressed the persistence of the past and the efficacy of insight. Putnam and a patient had traced his symptoms back to the age of four, "much as one sees at one glance in a transparent microscopic-section . . . of the brain the whole course of a great neurone tract." [78] As his patient's insight increased so did his rational self-control. In the history of psychiatry, it has often been observed that enthusiasm for a new therapy contributes to its initial success.

In attempting to arouse enthusiasm for psychoanalysis, however, Putnam encountered a major obstacle — the "taboo of silence" and the disgust often aroused by Freud's sexual theories, both reflections of the existing norm of what Freud termed "civilized" sexual morality. This later-nineteenth-century moral system, medical and religious, restricted sexual expression to intercourse within monogamous marriage and, according to some authorities, solely for the purpose of procreation. As a mode of control, "civilized" morality exacted, especially from women, reticence about all sexuality. Freud believed that the American version of this western moral code was unusually strict, and many Americans would have been proud to agree.

Putnam's attack on "civilized" morality, begun in July of 1909, was for him a daring novelty. He and a growing number of Americans, such as G. Stanley Hall, wished to discard the code's most repressive restrictions — reticence and the limiting of intercourse within marriage solely to procreation. Thus, they hoped to preserve the code's deepest core — faithful, monogamous marriage. This conservative attack on "civilized" morality marked a massive social change in the mores, in which psychoanalysis played an early and complex role. In a letter to Freud of September 30, 1911, Putnam described his own struggles with his strong sexual drives. The following spring, he eloquently attacked the extremist posi-

[78] Putnam, "Personal Experience with Freud's Psychoanalytic Method," p. 673; Ad Psa, 47.

tion: "It is another offense against freedom, and another well meant but injurious attempt to cast a slur of shame over what should be pure, for society to step into the home, and, in the name of continence, to attempt to impose the principle that sexual relations between man and wife are in themselves self-indulgent and wrong, and something to be tolerated only in so far as they subserve their strict needs of race perpetuation." [79]

Putnam invoked a theme of his college years — the sacred right to oppose tradition and custom. Like Cromwell or the proponents of every true reform, such as the abolition of slavery, those who investigated sexuality were regarded by society as "disturbers of the peace." [80] But this growing band — Freud, Krafft-Ebing, and Havelock Ellis, among others — represented truths which the "upholders of the established order" already had divined but would not "formulate to themselves or listen to when adduced by others." [81]

Next he denounced medical prudery. Physicians were accustomed to studying the "bodily secretions" without a "trace of unpleasant feeling." But even psychoanalysts had to overcome their aversion to details such as those disclosed in Freud's study of "Little Hans." Physicians might object to this demonstration that we were once "little animals" and urge: "Let us rather press constantly forward into the free air and more abundant light, and let those who have had a dark history forget it. Look forward and not back.

"This is a fine cry, but unfortunately it has served the cause of ignorance, narrowness, and prejudice as well as that of progress. It was the cry of the church against Darwin, when he sought to 'introspect' the history of life, and its echoes have drowned the voices of those who have sought to talk about the problems of sex, no matter with what earnestness. The cause of formal modesty and reticence has indeed had many noble martyrs, both before the days of Paul and Virginia and since. But there is such a thing as paying too dear for this niceness, especially when, through the opposite course, we can have all that we should gain by this and more besides.

[79] Comments on Sex Issues from the Freudian Standpoint," *New York Medical Journal,* 95 (June 15, 1912), 1251; Ad Psa, 135.

[80] "Personal Impressions of Sigmund Freud" (part 2), pp. 372; Ad Psa, 22.

[81] "On the Etiology and Treatment of the Psychoneuroses," *Boston Medical and Surgical Journal,* 163 (July 21, 1910), 79; Ad Psa, 68.

"All this is wrong. A fool's paradise is a poor paradise. If our spiritual life is good for anything it can afford to see the truth. No investigation is wrong if it is earnest. Knowledge knows nothing as essentially and invariably dirty." [82]

Putnam placed Freud in the vanguard of the revolution in neurology begun by Charcot and Janet. Giving a comprehensive philosophical and social dimension to this revolution, Freud had extended it to character study, educational psychology, race-psychology, child-study, and folk lore. No future student of human character and motives could afford to ignore his work. Freud was so pleased with this address, "On the Etiology and Treatment of the Psychoneuroses," delivered to the Canadian Medical Association in June 1910, that he translated it himself for the *Zentralblatt*.[83]

Putnam's campaign aroused some sympathetic interest and considerable opposition. On April 14, 1910, a month before his address to the American Neurological Association he wrote to Freud that he was doing all he could to "help on the cause." The Washington address provoked a debate that ran for eight and a half pages in the *Journal of Nervous and Mental Disease*. Putnam and his colleagues fought over several issues that plagued the subsequent history of psychoanalysis: a psychological as opposed to a somatic approach to nervous diseases; the "sexual taint" of psychoanalysis; the "mystical" nature of dreams and the sub-conscious; the length of treatment; the "dangers" of "introspection." [84]

A Boston colleague, Phillips Coombs Knapp, observed that Putnam was an "invincible optimist," accustomed to finding the precious jewel in the head of even the "ugliest and most venomous toad." Surely he must have disinfected Freud's methods. A neurologist from Rochester, New York, recalled his own prescription for obsessive doubts. The patient was made to say aloud each time a doubt occurred, "What a damn fool I am!" [85] Charles L. Dana, a former assistant of George Beard and a famous New York neu-

[82] "Personal Impressions of Sigmund Freud" (part 1), pp. 306–307; Ad Psa, 17–18.

[83] Freud to Putnam, September 29, 1910; Putnam, "Über Ätiologie und Behandlung der Psychoneurosen," *Zentralblatt*, 1 (1911), 137–154. [The translator's name was not given.]

[84] See the discussion of Putnam, "Personal Experience with Freud's Psychoanalytic Method" in *Journal of Nervous and Mental Disease*, 37 (October 1910), 630–639.

[85] Discussion of "Personal Experience with Freud's Psychoanalytic Method," *ibid.*, pp. 635, 631, respectively.

rologist, argued that isolation in a private hospital with an intelligent nurse was a faster, more effective treatment than psychoanalysis. A few neurologists, although favorably inclined to psychotherapy, didn't like the "subconscious business"; another condemned the detailed study of dreams as a baffling, valueless exercise. Only a few were pleased by Putnam's paper, largely because of their high respect for him. Lewellys F. Barker, a professor at the Johns Hopkins University Medical School, was delighted that "a man in whom we have absolute confidence" had tested Freud's method, which already had excited "world wide interest." [86]

Putnam replied that he had brought up so unpopular a subject to raise the entire issue of a functional, psychological approach that now divided neurologists by bitter misunderstandings. "We all of us spend vast amounts of time on the anatomy of the nervous system," he remarked.[87] It was equally justifiable to study the anatomy of the mind. If physicians disliked the subconscious, they should realize that their patients in fact suffered from subconscious memories. Psychoanalysis prevented rather than encouraged morbid introspection. Finally, the patient, not the physician, brought up sexual material. "One does not take a young unmarried girl and begin to talk to her bluntly and tactlessly about her sexual relations as has been suggested . . . If sexual ideas come out it is because the patient brings them out." [88]

During the debate Putnam had gone far beyond the cautious and reserved acceptance of psychoanalysis in his first letters to Freud. Freud's view had never been a "hypothesis," he told his colleagues. "It was a generalization based upon observation. The facts forced themselves upon his notice." [89] On May 10, he wrote to Freud that he had had a "lively and interesting time" during the discussion. He forwarded the official notes of it, along with his addresses.

One of Putnam's most provocative tactics was to argue that "resistance" to Freud's sexual theories sprang from sexual preoc-

[86] Discussion of "Personal Experience with Freud's Psychoanalytic Method," *ibid.,* p. 632.
[87] Discussion of "Personal Experience with Freud's Psychoanalytic Method," *ibid.,* p. 638.
[88] Discussion of "Personal Experience with Freud's Psychoanalytic Method," *ibid.,* p. 637.
[89] Discussion of "Personal Experience with Freud's Psychoanalytic Method," *ibid.,* p. 637.

cupations. This argument provoked one of the bitterest attacks ever made against Freud. On April 4, 1912, Putnam delivered an address, "Comments on Sex Issues from the Freudian Standpoint," to the Section in Neurology of the New York Academy of Medicine: "Many of the most fair minded . . . [physicians] think it is an extra amount of broad mindedness which leads them to say that 'although there is a good deal of value in this movement, yet the importance of the sexual element is over-rated, etc.', whereas in my opinion, it is not broad mindedness, but a series of internal resistances that keep them, and all of us, from looking squarely at this particular class of facts, and that the force of these resistances is a measure of the importance of the subject, and of the insistence with which thoughts and emotions of which their holders are unconscious are lording it over those of which they are conscious." [90] One listener, Moses Allen Starr, a New York neurologist, argued that the sexual emphasis of psychoanalysis had compromised the cause of psychotherapy.

Starr went on to denounce Freud: "I knew Dr. Sigmund Freud well in Vienna some years ago. Vienna is not a particularly moral city, and working side by side with Freud in the laboratory all through one winter, I learned that he enjoyed Viennese life thoroughly. Freud was not a man who lived on a particularly high plane. He was not self-repressed. He was not an ascetic. I think his scientific theory is largely the result of his environment and of the peculiar life he led." [91]

In the confusion that followed Starr's attack, Putnam did not reply, but he wrote to Freud on June 4 that he had seen Starr and made him feel ashamed. Freud replied that Starr's information "about my early years amused me mightily. Would that it had been true!" But he had never known Starr.[92]

The next stage in the development of American psychoanalysis was the founding of formal organizations. In defending Putnam during the debate in 1910 before the American Neurological Association, Ernest Jones had invoked a thriving Freudian host. No opposition could now crush Freudism, because there was an important

[90] "Comments on Sex Issues from the Freudian Standpoint," pp. 1251–1252; Ad Psa, 137.

[91] The New York Times, April 5, 1912, p. 8, col. 2.

[92] Freud to Putnam, June 25, 1912. See Jones, The Life and Work of Sigmund Freud (3 vols.), I (New York: Basic Books, 1955), 202.

"International Society for Psycho-analysis with five sub-sections: there were some two hundred trained workers who had confirmed Freud's conclusions in most of the countries of Europe: there were four periodicals exclusively devoted to the work, not to speak of a mass of literature that had appeared . . . in the special journals." [93]

This was a considerable exaggeration. The International had been founded at the Psychoanalytic Congress in Nuremberg on May 30–31, 1910, but, as discussions at the Vienna Society indicate, it was then a delicate plant.[94] Its strength is less important than the psychological need for social reinforcement that Jones's argument disclosed.

Freud hoped that if psychoanalysts joined a formal organization, it then would be possible for them to repudiate practitioners of "wild" psychoanalysis, who sometimes prescribed sexual intercourse. A second motive was the need for training. Psychoanalysis could not be learned from books but only from those already proficient, Freud insisted. He hoped that local branches, drawing membership from a given area, could meet easily and often for "friendly communication" and "mutual support." [95] Jung had been chosen president and Zurich, headquarters, and the International published an official *Zentralblatt*, edited by Alfred Adler and Wilhelm Stekel.

The letters Putnam exchanged with Jones, Ferenczi, and Freud reflect these developments and provide some of the first detailed information about the American Psychoanalytic Association. The initial suggestion came from Ferenczi immediately after the Nuremberg Congress where he had presented, at Freud's request, a plan for the International Association. Ferenczi had visited Putnam with Freud at Keene Valley, and they already had corresponded. Ferenczi mentioned the new branch societies in Vienna, Berlin, and Zurich, and asked Putnam whether one or more such branches might be founded in America.[96]

---

[93] See *Journal of Nervous and Mental Disease*, 37 (October 1910), 636.

[94] Herman Nunberg and Ernst Federn, eds., *Minutes of the Vienna Psycho-Analytic Society, II, 1908–1910* (New York: International Universities Press, 1967), 463–471, 553, 573.

[95] "On the History of the Psycho-Analytic Movement" (1914), SE, XIV, 43–44; " 'Wild' Psycho-Analysis" (1910), SE, XI, 226–227.

[96] Ferenczi to Putnam, April 1, 1910.

Then on April 14, 1910, Freud suggested that Brill found a branch society in New York and Ernest Jones, another in Boston.[97] Freud probably soon heard from Jones about the Washington debates and the universal respect in which Putnam was held even by those who opposed his new Freudian views. Freud asked Putnam on June 16, 1910, to head the proposed American branch because no one else could so effectively defend psychoanalysis, and because he understood that all important intellectual movements in America began in Boston.

Putnam did not reply immediately. The American Psychopathological Association had been founded in Washington in May, with his friend Morton Prince as president and George Waterman, Putnam's former assistant, as secretary. It was to provide a forum for physicians and psychologists interested in psychotherapy. The psychopathologists still were few, those actively interested in psychoanalysis fewer still. Jones wrote to Putnam on July 12 that the American Psychopathological Association "fills the bill at present. We are too few to make it worth while to organize a new society. On the other hand it would please Freud if we simply got up a *formal* branch of the International Psychoanalytic Verein, and it might strengthen their hands a little . . . It might also be of service in co-ordinating our work a little and exchanging experiences and views." Jones sailed for Europe in July on the *Lusitania,* attended the International Congress of Medical Psychology in Brussels, and visited Freud, who was vacationing in Holland. Freud was a "little puzzled," Jones wrote, at not having heard from Putnam about the branch society. Freud argued that amateurs and charlatans were likely to damage the work, so that an official Verein "would be *some kind of* guarantee in a general way that the members knew what they were talking or writing about." Putnam already had written Freud that he and Jones would found the branch in connection with the next meeting of the American Psychopathological Association, scheduled for the spring of 1911.[98]

On September 9, 1910, Jones suggested to Putnam that, together

[97] The letter was dated by A. A. Brill as November 14, in my opinion mistakenly because it clearly concerns the Nuremberg Congress, which took place at the end of March, and mentions Freud's handing over leadership of the Vienna Society to Adler, which occurred on April 6, 1910. See Herman Nunberg and Ernst Federn, eds., *Minutes of the Vienna Psycho-Analytic Society, II, 1908–1910,* 470–471.

[98] Jones to Putnam, August 14, 1910; Putnam to Freud, [late July 1910].

with Brill they send an invitational circular to the following psychologists and physicians: G. Stanley Hall; August Hoch, who had succeeded Adolf Meyer as Director of the Psychiatric Institute of the New York State Hospitals for the Insane; C. Macfie Campbell, a Scottish physician trained in Edinburgh, who worked with Meyer; Edwin Bissell Holt assistant professor of psychology at Harvard; William Alanson White; Isador Coriat, a psychopathologist who also had worked with Meyer; and Bernard Hart, a British medical psychologist. Meyer could join if he wished, but need not be asked. Jones proposed himself as secretary and Putnam as president.

The proposal for an American psychoanalytic organization, so casually initiated, and a bitter controversy over the significance of Freud's method sharpened the lines between the psychoanalysts and their opponents, even among the psychotherapists. In early 1911 Morton Prince observed with some disdain that Freud's followers were "styling themselves psychoanalysts," one sign of a cult of "believers." [99] Prince had published an article on dreams in which he had gone far toward accepting important aspects of Freud's theories — the difference between manifest and latent content, the function of symbolism, the relation of dreams to past experience.[100] But his investigations had relied primarily on hypnosis, and he could not confirm Freud's view that every dream represented the fulfillment of a repressed wish. On October 13, 1910, Jones had proposed that he or Putnam write a critique for the next issue of the *Journal of Abnormal Psychology*, and Prince was informed of their intention.[101] He wrote to Putnam on October 21, welcoming the criticism, but cautioning against making public a sexual interpretation of his patients' dreams. He implored Putnam not to get "so far involved with Jones and his crowd as to unconsciously slide into 'the attitude' — largely I am afraid from a mistaken sense of duty and loyalty." The "attitude" to Prince meant fanaticism.[102]

[99] "The Mechanism and Interpretation of Dreams — A Reply to Dr. Jones," *Journal of Abnormal Psychology*, 5 (February–March 1911), 349. See Jones, "Remarks on Dr. Morton Prince's Article: 'The Mechanism and Interpretation of Dreams,'" *ibid.*, pp. 328–336.
[100] "The Mechanism and Interpretation of Dreams," *Journal of Abnormal Psychology*, 5 (October-November 1910), 139–195.
[101] Jones to Putnam, October 13, 1910.
[102] Prince to Putnam, October 21, 1910, March 3, 1911.

Jones undertook the criticism, insisting that because Prince had not used Freud's psychoanalytic technique he had not gotten Freud's results. The term "psychoanalysis," by 1908 and 1909 was used relatively often by psychotherapists to describe any attempt to discover the origins of a given symptom, largely in accordance with the theories of French psychopathology. To this Ernest Jones made strenuous objections. The term psychoanalysis should be reserved for Freud's method alone. Jones wrote to Putnam on April 9, 1910, that "all sorts of amateur claims and confusions" would result if the term were not thus restricted. He developed the point further in his critique of Prince's article on dreams, arguing in effect that Prince's work with hypnosis was irrelevant and useless because it did not reveal resistances. Moreover, he observed to Putnam that Prince had not read the *Traumdeutung* before writing his article.[103] Jones developed a psychoanalytic critique of hypnosis and suggestion, borrowing from Ferenczi and arguing that they depended on sexual and Oedipal feelings.

Not only was Prince's work brushed aside but it seemed to him that the solidarity of the psychotherapists, who before had been relatively united against a hostile medical profession, would now be broken. In obedience to what Putnam called his "unity complex" he tried to reconcile his old friend with Jones. On January 5, 1911, Putnam urged Jones to refrain from criticizing the value of other methods and proposed a set of fundamental principles, whose major point was that Freud's views were not a theory to which each psychoanalyst must entirely subscribe. Rather, they were tentative conclusions, in much the spirit Freud had conveyed in his first letter.[104]

Then, in the *Journal of Abnormal Psychology* for February–March, 1911, Prince published his own rejoinder to Jones as well as a harsh criticism of psychoanalysis by A. Friedländer, a German psychiatrist, and another by Boris Sidis. Jones threatened to resign as an editor of the *Journal* and proposed to Putnam that the psychoanalysts found a publication of their own.[105]

Putnam wrote to Jones on February 24, 1911, expressing his sorrow and dismay and suggesting that it would be "utterly un-

---

[103] Jones to Putnam, October 20, 1910.
[104] Freud to Putnam, December 5, 1909; Putnam to Jones, January 5, 1911.
[105] See n. 99 above and Jones to Putnam, February 19, 1911.

fortunate if those of us who really care about psychopathology in the large sense, should drift apart, no matter what the provocation." Jones sent the letter to A. A. Brill and stayed on as an editor of the *Journal*. To Putnam, Jones had argued that he himself had a "truth for truth's sake complex" and urged that unity should not be bought at the "price of self-respect and honest convictions. I suppose no big movement can proceed harmoniously, without involving some alienation."

Despite Jones's plan to issue a common invitation to join an American branch society, Brill founded the New York Psychoanalytic Society independently on February 12, 1911. Membership was restricted to physicians practicing psychoanalysis, and ten of the fifteen were drawn from the staff of the Manhattan State Hospital on Ward's Island, also the location of the Psychiatric Institute. The founders included August Hoch, then the Institute's director; Edward W. Scripture, a psychiatrist at Columbia University; C. P. Oberndorf, the first historian of psychoanalysis in America; and Horace W. Frink, whom Freud came to regard as one of the most promising American analysts. The Society functioned as a real working group, met once a month, and under Brill's leadership became the center of orthodox psychoanalysis in the United States.

Brill did not become a member of the American Association until a year after it was organized in Baltimore on May 9, 1911. It was open to anyone who had given "evidence of a competent knowledge of psychoanalysis"; its members were highly eclectic in outlook and met only once a year. Putnam was elected president and Jones, secretary; the five other founders were Trigant Burrow, who had studied with Jung and was an assistant in clinical psychiatry at the Johns Hopkins University Hospital; Ralph Hamill, who had studied in Vienna and was an assistant to Hugh T. Patrick; John T. MacCurdy, then in the Johns Hopkins University Medical School; G. Alexander Young, an Omaha neurologist who also had worked at the Burghölzli.[106]

The New York Society had voted to remain independent, and the Weimar Congress officially accepted both American groups as

---

[106] See "The New York Psychoanalytic Society," *Journal of Abnormal Psychology,* 6 (April–May 1911), 80, and "The American Psychoanalytic Association," *ibid.* (October–November 1911), 328; *Zentralblatt,* 2 (1912), 236, 241–242.

entirely separate organizations.[107] Jones's "General Association" was an exception to the custom that branch members come from the same city, for members were "dispersed throughout America and Canada."

In 1914 the Boston Psychoanalytic Society was founded, with Putnam as president. He wrote to Freud early in 1915 that a group met every Friday afternoon at his house, "and although we are not geniuses, yet we do fair work, and, I think, keep our heads level." [108] They probably included Coriat, Louville Eugene Emerson, a psychologist who worked as a psychoanalyst at the Massachusetts General Hospital, and James Van Teslaar, a Romanian immigrant who was on the staff of the Massachusetts Mental Hygiene Society. Prince may have met with them occasionally.

The founding of psychoanalytic organizations and of the *Psychoanalytic Review* in 1913 by William Alanson White and Smith Ely Jelliffe confirmed the emergence of psychoanalysis as a profession. Although membership in the psychoanalytic organizations was intended as a "minimum guarantee" of knowledge and competence, the training of psychoanalysts was not formalized for at least another decade. The first members of the analytic organizations were in fact largely self-selected and self-trained. Psychoanalysis, as Ferenczi wrote to Putnam, was still a "young science," highly experimental and individual.

Putnam became deeply interested in the interpretation of dreams. To William James, Putnam observed in his first address on psychoanalysis, dreams were "phantasmagorias of the fancy, sparks leaping to and fro on burnt-out paper." Freud had demonstrated that they occupied a "definite and useful place in the economy of life." Freud and Jones interpreted several of Putnam's dreams from the accounts he gave of them.[109] Putnam also was troubled by the problem of defining the unconscious. He wrote to Freud on February 15, 1910, that he agreed with the view of the French philosopher and psychologist Henri Bergson, that memories

---

[107] See n. 106 above and "Minutes of the New York Psychoanalytic Society," February 12, 1911, and June 27, 1911.

[108] Putnam to Freud, [early 1915]; Putnam to Jones, November 1, 1914; "Notes," *Journal of Abnormal Psychology,* 9 (April–May 1914), 71.

[109] Putnam to Freud, September 30, 1911; Freud to Putnam, October 5, 1911; Jones to Putnam, October 29, 1911.

were not brain-residua. Freud promptly replied that from the beginning he had agreed with Bergson's view of the unconscious, and cautioned that terminology didn't have to fit perfectly.[110] More important than theoretical understanding was actual training in the technique of analysis.

During Putnam's trip to attend the Weimar Congress, he spent six hours in analysis with Freud in Zurich, where the latter was visiting Jung. Putnam returned home with a keen sense of the importance of the analysis of the analyst, an innovation that the Zurich School had introduced and Freud had endorsed. The analyst, Freud insisted, must be purified of his own "complexes." The first analysts also continued to emphasize self-analysis, the analyst's exploration of his own unconscious. Freud had made some of his major discoveries, including the Oedipus complex, in this way. After Weimar, Putnam began to pursue self-analysis assiduously. Freud informed him that it was an interminable process and that each attempt brought its own surprises.

From 1911 on the psychoanalytic movement was troubled by schisms, and Freud worried lest Putnam desert the cause. Differences arose over fundamental aspects of Freud's theories, notably infantile sexuality and the unconscious. Freud expressed himself freely to Putnam about these developments, giving his unvarnished opinions of Jung and Adler.

Although Putnam hoped for a time that the dissidents could be reconciled, he remained entirely loyal to Freud.[111] He rejected Jung and Adler for ethical and clinical reasons, although both enjoyed a vogue among such eclectic American analysts as Jelliffe and White. First, Putnam argued that Freud's former followers were usurping the leadership and claiming insights that in fact were Freud's alone. Second, Putnam completely opposed their desexualization of psychoanalysis. He had come to insist that a thorough psychoanalysis entailed discovery of the patient's infantile sexual goals. To disregard them was to accede to the patient's resistances, yet this was precisely what Adler and Jung proposed.

Adler's special emphasis on organ inferiority and the will to power was far too narrow, vague, and exclusive. Putnam agreed

---

[110] Freud to Putnam, March 10, 1910.
[111] Putnam to Adolf Meyer, January 9, 1913, the Meyer Papers, the William H. Welch Library of Medicine, The Johns Hopkins University.

with Freud that Adler's dismissal of love as a fundamental motive was one more attempt to eliminate the "sex problem." Surely patients "are not torn and thrilled by their desire for supremacy (regarded as freed — if one can so regard it — from the sex feelings that attend it) at all as they are torn and thrilled by their (unrecognized and unacknowledged) sex passions. Neither is the repression discoverable in the one case at all comparable to that met with in the other." [112] For years, Freud had been aware of the role of self-assertion, and Adler's contributions were hardly original. As a careful neurologist, Putnam judged Adler's neurological speculations to be entirely unproven, especially such flights as the assertion that cancer was unusually prevalent in erogenous zones. Adler was at once too simplistic and too speculative. Ultimately Adler's goal receded in a "never-ending procession of super and super-super men."

Putnam dismissed Jung on clinical grounds, and he shared in part Freud's estimate of Jung's personality. He had sent the daughter of his old friend and colleague Henry P. Bowditch to Zurich for treatment. To Putnam's astonishment, Jung's therapeutic methods seemed to exacerbate her sense of abnegation and self-reproach. He counseled her to be wary of Jung's assertive "masterful ways." He contrasted his own reaction to his psychoanalysis with Freud to hers with Jung: "I remember that Dr. Freud pointed out to me, in the very first of our few conferences in Zurich, that I was a murderer! Think of that. But did he mean, or did I suppose he meant, that I was to go and jump overboard, or give myself up to the hangman? Not a bit of it. I was to be healthier minded from then on, and happier, and better able to stop being a murderer." Psychological change, he wrote, could only come about "through a process of slow, intelligent and quiet growth." [113]

Jung had expressed his disagreement with Freud's sexual emphasis as early as the monograph on dementia praecox. In 1912 he was invited to lecture at Fordham University and there publicly

[112] Putnam, "The Work of Sigmund Freud," *Journal of Abnormal Psychology*, 12 (August 1917), 156; Ad Psa, 360; see also Putnam, "The Work of Alfred Adler, Considered with Especial Reference to That of Freud," *Psychoanalytic Review*, 3 (April 1916), 121–140; Ad Psa, 312–339.
[113] Putnam to Fanny Bowditch, December 10, 1913; see also Putnam to Fanny Bowditch, October 12, 1912, December 1, [1912], December 9, [1912].

rejected Freud's major theories. Jung denied the significance of the Oedipus complex and of infantile sexuality in general. Putnam heard the last part of the speech and described his reactions to Ernest Jones: Jung was rejecting precisely the most valuable element in Freud's theories. In 1917 Putnam summed up his impressions. The defections of both Jung and Adler partly occurred as a result of Freud's brilliant but one-sided genius. Putnam could sympathize with Jung's wish to help with his patients' present problems. But this "would often be to impose one's own personality upon the patient, and would lead inexperienced students of psychoanalysis to abandon methods in the use of which more rigid studies might have made them competent." Jung's departure in this respect represented a return to pre-Freudian therapeutics, to the old relationship of "mentor and advisor," when the therapist was too "masterful or too intimate" in a way that was strongly tinged with sexual feelings. Freud's discovery of the transference had obviated this earlier dependent relationship. "Furthermore, I cannot in the least sympathize with the rejection by Jung of Freud's theories of regression, infantile sexuality, and fixation." [114]

Freud was grateful for Putnam's support and assured him that despite philosophical differences, the psychoanalysts paid close attention to his ideas and that after them would come other, less limited analysts who would be more receptive to his stimulus.[115] Putnam, however, remained deeply troubled by aspects of psychoanalytic therapy and above all by Freud's Weltanschauung.

Differences, 1909–1918

Despite unswerving loyalty to the psychoanalytic cause and to Freud, Putnam did not gloss over their growing differences. In correspondence they worked through some of these nearly irreconcilable conflicts, which threatened, but did not disrupt their mutual respect and friendship.

In some ways Freud was more deeply affected than Putnam. Putnam insisted all the more vehemently on the importance of

---

[114] Putnam, "The Work of Sigmund Freud," p. 158; Ad Psa, 363; Putnam to Jones, October 24, 1912.
[115] Letter of January 1, 1913.

values. Partly because of Putnam's persistence, Freud took up the study of the psychological origin of Putnam's preoccupations — religion and man's "higher nature."

Putnam's criticism and his therapeutic principles often anticipated the course of later psychotherapeutic developments both inside and outside the psychoanalytic movement. His insistence on "will" is reminiscent of Otto Rank's work in the 1920's. Putnam's emphasis on philosophy and values anticipated Erich Fromm and the neo-Freudians. His belief in creativity, conscious decision, and conflict-free spheres of action anticipated the later psychoanalytic ego-psychologists. If Putnam's criticisms and his therapeutic aperçus were prescient, his philosophical formulations were less apt. He was an amateur, not a professional philosopher, and the idealist principles he attempted to expound were derived from one of the most obscure formulations of an intensely complex tradition.

At the level of the cultivated American's fundamental assumptions, the popular moral idealism Putnam represented began to pass out of American life in the years before the Great War. Nevertheless the issues he raised, if not the terms in which he raised them, have remained significant.

In a paper Putnam was revising at the time of his death, he recalled that the essence of his disagreement emerged clearly in conversation after one of the Worcester lectures. Freud had been arguing that causality applied alike in physics and in human thought. People were the products of "biologic evolution, personal experience and social education," but not of "spontaneous choice, with reference to an ideal aim consciously conceived." Putnam asked whether such determinism ruled out all moral estimates so that one could no longer judge one person better or worse, nobler or ignobler than another. Freud replied "with impressive earnestness, that it was not moral estimates that were needed for solving the problem of human life and motives but more *knowledge*." [116]

Putnam rejected this conclusion along with Freud's materialism and determinism, the unquestioned postulates of much nineteenth-century science. Putnam essentially asked whether value

---

[116] Putnam, "Elements of Strength and Elements of Weakness in Psychoanalytic Doctrines," *Psychoanalytic Review,* 6 (April 1919), 118–119; Ad Psa, 449–450.

judgments were relevant to Freud's therapy and implicit in his Weltanschauung. Putnam believed that philosophy provided insights as valid as those of science. He refused to reduce motives, including religious motives, to human necessity, and he rejected the theory that evolution represented nothing more than adaptation to environment. Steeped in a powerful Unitarian and idealist tradition, he argued that the human being was a creative center, ruled by an inherent principle of growth.[117] With increasing firmness he insisted that Freud was a brilliant scientist but a weak philosopher and that the attitude of the persistent agnostic required examination as much as did that of the believer.[118]

A slight note of qualification began to appear in Freud's affectionate appraisals after 1914. "That old man is altogether a wonderful acquisition," he wrote to Karl Abraham in 1910.[119] Four years later he described Putnam as the "chief pillar" of the psychoanalytic movement in America. His addresses were rich in content and brilliant in form; he had contributed immensely toward creating the high esteem psychoanalysis enjoyed among psychiatrists and the public. Only one thing in Putnam was disquieting: his wish to place psychoanalysis "in the service of a particular philosophical outlook on the world" and to "urge this upon the patient for the purpose of ennobling his mind. In my opinion, this is after all only to use violence, even though it is overlaid with the most honorable motives." Freud explained this "ethical bias" as a "reaction against a predisposition to obsessional neurosis. His closer personal acquaintances could not escape the conclusion that he was one of those happily compensated people of the obsessional type for whom what is noble is second nature and for whom any concession to unworthiness becomes an impossibility." [120] Possibly this neurosis represented a conflict over aggressive drives, as Freud had indicated to Putnam at Zurich in 1911. Like Freud and many other neurologists, Putnam, too, suffered from nervous symptoms,

---

[117] "The Philosophy of Psychotherapy, II," *Psychotherapy: A Course of Reading in Sound Psychology, Sound Medicine and Sound Religion*, vol. 3, no. 4 (New York: Centre Publishing Co., 1909), pp. 37–38.

[118] *Human Motives* (Boston: Little Brown and Co., 1915), p. 46; Putnam, "The Work of Sigmund Freud"; Ad Psa, 352.

[119] Letter of December 16, 1910, in Jones, *Sigmund Freud*, II, 165.

[120] "James J. Putnam" (1919), SE, XVII, 271; "On the History of the Psycho-Analytic Movement" (1914), SE, XIV, 31–32; "Advances in Psycho-Analytic Therapy" (1918), SE, XVII, 165; "An Autobiographical Study" (1925), SE, XX, 51.

chiefly neuralgia, and occasional depression. He once wrote to his friend Storey that he felt inconsequential, and later he was cautious in rejecting Adler's theories of inferiority and compensation because of his own "complexes." [121]

Yet Putnam's "ethical bias" was more than "compensation" and represented an aspect of the same New England character that first had led him to defend psychoanalysis. His Weltanschauung had been formed by powerful forces, of which Freud could have known very little — his social world, his parents, his intellectual companions, his patients, his educational and religious tradition, his earlier approach to psychotherapy.

Putnam's discussions of his Weltanschauung provide the obscurest passages in his letters to Freud and Ernest Jones. What did Putnam mean by the "necessary presuppositions of all thinking," the "study of humanity at its best," the "necessary connection between progress and freedom," a "personal universe"?

In 1910 Putnam informed Freud that until recently he had had "no religion at all, properly speaking, and was ready to let 'natural science' be the arbiter of all." But in fact religion and his mother's piety had played an important role in his early life, and the views he proposed to Freud were close to those of his youth. In 1864 his mother had written:

"While you are studying wisely, no doubt, the external historical evidences of the peculiar life of Christ, look a little at what has been always enough for me and other 'babes' the internal Evidence, leaving the Miracles to work their effects upon us, sooner or later, when they may be needed or *never* with some people . . . It seems to me, I could have believed had there been nothing done so wonderful — but the heavenly sentiment 'the Grace' shown out so charmingly in the Life. We trust to the effect of it upon us in other human creatures, surely we may in this Holy One, giving out as it never was given before or since the 'spirit of the father.' " [122]

This emphasis on the inner life was reinforced by reading Emerson, whom Putnam quoted all his life. At Harvard, he mocked at

[121] Putnam to Storey, December 6, [1867], in the possession of Charles Moorfield Storey; Putnam to Freud, September 30, 1911; Putnam, "The Work of Alfred Adler, Considered with Especial Reference to That of Freud" (1916), Ad Psa, 312.
[122] Letter of Sunday noon, [1864].

old-fashioned Calvinism, the divinely ordained Sabbath, and Original Sin. He insisted that the "untrained impulses of the human mind inclined more to good than to evil." The "marks of depravity in children that are pointed out by believers in 'original sin' can, I believe, be all shown either to exhibit the remarkable purity of that early age or else to exist really only in the imagination of observers." Later he took pains to argue that Freud's theories of infantile sexuality bore no relation to doctrines of innate depravity.[123]

While in medical school Putnam informed Moorfield Storey that he agreed with one of the popular Unitarian tracts of the day, James Freeman Clarke's *The Christian Doctrine of Prayer.* In terms surprisingly close to those Putnam used in writing to Freud, Clarke, who was sympathetic to Transcendentalism, argued that every soul had its own "law of development and growth," and that although the soul depended on the body it was not the same as the body.[124] Putnam informed Storey that he did not believe in a "concrete being with senses and passions, that watches over this mundane sphere." [125] But he did believe that "temporal things only exist as supplementary and dependent on spiritual things and are subject to change the moment that a corresponding change takes place in the spiritual world to which they are subject." [126]

Putnam modified this Transcendentalist view during his trip to Europe and entered a period of militant scientific determinism, at least in medicine. He judged the philosophy of his friend William James "too mystical" and preferred the materialistic cosmology of Herbert Spencer.[127] From medical school days James and Putnam had remained close friends, and James spent summers at Keene Valley with the Putnam and Bowditch families. Putnam described for Frances Morse, what he took to be James's increas-

[123] "Whether the Untrained Impulses of the Human Mind Incline More to Good or Evil?" [undated], pp. 1, 7; "The Authority for the Religious Observance of One Day in Seven," no. 1, [undated]; Putnam, *Human Motives,* pp. 95–96.

[124] *The Christian Doctrine of Prayer* (Boston: American Unitarian Association, 9th ed., 1880), pp. 229–231; Putnam to Moorfield Storey, April 20, [1864], in the possession of Charles Moorfield Storey.

[125] Letter of April 20, [1864], in the possession of Charles Moorfield Storey.

[126] Putnam to Moorfield Storey, September 7, 1867, in the possession of Charles Moorfield Storey.

[127] See n. 29 above and Putnam to "My dear cousins" [Frances and Mary Morse], May 31, 1871.

ingly scientific attitude, displayed in his first public lectures on the "Mind and the Brain": "When his tongue is stimulated by the difficulties of a complicated psychological explanation he becomes as usual, brilliant, and bursts out into almost a redundancy of flowery metaphors, or pithy homely illustrations. It seems to me that he has been doing more close scientific thinking the past year or two than before, or at any rate I have never got hold of his ideas until within that time. I now amuse myself by fancying that I have discovered his mission, so far as he has one, as an indendant[128] philosopher, and that is, to establish what he calls the 'common sense' doctrines — the belief in free-will, in the efficacy of consciousness, the discoverability of the relation between mind and matter, etc., on a scientific basis." [129]

James's early attack on materialistic causality bore directly on psychotherapy and ethics. To James and other critics, materialists assumed a mechanical, totally determined universe, without freedom to choose good from evil. Physical nervous processes were the supreme reality; feelings, thoughts, and consciousness were mere collateral products of neurological events and could not alter them significantly.

The mind, including the feelings, James insisted, played a more important role than this. The more complex the brain, the less determined and reflex were the organism's reactions. Consciousness permitted not only new and unforeseen responses to environment but, even more important, resistance to immediate impulse in favor of a distant end. Only this capacity for postponement made ethical conduct possible. Resistance to impulse constituted the essence of human will.[130]

The power of consciousness to alter bodily and emotional states and of the will to resist impulse were at the heart of James's own lifelong struggle against neurotic depression. Putnam admired this brave fight and believed that it fundamentally changed James's personality and outlook. James adopted with a large measure of

[128] "Independent" was probably intended.
[129] Letter of October 29, [1878].
[130] "Remarks on Spencer's Definition of Mind as Correspondence," *Journal of Speculative Philosophy*, 12 (January 1878), 1–18; James's unsigned review of Herbert Spencer's *Data of Ethics*, *Nation*, 29 (September 11, 1879), 178–179; William James, "Are We Automata?" *Mind*, 4 (January 1879), 20–21.

success, the "bearing, the expression, and the sentiments that go with health." [131]

The qualities Putnam most admired in James, "personal courage," rejection of "physico-chemico positivism," "belief in the creative power of a voluntary act," recur often in Putnam's letters to Freud. James's last years reflected his courageous voluntarism. In 1898 James consulted Putnam for chest pains, symptoms of angina pectoris, partly brought on by a strenuous hike at Keene Valley. James saw other specialists, took the waters at Bad Nauheim, which seemed only to make him worse. Despite his health, much of his most important work was completed between 1898 and 1910, including *The Varieties of Religious Experience* and the essays on pragmatism and radical empiricism. Impatient with the limitations of experimental academic psychology, James kept up his interest in the "vaguer" but more "adequate" psychological work of the clinicians. In 1894 he had reviewed Breuer's and Freud's "Preliminary Communication" on hysteria and referred to their work again in *The Varieties*.[132] His general interest in functional psychology rather than any special fondness for psychoanalysis probably inspired his parting words to Ernest Jones at the Clark Conference: "The future of psychology belongs to your work." Freud recalled his meeting with James at Clark: "I shall never forget one little scene that occurred as we were on a walk together. He stopped suddenly, handed me a bag he was carrying and asked me to walk on, saying that he would catch me up as soon as he had got through an attack of angina pectoris which was just coming on. He died of that disease a year later; and I have always wished that I might be as fearless as he was in the face of approaching death." [133] This was the kind of example Putnam probably had in mind when he insisted to Freud that for a truly rounded view of man, the best should be studied along with the worst.

After the Clark Conference, Putnam wrote to James that he hoped Freud's "terribly searching psychogenetic explanations" offered but one pole of human life and that there was another in

[131] Putnam, "William James," *Atlantic Monthly,* 106 (December 1910), 839.
[132] See Breuer and Freud, "On the Psychical Mechanism of Hysterical Phenomena: Preliminary Communication" (1893); SE, II, 3–17, n. 33 above, and *The Varieties of Religious Experience* (New York: Longmans, Green and Co., 1902), pp. 234–235.
[133] "An Autobiographical Study"; SE, XX, 52.

which he took no interest. "The alternative is surely between a gross materialism and a truly personalistic universe with love and hope in it from the start." [134] James died August 26, 1910. In the December *Atlantic Monthly,* Putnam praised James's "truly radical empiricism" which "enabled him to maintain his stout adherence to scientific accuracy and to assert the necessity for taking experience as the court of last resort, yet at the same time to recognize the existence of influences that transcend the evidence of the senses, kept him in touch at once with science and with religion, and made it possible for him to believe in a spiritual freedom." [135]

Indeterminacy and the reality of the spiritual world were confirmed for Putnam by the vitalism of Henri Bergson, the French philosopher-psychologist. In *Matière et Mémoire,* published in 1896, Bergson attempted to re-examine the relation of mind and brain, partly through a careful study of the literature of aphasia, including Freud's monograph. Bergson argued that memory images were not "stored" in the brain, but were called up by the entire sensori-motor system as it became set for action in the present. Putnam insisted with Bergson that the effective meaning of mental activity could not be described in terms of cerebral physiology. Bergson argued that the mental state was "immensely wider than the cerebral state." [136]

These were the arguments Putnam had in mind when he wrote to Freud that memories were not "brain residua," but a "possession of the mind, having as such a real existence independent of physical laws." Actually, Putnam had extended Bergson's position. Bergson had left extremely vague the relation of what he called "pure memory," that is, perceptions as they occurred, to the organism. James had accused him of conjuring up a "soul" in which these pure memories were stored. To Bergson it seemed as if the mind did not fulfill Descartes' description of the properties of matter: extension, measurement, law, and passivity. Rather, the mind was indivisible, active, and free.

Bergson argued that personality and character, and all present

---

[134] Letter of June 25, 1910.

[135] "William James," p. 846.

[136] Henri Bergson, *Matter and Memory,* trans. Nancy Margaret Paul and W. Scott Palmer (New York: The Macmillan Co., 1912), p. xvii; Putnam, "The Bearing of Philosophy on Psychiatry," pp. 1021–1022; Bergson, *Creative Evolution,* authorized trans. by Arthur Mitchell (New York: Henry Holt and Co., 1911), pp. 181, 262–263.

perceptions, were formed largely by unconscious memories. In dreams and in insanity, the attention became relaxed, and pure memories, including childhood perceptions, detached from realistic sensori-motor adaptations, crossed into consciousness once more. Putnam's first paper on psychoanalysis, delivered before the American Psychological Association meeting in Boston in December 1909, was devoted to a comparison of Bergson's and Freud's views of the unconscious. G. Stanley Hall wrote to Freud that he had been unable to understand it, and it has not survived among Putnam's papers.[137]

Bergson added another element to Putnam's approach to psychoanalysis—the poussée vitale, or life force, an original impetus, "an internal push that has carried life, by more and more complex forms, to higher and higher destinies." With James, Bergson believed that indetermination was an essential aspect of the life force. "Throughout the whole extent of the animal kingdom," Bergson wrote, "consciousness seems proportionate to the living being's power of choice." [138] Putnam, and several other American psychoanalysts, notably William Alanson White and Smith Ely Jelliffe, saw in Freud's libido, one manifestation of Bergson's élan vital.

Putnam's view of the intellect, the most obscure aspect of his philosophy, came from American Hegelianism, to which he was introduced by his former patient Susan Blow. Although Putnam did not once mention Miss Blow in his surviving letters to Freud, she furnished much of the material for his debate with the psychoanalysts. She acquainted Putnam with the "necessary presuppositions of all thinking," her personal distillation of Friederich Froebel and William Torrey Harris. Putnam had treated Miss Blow successfully in 1894 after she had been a nervous invalid for a decade. A member of a well-to-do St. Louis family, Miss Blow had founded one of the country's first Froebelian kindergartens. As Putnam became even more deeply interested in psychotherapy around 1906, he also became more interested in Miss Blow's philosophy.[139] Until her death at 76 in 1916 they spent many hours

[137] G. Stanley Hall to Freud, December 30, 1909, Clark University Papers.
[138] *Creative Evolution*, p. 179.
[139] Susan Blow to Putnam, March 1, 1894, June 15, 1906, November 14, 1909, November 17, 1910, September 17, 1913; Putnam to Susan Blow, July 19, 1912, March 5, 1913.

discussing the mental life of the child and the ideas of the latest luminaries — Bertrand Russell, Royce, Bergson — and Freud. Putnam cancelled a visit to Miss Blow to hear Freud at Clark in 1909.

At first Miss Blow suggested that Freud was only rediscovering man's "total depravity." A relic of her childhood Calvinism, total depravity was for her a comforting article of faith along with her belief in man's divinity. Reflecting the "civilized" norm of womanly reticence, Miss Blow argued that psychoanalysis attacked the modesty of the soul. After reading more deeply in the Freudian "sloughs," guided by Dr. Putnam, she concluded that psychoanalysis fostered integration. But the mere recall of the past was not enough. Patients needed ideals to direct their sublimation and their management of themselves.

A fierce opponent of Rousseau, John Dewey, and G. Stanley Hall, Miss Blow insisted that only native impulses in the child that conduced to virtue should be permitted expression. In Putnam's popular book on psychoanalysis, *Human Motives,* he softened her view. The child's play was a pure and glorious self-forgetting spontaneity. Nevertheless, he should be gently guided toward a consciousness of his social obligations.[140]

Miss Blow did not believe that logic was a set of formal conventions but rather a revelation of the "form and structure of the intellect." This view she derived from Harris, Hegel's foremost American disciple, and Putnam suggested Freud read Harris instead of Sir James Frazier while writing *Totem and Taboo.* Harris argued that everything was known through concepts. Some were derived from experience; but others, such as "causality," "space and time," were "furnished by the mind itself, as the a priori conditions necessary to all experience." These thought forms expressed ultimate, true Being.[141]

Far more mystical than Harris, Miss Blow argued that "self-activity," the heart of the logical process, expressed the self-determining" energy of life. Man mirrored the divine, and the universe was evolving toward an "infinite community of souls." Putnam discarded Miss Blow's sentimentality, but kept many of her "presuppositions" — self-activity, the idealist view of mind, the transcend-

[140] *Human Motives*, pp. 96–97, 110.
[141] William Torrey Harris, *Hegel's Logic: A Book on the Genesis of the Categories of the Mind* (Chicago: S. C. Griggs and Co., 1895), pp. 19–20.

ental relation between the individual and the divine. These were the conceptions Putnam had in mind when he wrote to Freud that one must "study the mind itself à la Hegel," or that philosophy dealt with the "essential laws of thinking," or that the "only *reality* is the nature of *personal consciousness.*"

The final elements in Putnam's intellectual exchange with Freud came from Josiah Royce's examination of the relation between the individual and the community. Putnam and Royce sustained an uneasy balance between the claims of conscience and those of society. Unlike conservative Hegelians, they did not proclaim an unquestioned faith in existing institutions. Rather, tension between present reality and the envisioned ideal was a major spur to change and progress. Royce and Putnam, as well as Miss Blow, insisted that there were always "heights yet to ascend," that one must "hitch one's wagon to a star." [142] The very difficulty of attaining an ideal was part of its leavening value.

Sometimes overstrained idealism could sour into morbid self-criticism. Putnam combined Royce's insights on the origins of the self-image with his clinical experience to elaborate in the early 1900's a theory of internal conflict and alienation as major factors in nervous disorder. Like many New England physicians, Putnam often encountered the morbidly sensitive conscience that drove patients to pathological self-reproach. Royce had suggested clues as to how one aspect of this conscience might be formed. The child developed his sense of himself and of society through imitation. When he learned to speak, he became a self-conscious moral agent because he learned to look upon himself through the eyes of others. Yet this process, Putnam wrote, could result in a painful sense of isolation. This might begin in the "thoughtless ostracism by children of playmates." Then physical weakness, "inability to conform to social standards, to compete in occupations, to take part in sports and games" exacerbated the loneliness.[143]

Gradually a person might begin to stand apart from "himself and see or hear and criticize himself." He might develop a "vague

[142] Josiah Royce, "The Recent Psychotherapeutic Movement in America," *Psychotherapy: A Course of Reading in Sound Psychology, Sound Medicine and Sound Religion,* vol. 1, no. 1 (New York: Centre Publishing Co., 1909), p. 32; Susan Blow to Putnam, March 11, 1910.

[143] "The Treatment of Psychasthenia from the Standpoint of the Social Consciousness," *American Journal of the Medical Sciences,* 135 (January 7, 1908), 78–83.

sense of himself as surrounded by an imagined circle of critics, enemies, or admirers, toward whom he must adopt an attitude of secrecy, shame, hostility or superiority. His diverse mental states may even become personified in his own eyes so as to reproduce the community in miniature. He then sets himself against himself." [144] The restoration of social ties, and an ending of alienation, were integral parts of this therapy. Each person had to "feel his social obligations at their full value," and this sometimes required overcoming a "cramp-like dread" of change.[145] Putnam's later psychoanalytic emphasis on sublimation came from this earlier therapeutic development.

Putnam had shaped each major influence in accordance with his clinical experience and unconsciously, according to his early Transcendentalism. Thus he had interpreted James as a believer in the reality of spiritual freedom. He had used Bergson to suggest that the mind transcended the brain, and Miss Blow to reinforce his faith in the existence of constructive innate impulses. He had been reassured by Royce's faith in the unseen ideal. Putnam was not a logician, given to rigorous exposition. His idealism was more a reincarnation of his youthful Unitarianism than a sophisticated version of Harris or Royce. Rather Putnam was a sensitive clinician, who fought the depression he saw in his patients and sometimes sensed in himself. Without faith in free will, therapeutic effort seemed vain, and the fate of nervous invalids darker than it should be.[146]

There were many reasons why Putnam should regard philosophy as a true science of the mind. It enjoyed high prestige at his university and in his social and intellectual worlds. Despised by many scientists, as Putnam realized, metaphysics yet was of consuming interest to his Harvard friends James and Royce. Putnam urged physicians to study philosophy because it alone gave insight into the nature of consciousness.[147] Putnam renewed his interest in

[144] "The Treatment of Psychasthenia," p. 79.
[145] "The Treatment of Psychasthenia," pp. 82–83, 87, 91. Putnam treated Royce after a stroke in 1912, see Royce to Putnam, March 24, 1913. See Royce, "The Case of John Bunyan" and "Some Observations on the Anomalies of Self-Consciousness," in *Studies in Good and Evil,* and Putnam, "Remarks on the Psychical Treatment of Neurasthenia," p. 507, and "The Bearing of Philosophy on Psychiatry," p. 1021.
[146] "The Philosophy of Psychotherapy, I," *Psychotherapy,* vol. 3, no. 3 (1909), pp. 15–16.
[147] "The Bearing of Philosophy on Psychiatry," pp. 1021–1022.

John Hughlings Jackson, the most philosophical of neurologists, with whom he had studied in 1877 and who interpreted many symptoms of disease as representing the organism's positive attempts at readjustment.[148]

By 1906 James, Putnam, and many others believed they were riding a wave of renewed spirituality and idealism and that Bergson's was the philosophy of the future. The whole gloomy determinist outlook was giving way to the faith that men could change themselves and their society. The prestige of idealism was high in England and the United States, and to a lesser extent in Germany. But Austria never had enjoyed a strong Hegelian vogue and did not see a revival of idealism or of vitalism of the kind that excited some American intellectuals. Many of these connected idealism and vitalism with new movements for social reform. Putnam, for one, concluded that only philosophy treated man "as a free and responsible creator of a better order in the world."

Putnam became caught up, as were other Americans, in that search for community that formed an important aspect of progressivism. A founder of the charity organization movement in Boston, he had once been concerned with fostering Emersonian self-reliance among the poor. Around 1906 he was becoming more aware of the need to extend social services in the treatment of nervous disorders. Seeing the success of a group program for tuberculosis patients at the Massachusetts General Hospital he organized one for nervous patients conducted by social workers who themselves had "been through the purgatory of nervous invalidism."

At the beginning of his professional life he had founded a public clinic as well as carrying on a private practice. By birth, by marriage, and by social and professional ties he was part of a powerful establishment. His professional life and social status contrasted profoundly with Freud's, whose isolation and Jewishness may have exacerbated his sense of the conflict between the individual and society. For Putnam, the recognition of social duties and the fulfillment of patrician obligations were paramount. A note of snob-

[148] "Certain Features of the Work of the Late J. Hughlings Jackson of London," *Boston Medical and Surgical Journal*, 169 (July 17, 1913), 73–75; Putnam, "The Value of the Physiological Principle in the Study of Neurology," *Boston Medical and Surgical Journal*, 151 (December 15, 1904), 641–647; John Hughlings Jackson to Putnam, November 29, 1876.

bery about the uneducated and the urban and rural masses, evident in his early years, gradually became muted in his writing,
public and private. By 1911 he was expressing sympathy with so-
cialism.[149]

Putnam's concern for community and for philosophy and religion provided the ground for his prolonged debate with Freud.
From the first, Putnam rejected decisively Freud's attempts to reduce God to nothing but the infant's helplessness and need for a
protecting father. Putnam also rejected Freud's efforts to explain
the philosopher's desire to know the essential nature of things by
what Putnam euphemistically called "infantile curiosity about
fundamental facts in physiology." These explanations might be
partial truths, Putnam insisted, but, like science itself, they failed
to explain some of the most significant phenomena of life.

In 1911 Putnam gathered his courage to express his convictions
to the Psychoanalytic Congress at Weimar. He argued, using some
of Miss Blow's material, that the "very constitution of the mind"
included an intuitive recognition of moral distinctions and a sense
of social loyalty and obligation. Thus the "unconscious" contained not only the "shady" side of human nature, but an implicit recognition of the good. Analysts should sympathize with and
occasionally encourage these dim, innate aspirations. The Biblical
assertion that "the people who do not see visions shall perish from
the face of the earth," he warned, was an "accurate expression of
the truth."

The insights of psychoanalysis had a moral function, the discovery beneath conventional appearances of infantile tendencies
that prevented "progress" and maturity: "It is truly remarkable
what a touchstone has been put into our hands wherewith to
recognize the real motives which underlie apparent motives, and,
underneath the faults and failings, the fears and habits of adult
life, to see the workings out of the instinctive cravings of imaginative, pleasure-seeking, and pain-shunning infancy, dragging back
the adult from the fulfillment of his higher destiny." [150]

The acknowledgment of these "repressed devils" implied the

[149] Putnam to Frances Morse, Hotel Kurhaus Honegg, Bürgenstock, September 1,
1911.
[150] "A Plea for the Study of Philosophic Methods in Preparation for Psychoanalytic
Work," *Journal of Abnormal Psychology,* 6 (October–November 1911), 249–250, 263;
Ad Psa, 79–80, 95.

intuitive recognition of a standard of the good. It was over the nature of this standard that Putnam's disagreement with the psychoanalysts was deepest. He insisted that "belief in 'the good' was one of the most real of all our intuitions," because each individual contained a "permanently abiding element which partakes of the nature of the real, permanently abiding energy of which the life of the universe itself is made." The unseen world of spirit was the eternal reality. "Ultimate truth, like motion, hope, love and the sense of beauty" were unpicturable, yet were the only true life. Putnam argued that in each act, "the mind goes out as it were, from itself, only to return to itself and rediscover itself." [151]

Putnam's address was a disaster. Freud remarked to Ernest Jones, "Putnam's philosophy reminds me of a decorative centerpiece; everyone admires it but no one touches it." [152] Oscar Pfister suggested that Putnam arrogantly was dictating laws to natural scientists.[153] Putnam debated the issue with Ferenczi in *Imago* and with Theodor Reik in the *Zentralblatt*. Theodor Reik argued that Putnam's idealism was "only a matter of faith . . . an artistic creation," which psychoanalysts were under no obligation to adopt, because Freud's metapsychology was uncovering the "psychogenesis of philosophical systems as they arise out of a combination of constitution and experience." [154]

Putnam replied that psychoanalysts were by no means neutral about philosophy. They were positivists. When they left the firm ground of the "purely therapeutic task," they were functioning as philosophers without recognizing that they were doing so. They should examine the discipline they were thus covertly taking up.

[151] "A Plea," p. 96.

[152] Jones, *Sigmund Freud*, II, 86.

[153] *Some Applications of Psychoanalysis* (New York: Dodd, Mead & Co., 1923), pp. 178–179.

[154] Sandor Ferenczi, "Philosophie und Psychoanalyse. (Bemerkungen zu einem Aufsatze des H. Professors Dr. James J. Putnam von der Harvard-Universität, Boston, USA)" [Philosophy and Psychoanalysis (Comments on a Paper of Dr. James J. Putnam of Harvard)], *Imago*, 1 (December 1912), 519–526; Putnam, "Antwort auf die Erwiderung des Herrn Dr. Ferenczi" [A Rejoinder to Dr. Ferenczi's Reply], *Imago*, 1 (December 1912), 527–530; Theodor Reik, "Putnam, J. J.: 'Über die Bedeutung Philosophischer Anschauungen und Ausbildung für die weitere Entwicklung des psychoanalytischen Bewegung'" [Putnam, J. J.: 'The Role of Philosophical Views and Training in the Further Development of the Psychoanalytical Movement'], *Zentralblatt*, 3 (1913), 43–44; Putnam, "Psychoanalyse und Philosophie (Eine Erwiderung auf die Kritik von Dr. [Theodor] Reik)" [Reply to the Criticism by Dr. Reik], *Zentralblatt*, 3 (1913), 265–269.

If they remained positivists, they were turning back to that "terrible form of individualism and indifference of the so-called scientific age from whose all too-confining embrace we have just now freed ourselves." They had an obligation to study "all other methods of interpretation with open minds by which the actions and motives of normal people have been explained in previous times." [155]

Moreover, even the therapeutic task, that educational process of which psychoanalysis was one phase, inevitably took into account the "will, the ethical insight," the "social conscience" of the patient, for only thus could a true and useful sublimation be achieved. Putnam suggested that Jung's libido represented nothing more than Hegel's "self-activity" or Bergson's poussée vitale, and thus an implicit admission of idealism.

Freud reacted to Putnam's Weimar address in what he called a "very strange way" — by attempting to understand the psychogenesis of religion and his own lack of a religious need. The first result was *Totem and Taboo*.[156] However, Freud did not mention Putnam in the preface, where he stated that the first stimulus for the essays had come from Wilhelm Wundt's studies of folk psychology and from the writings of the Zurich school. Putnam read *Totem and Taboo,* he informed Freud, with "pleasure and admiration." [157] He was not convinced by Freud's "Just-So-Story" of patricide as the historical basis of social cohesion.

Social ties were an inherent aspect of existence, Putnam argued in *Human Motives,* a book that aroused a far more emotional reaction in Freud than the Weimar address. At once naïve and profound, archaic and surprisingly modern, *Human Motives* resolved Putnam's conflict with the psychoanalysts, summed up the major influences in his intellectual life, and uncompromisingly reasserted his early Unitarianism. It was obviously addressed to a lay audience of New Englanders, steeped like himself in Emerson, Wordsworth, and an influence Putnam perhaps had forgotten — the Unitarian minister James Freeman Clarke. Where Emerson held that our "best selves," rush to meet us, Putnam insisted, as had Clarke, on the inescapability of moral conflict.[158] Men were

[155] "Psychoanalyse und Philosophie," pp. 265, 267.
[156] Freud to Putnam, November 5, 1911, and March 28, 1912.
[157] Letter of November 29, [1913].
[158] *Human Motives*, pp. 5–6, 170–171.

torn by two sets of motives, those of constructiveness, ultimately expressible only in ideal and religious terms, and those of "adaptation" which reflected biological instincts and social pressures. Often the second held men back from realizing the first. Analogous disciplines, philosophy and psychoanalysis provided insights respectively into the constructive and the genetic drives. But if one were to choose, Putnam concluded, the superiority of philosophy was obvious.

At the heart of Putnam's concern lay the relation of philosophy to those "moral crises" he had discussed with Moorfield Storey in 1867. Self-interest or hedonistic calculations never provided sufficient motives to resolve them. In fact, men often relied on moral obligations and on ideals that could not be defined or defended in strictly scientific terms. To study such decisions was supremely important, and Putnam cautioned his readers: "To accustom ourselves to the study of immaturity and childhood before proceeding to the study of maturity and manhood is often to habituate ourselves to an undesirable limitation of our vision with reference to the scope of the enterprise on which we enter." [159]

Freud acknowledged that this passage applied to him, and admitted that he was intrigued with the question Putnam posed of how and why people were virtuous. Freud could not explain why he and his six adult children were "thoroughly decent human beings." [160]

Putnam pushed far beyond his argument based on the performance of moral acts. "We cannot assert our power of disinterested love and will and at the same time deny that love and will exist," he wrote.[161] If men conceived of the existence of a perfect Being, they affirmed that Being's existence. Like many nineteenth-century Americans raised in a religious faith, Putnam found it impossible to abandon the belief that the moral order reflected the nature of the universe. Perhaps unconsciously alluding to his own tradition, he argued that to feel a relationship to the universe as a whole was to find moral obligations as coercive as the "noblesse oblige" of a noble family. Moreover, modern scientists were redefining the nature of the universe and of scientific laws. The

[159] *Human Motives*, p. 20.
[160] Freud to Putnam, July 8, 1915.
[161] *Human Motives*, pp. 42–43, 57–66.

"laws" of physics were symbolic expressions of the thought of the observer, just as religious statements were. Those who feared religion were acting as if behind its symbolic statements there actually lurked a god to be loved or a devil to be feared. Putnam's God was not a personage, but a transcendental energy, self-activity, the élan vital. It could be observed in the individual and in the ascending spiral of evolution. Each person's conscious sense of unity within constantly changing selves could be expressed only in constantly new forms and possibilities. The primal energy also was reflected in the laws of physics, in the vegetable and animal worlds, and in the history of the "growth of freedom." Putnam had touched one of Freud's most sensitive areas.

The religious element in *Human Motives* repelled Freud. During the night after he had been reading the book he dreamed of the death of his son Martin at the front. Freud believed that the dream "was a defiant challenge to occult powers to test whether they could be as destructive as he often feared." [162] He wrote to Ferenczi, "It is a good and loyal book, but filled with the sense of religion which I am irresistibly impelled to reject. From the psychical reality of our ideas he directly infers their material reality and therefore God." [163]

The reception of *Human Motives* at home was disappointing. Putnam's colleague Richard Cabot dismissed it in the social workers' magazine *Survey,* as a murky, expurgated mélange of Emerson, Bergson, and Freud, in 175 pages. The *Dial* found it "consoling when not convincing." In the *Psychoanalytic Review,* William Alanson White argued, however, that it disproved the "silly criticisms" current against psychoanalysis. Putnam wrote to Frances Morse, "I am very much in doubt whether anyone outside of a small group will take the slightest interest. You speak with doubt of your understanding it. But Goodness me!!!, if that were or is so, then the small group becomes vanishingly smaller." [164] One member of that group, Moorfield Storey, found *Human Motives* helpful, "It is the same Jim with whom I used to discuss the problems of the universe, with his ideals unspoiled by the experiences of life, but on the contrary held more firmly and intelligently. You

[162] Jones, *Sigmund Freud,* III, 390.
[163] Jones, *Sigmund Freud,* II, 416.
[164] *Survey,* 36 (June 1916), 292; *Dial,* 59 (August 15, 1915), 114; *Psychoanalytic Review,* 3 (January 1916), 116; Letter of [1915].

do not realize what a missionary you have been all your life, and what an example to us all. Not every one holds so closely through life the faith of his youth, indeed there be very few who do." [165]

The general reaction depressed Putnam, and he informed Ernest Jones that he was in no mood to write anything more. However, the mood passed. Putnam helped with a translation of the first psychoanalytic monograph on the sexual life of the child, Dr. H. von Hug-Helmuth's *Aus dem Seelenleben des Kindes.* He wrote eight more papers on psychoanalysis, including "Sketch for a Study of New England Character," and "The Work of Sigmund Freud," which are among his best.

He lived to see a rapidly growing interest in psychoanalysis in the United States and in 1917 observed: "Who would have dreamed, a decade or more ago, that to-day college professors would be teaching Freud's doctrines to students of both sexes, scientific men turning to them for light on the nature of the instincts, and educators for hints on the training of the young?" [166]

Given Putnam's principles, what was the nature of his psychoanalytic practice? Did he reinforce the pathological elements of conscience in a search for infantile impulses and ethical ideals? Was he a proponent of conformity and adjustment? The exact nature of his therapeutic must remain uncertain, partly because all his case notes, kept in cipher, were destroyed. However, his letters and published papers provide clues.

At first Putnam argued that complete sublimation, in the sense of overcoming all infantile tendencies, must be the analyst's goal for himself and for his patient. It was legitimate to help a patient attain his own sense of values, including ideals of loyalty to the community. Freud disagreed with both aims. Sublimation, he cautioned, was impossible for many patients because of their strong drives and inferior constitutions. To foster a patient's ethical aspirations could mean the neglect of the far more difficult task of analysis. By 1916 Putnam reserved discussion of the patient's ethical impulses for the close of treatment and insisted time and again on the thorough carrying out of the analysis itself.[167]

[165] Moorfield Storey to Putnam, August 7, 1915.

[166] "The Work of Sigmund Freud," p. 146; Ad Psa, 348.

[167] Freud to Putnam, May 14, 1911; Putnam, author's abstract of "On the Place of Sublimation in a Psychoanalytic Treatment," *Psychoanalytic Review,* III (1916), 463.

He also wrote to Ernest Jones that he could not separate men's "symptoms" from their faults and shortcomings. To Freud he observed that many patients lacked a sense of purpose. Callous ones did not suffer under the "disillusionment" of analysis; still others improved in character while their health deteriorated. This suggests a reinforcement of guilt. Yet, it is absurd to suppose that like G. Stanley Hall, Putnam believed that psychoanalysis cured because of the embarrassment the patient experienced when he learned the nature of his unconscious impulses. Again and again Putnam emphasized in *Human Motives* and elsewhere that psychoanalysis worked by removing the inhibitions that resulted from childhood fixations.

In Putnam's theoretical discussions he defended the positive aspects of conscience. Yet in practice, he was keenly alive to morbid self-blame and to rigid, false ideals. In his subtle and masterly "Sketch for a Study of New England Character," he emphasized the interplay between the Oedipus complex, desires to submit and to dominate, to suffer and inflict pain and what he called the "old-fashioned" religion of hell-fire and damnation. His letters to Fanny Bowditch stressed self-acceptance against what he interpreted as Jung's reinforcement of her sense of guilt. A suicidal and depressed man has recalled that Putnam calmly observed that he, too, sometimes felt like killing someone. Putnam also stressed this patient's positive capacity for growth. Moreover, Putnam's idealist critique of society precluded the mere "adjustment" of the patient to a world Putnam argued should be improved. His ideal was not conformity but the change of both society and the patient. More important than Putnam's theoretical views were his personal qualities, the warmth, sympathy, sincerity, and generosity to which not only Freud and Ernest Jones but letters from grateful patients attest.

The Great War that had begun in August of 1914 drew from Freud and from Putnam characteristic responses. Together with the bitter splits within the psychoanalytic movement, the war reinforced a darker aspect of Freud's outlook. In "Thoughts for the Times on War and Death," about which he wrote deprecatingly to Putnam, Freud expressed his disillusionment: "Well may the citizen of the civilized world of whom I have spoken stand helpless in a world that has grown strange to him — his great fatherland disintegrated, its common estates laid waste, his fellow-citizens divided and debased!" [168]

Putnam found the war so depressing as to interfere seriously with work and sleep at times. In early February, 1915, Putnam sent Freud a postcard with a drawing of clasped hands. Freud wrote back, expressing some of the depression and lassitude he felt.

The final item of their correspondence was a card from Freud on October 1, 1916, two years before Putnam's death. He had tried to send the first volume of his introductory lectures, but the Austrian post office would accept no mail for America. "Let us hope for better times," he concluded.

Putnam's death on November 4, 1918, was one of the first pieces of news to reach Freud from England and America after the war. He wrote a generous obituary notice and a preface to a volume of Putnam's addresses in 1921, the first publication of the new International Psycho-Analytical Library.

In a paper Putnam was revising at the time of his death, he had appraised the significance of psychoanalysis: "It is certain that the chance, made possible by the researches of Freud and his colleagues, to substitute knowledge of some sort for unreflective emotional reaction, and thus to eliminate passion, misunderstanding and misery, even if only in somewhat greater measure than before, and withal, to look more deeply into the motives of men no longer living, came to me, as to many persons, as a refreshing breeze . . . Before the days of Freud it was simply impossible to realize what hosts of hidden feelings inspired such designations as 'mean,' 'cowardly,' 'selfish,' 'criminal,' 'perverse,' and thus to exchange them for terms suggestive of their causes, or to take them as indications that the motives of those who used them might need scrutiny. How many persons are there who have felt themselves crushed and isolated under such epithets — often self-applied — and yet who, in the light of psychoanalytic study, have learned to regain their own sense of companionship and self-respect, at the sole cost of a willingness to break away from illusion and self-deceit." [169]

---

[168] (1915), SE, XIV, 280.
[169] "Elements of Strength and Elements of Weakness in Psycho-analytic Doctrines"; Ad Psa, 453.

Thus psychoanalysis had contributed to human progress, in which Putnam still believed in 1918 despite war and sickness, almost as firmly as he had in 1865. Indeed, Freud wrote of Putnam to Lou Andreas Salomé, "That man can't be helped, he must become a pessimist." [170]

Ernest Jones suggested that Freud's prediction about understanding the genesis of "nobler feelings," in his earlier letter to Putnam was borne out a few years later in the studies of the superego.[171] Putnam persistently had raised three issues: what accounted for man's higher nature — for his conscience, his religion and philosophy, and his sense of social obligation? Precisely these vexing questions were explored in 1923 in Freud's "The Ego and the Id."

Elements of Freud's answer had been foreshadowed especially in the studies of the neuroses of defense in 1896 and in the essay on "Narcissism" of 1914. The essay of 1923 explored sublimation, which he had informed Putnam he did not understand. Freud concluded that sublimation arose from the transfer of object to narcissistic libido. Behind the ego ideal lay the hidden identification with the parents. "Now that we have embarked on the analysis of the ego we can give answer to all those whose moral sense has been shocked and who have complained that there must surely be a higher nature in man: 'Very true,' we can say, 'and here we have that higher nature, in this ego ideal or super-ego, the representative of our relations to our parents. When we were little children we knew these higher natures, we admired them and feared them; and later we took them into ourselves' . . . Religion, morality, and a social sense — the chief elements in the higher side of man — were originally one and the same thing." [172]

Putnam would have found Freud's solution one more daring and clinically useful but still only partial truth. Indeed, some of the objections Putnam raised have been repeated by later critics: the limitations of Freud's nineteenth-century determinism based on extrapolations from physics and economics and of his reductive explanations of religion and ethics.

If Putnam agreed with some of Freud's critics he also raised

[170] Letter of July 30, 1915, in *The Letters of Sigmund Freud,* ed. Ernst L. Freud (New York: McGraw-Hill Book Co., 1964), p. 311.

[171] Jones, *Sigmund Freud,* II, 181–182.

[172] "The Ego and the Id" (1923), SE, XIX, 36–37, 30–31.

other problems that later psychoanalysts and psychotherapists have attempted to work out. When he insisted that conflict did not account adequately for the totality of human functioning, he anticipated some of the psychoanalytic ego psychologists. When he insisted that the aim of treatment was the "recovery of a full sense of one's highest destiny and of the bearings and meanings of one's life," he was anticipating the existentialist schools. When he insisted on an inherent principle of growth within each human being, he expressed something of the attitude of the gestalt therapists. Although he clearly saw these therapeutic and human problems, his solution of them was shaped by his own Transcendentalist tradition. His idealist philosophy now seems light years away, the conviction of a man living in an intellectual world very different from our own.

Yet some of the issues he posed, if not the form in which he posed them, have remained in his sense "eternal" and "recurring": the necessity of commitment, the ethical implications of therapy, the need for a sense of values invulnerable to reductive explanations.

I

James–Putnam Correspondence

Letters 1–9

William James, 1877–1910

It is possible that Putnam would not have taken up psychoanalysis without the influence of William James, whom he admired to the point of adoration. The two remained close friends after they met at Harvard Medical School in 1866, and Putnam was one of five men whose intellectual companionship inspired the *Principles of Psychology*.

Perhaps the first American to notice the work of Breuer and Freud on hysteria, James published a short abstract of their "Preliminary Communication" in the *Psychological Review* in 1894. James also probably led Putnam to take psychotherapy seriously, a prerequisite to his interest in psychoanalysis. In 1876 Putnam had dismissed the experiments in mental therapeutics of the famous American neurologist George Beard as "unscientific" because the emotions could not be "isolated." On the other hand, James insisted that thoughts and feelings, that is, consciousness, were too important to be ignored and played a central role in human adaptation. It is this position that he defended in his first letter to Putnam.[1]

James's own occasional anxiety and depression gave him an abiding interest in medical psychology. He was one of the first Americans to review sympathetically the new literature of hypnotism and the subconscious, beginning with Liébault's classic, *Du Sommeil*, in 1868. In 1893 James's insomnia was benefited by a mind-cure practitioner; five years later he testified against a bill

[1] W. J. [William James] review of J. Breuer and S. Freud, "Uber den psychischen Mechanismus hysterischer Phänomene" [On the Psychical Mechanism of Hysterical Phenomena], *Psychological Review*, 1 (March 1894), 199; discussion of George M. Beard, M.D., "The Influence of the Mind in the Causation and Cure of Disease — The Potency of Definite Expectation," *Journal of Nervous and Mental Disease*, 3 (July 1876), 433.

that would have required all persons in Massachusetts who treated the sick to pass an examination and be licensed.

Putnam's growing interest in psychotherapy after 1890 was accompanied by a renewal of his youthful concern for philosophy. James congratulated his friend for planning a series of articles, based partly on the views of Henri Bergson, whose *Creative Evolution* James introduced to Americans in 1907. Putnam's efforts were met by a fierce blast from the ultra scientific psychologist at the University of Pennsylvania, Lightner Witmer, who regarded James, Royce, hypnotism, and much psychotherapy as full of moonshine. Putnam's excursion into philosophy, Witmer wrote, was a naive, obscurantist "museum specimen," a "perspicacious display of absurdities." [2] Despite the opposition of such psychologists as Witmer, medical and lay interest in psychotherapy grew rapidly in the United States, and James continued to follow the new developments.

Ill with angina pectoris, James nevertheless traveled to Worcester in September of 1909 to see "what Freud was like." In June 1910 he wrote from Bad Nauheim of his failing health and the news of Putnam's "ovation" after his first major address on psychoanalysis in Washington, D.C. Putnam replied on June 25, describing his growing confidence in Freud's method as well as the basis for his disagreement with Freud's philosophical assumptions. James died a month later, on August 26, 1910.

[2] [Lightner Witmer], "Mental Healing and the Emmanuel Movement," *The Psychological Clinic*, 2 (February 15, 1909), 296–297.

1

James to Putnam

[May 26, 1877]

May 26

Dearest Jim

Your insolent card of May 13 reaches my eyes (by a strange coincidence) just as I return from the last crowning lecture of the course in wh. poor Spencer has been shaken in my jaws as a mouse is shaken by a tiger (as soon as the latter can conquer his

native timidity and once fairly take hold of the mouse).[1] The
course (I need not say) closed amid the tumultuous, nay, delirious,
applause of the students. Poor Spencer, reduced to the simple
childlike faith of merely timid, receptive uncritical, undiscrimi-
nating, worshipful, servile gullible, stupid, idiotic natures like
you and Fiske! [2] Would *I* were part of his environment! I'd see
if his "intelligence" could establish "relations" that would "correspond" to me in any other way than by giving up the ghost before
me! [3] He and all his myrmidons, disciples and parasites! Down with
the hell-spawn of 'em! Of all the incoherent, rotten, quackish hum-
bugs and pseudo-philosophasters which the womb of all inventive
time has excreted he is the most infamous and "abgeschmackt" [4]
— but even *he* is better than his followers. Go! child of perdition,
fill thy belly with the East wind, froth at the mouth in doubly-
re-relational-compound-coördinated Spencerian phraseology, subscribe to the Popular Science Monthly, hang at the breasts of "Cos-
mism" (— breasts yclept "falsehood" and "inanity,") go to bed
with the Persistence of Force the unknowable, the Realism, the
Empiricism, the Substantialism the correspondences, the fatalism,
and all the other brats of the chromo-philosophy, and if you can
sleep quiet through their fratricidal strife, be it so, you are not
fit for better things! *I am.* If you were here I would prove to you
in a course of 24 lectures that your state of mind is even more
ignominious than I imply, but you are not, and when you return
I shall have forgotten my arguments.

Affectly yours

W. J.

[1] Probably James's lectures on Herbert Spencer delivered while Putnam was in
Europe for the six months beginning in January 1877. See James, "Natural History
2, 1876–1877," in William James Papers, The Houghton Library, Harvard University;
John Hughlings Jackson to Putnam, November 29, 1876, and Putnam to Trustees
of the Massachusetts General Hospital, December 6, 1876, Putnam Papers, the
Francis A. Countway Library of Medicine.
[2] John Fiske (1842–1901), American philosopher and historian, a popularizer of
Herbert Spencer.
[3] See William James, "Remarks on Spencer's *Definition of Mind As Correspondence*," *Journal of Speculative Philosophy*, 12 (January 1878), 1–18.
[4] Insipid, absurd.

2
James to Putnam
[January 17, 1879]

387 Harvard Street
Jan. 17. 1879

Dear Jim,

Your flattering note rec'd with thanks and its well-expressed phrases about universal determinism appreciated. Allow me to make one remark, which is that you Pop. Sc. Monthlyites always go off at half-cock and if one criticizes Spencer think he must do so in the interests of the New England Princes and catechism, or if he objects to leaving out desires etc. from the chain of causation, you think that he must needs mean to bring in the supernatural and miraculous.[1] To drop this shrewish style, I would say that I did not pretend in my article to say that when things happen by the intermediation of consciousness they do not happen by law. The dynamic feelings which the nerve processes give rise to, and which enter in consciousness into comparison with each other and are selected, may in every instance be fatally selected. All that my article claims is that this additional stratum which complicates the chain of cause and effect also gives it determinations not identical with those which would result if it were left out. If a hydraulic ram be interposed in a watercourse, a pendulum and escapement on a wheel-work the results are altered but still obey the laws of cause and effect. Free-will is in short, no necessary corollary of giving causality to consciousness. My phrase about choosing one's whole character is perfectly consistent with fatalism. I don't see if one has a fatalistic faith how it can ever be driven out, even from applying to the phenomena of consciousness. I equally fail to see on the other hand how free-will faith can be forcibly driven out, but I meant expressly to steer clear of all such complications in my article. I am sorry I did not make my purpose sufficiently manifest. My heart over flows with love for you but I must write briefly and consequently without sweet dalliance and compliments.

Ever,

W. J.

[1] See William James, "Are We Automata?" *Mind* (January 1879), 1–22.

3
James to Putnam
[March 2, 1898]

Mch:2 –98 [1]

Dear Jim,

On page 7 of the Transcript[2] tonight you will find a manifestation of me at the State house, protesting against the proposed medical license bill.

If you think I *enjoy* that sort of thing you are mistaken. I never did anything that required as much moral effort in my life. My vocation is to treat of things in an allround manner and not make *ex parte* pleas to influence (or seek to) a peculiar jury. *Aussi* why do the medical brethren force an unoffending citizen like me into such a position? Legislative license is sheer humbug — mere abstract paper thunder under which every ignorance and abuse can still go on. Why this mania for more laws? Why seek to stop the really extremely important experiences which these peculiar creatures are rolling up?

Bah! I'm sick of the whole business, and I well know how all my colleagues at the medical school, who go only by the label, will view me and my efforts. But if Zola and Col. Piquart can face the whole French army, can't I face their disapproval? — Much more easily than that of my own conscience!

You, I fancy are not one of the fully disciplined demanders of more legislation. So I write to you, as on the whole my dearest friend hereabouts, to explain just what my state of mind is.

Ever yours

W. J.

---

[1] The letters from James to Putnam of March 2, March 3, and March 4 and Putnam's of March 9, 1898, were published in *The Letters of William James*, edited by his son Henry James (Boston: The Atlantic Monthly Press, 1920).

[2] See the *Boston Evening Transcript*, March 2, 1898, p. 7. James argued that the state of medical knowledge was too imperfect to rule out contributions from any source. "Do you feel called on," he said, "do you dare, to thrust the coarse machinery of criminal law into these vital mysteries, into these personal relations of doctor and patient, into these infinitely subtle operations of nature, and enact that a whole department of medical investigation (for such it is), together with the special conditions of freedom under which it flourishes must cease to be?"

4
James to Putnam
[March 3, 1898]

Dear Jim

Thanks for your noble hearted letter which makes me feel warm again. I am glad to learn that you feel positively *agin* the proposed law, and hope that you will express yourself freely towards the professional brethren to that effect.

Dr. Russell Sturgis[1] has written me a similar letter.

Once more, thanks!

W. J.

March 3

P. S. March 3. The "Transcript" report,[2] I am sorry to say was a good deal cut. I send you another copy, to keep and use where it will do most good. The rhetorical problem with me was to say things to the Committee that might neutralize the influence of their medical advisers who, I supposed, had the inside track, and all the *prestige*. I being banded with the spiritists, faith curers, magnetic healers, etc., etc.

Strange affinities!

W. J.

Cambr. March 3. 98

[1] Russell Sturgis, Jr. (1856–1899), Boston pediatrician and psychotherapist. See Sturgis, "The Use of Suggestion during Hypnotism in the First Degree, as a Means of Modifying or of Completely Eliminating a Fixed Idea," *Medical Record* (New York), 45 (February 17, 1894), 193–197.

[2] For James's testimony, see the *Boston Evening Transcript,* March 2, 1898, p. 7.

5
James to Putnam
[March 4, 1898]

Dear Jim,

Pray send me your letter to the Transcript, of which you must have kept a copy. It is too bad that you should have spent infinite labor for nothing.

It seems to me it is not a question of fondness or non-fondness for mind-curers [heaven knows I am not fond, and can't understand a word of their jargon except their precept of assuming yourself to be well and claiming health rather than sickness which I am sure is magnificent] but of the *necessity* of legislative interference with the natural play of things. There *surely* can be *no* such necessity. From the general sea of medical insecurity, a law can hardly remove an appreciable quantity. Are the vital statistics of N. Y. State so much better than those of Mass. as to demand a law like theirs? — I don't notice that this is urged. If not, then a law can only do harm. The profession claims a law simply on grounds of personal dislike. It is antisemitism again. It is the justification of Armenian massacres, which we have so often heard of late, on the ground that the Armenians are so "disagreeable." The one use of our institutions is to force on us toleration of much that *is* disagreeable.

Send your letter!
W. J.

6

Putnam to James

[March 9, 1898]

Dear William, —

We have thought and talked a good deal about the subject of your speech in the course of the last week. I prepared with infinite labor a letter intended for the Transcript of last Saturday, but it was not a weighty contribution and I am rather glad it was too late to get in.

I think it is generally felt among the best doctors that your position was the liberal one and that it would be a mistake to try to exact an examination of the mind healers and Christian Scientists. On the other hand I am afraid most of the doctors, even including myself, do not have any great feeling of fondness for them, and we are more in the way of seeing the fanatical spirit in which they proceed and the harm that they sometimes do than you are. Of course they do also good things which would remain otherwise not done, and that is the important point, and sincere fanatics are almost always, and in this case I think certainly, of real value.

Always affectionately,
James J. P.

March 9, 1898

7
James to Putnam
[August 19, 1908]

Rye, Aug 19. 08
Address: Coutts & Co, W.C.

Dear Jim,

Your splendid letter of (no date) roused me this a.m. I agree with all you say about the english. They are so *wholesome* too— 100 unwholesome people with us for every 1 in England, — and so handsome! But we have to work out our own destiny, the which I doubt not will be a *greater* thing and a greater success than england's success, — if we *do* succeed!

Your program for Parker[1] takes my breath away. It is truly grand to see you in extreme old age renewing your mighty youth and planing yourself for flights to which those of the newest airships are as sparrows fluttering in the gutter! Go in, dear Jim! It is magnificent. It won't be easy work, but it has got to be done by someone. The program you sketch is, I think, the form which the more spiritualistic philosophy of the future is bound more and more to assume, tho I fancy it will always be dogged more or less by a more materialistic or mechanistic-deterministic enemy. Bergson[2] will have been the decisive initiator, but the necessary vagueness from the conceptual or intellectualistic point of view of so many of his ideas will make it long ere the *general* mind swings over to his doctrines. Meanwhile you are surely making the best possible use of your life in boldly coming out as his disciple & promulgator. I place myself alongside of you in these Oxford lectures,[3] confining myself, however, to his anti-intellectualism, while you swim after him in his adventurous voyage of construction.

I have been ready to return for a fortnight — only marking time here on Peggy's[4] account. I go to meet Alice[5] & her at Antwerp tomorrow, they having been a fortnight or more in Switz., I here. We all sail on the 22nd. I should infinitely rather from today on, be with you and the family crowd, (to each and all of whom my love!) at the Shanty.[6]

Yours affectionately,

W. J.

[1] William Belmont Parker (1871–1934), editor of the magazine *Psychotherapy: A Course of Reading in Sound Psychology, Sound Medicine and Sound Religion* (New York: The Centre Publishing Co., 1908, 1909). Putnam contributed a series of articles on philosophy and psychotherapy to the magazine that summed up the outlook he expressed in his dialogue with Freud. See Putnam, "The Philosophy of Psychotherapy," *Psychotherapy*, vol. 1, no. 1 (1908), pp. 17–37, reprinted in *ibid.*, vol. 3, no. 3 (1909), pp. 13–24, and *ibid.*, vol. 3, no. 4 (1909), pp. 28–38; "The Psychology of Health, I," *Psychotherapy*, vol. 1, no. 2 (1908), pp. 24–32; "The Psychology of Health, II," *ibid.*, vol. 1, no. 3 (1908), pp. 5–13; "The Psychology of Health, III," *ibid.*, vol. 1, no. 4 (1908), pp. 37–49; "The Psychology of Health, IV," *ibid.*, vol. 2, no. 1 (1909), pp. 35–44; "The Nervous Breakdown," *ibid.*, vol. 3, no. 2 (1909), pp. 5–13. See also the correspondence with Parker in the Putnam Papers.

[2] Henri Bergson (1859–1941), French philosopher-psychologist. Putnam sought an existential position that would encourage a sense of meaning and hope in patients. He raised this issue in his first letter to Freud, of November 17, 1909. Bergson reinforced Putnam's faith in spontaneity, the role of mind, and evolutionary progress. See the articles cited in n. 1 above.

[3] James delivered the Hibbert lectures at Manchester College, Oxford University, in the spring of 1908, and later visited Henry James at Rye. See *A Pluralistic Universe: Hibbert Lectures on the Present Situation in Philosophy* (New York and London: Longmans, Green, and Co., 1909).

[4] James's daughter Margaret Mary (1887–1947).

[5] James's wife, Alice Howe Gibbens James (1849–1922).

[6] Putnam Shanty, the Adirondack camp founded by Henry Bowditch, Charles Putnam, and James Jackson Putnam.

8
James to Putnam
[June 4, 1910]

Nauheim,
June 4, 1910

Dear Jim —

It seems to me high time for me to be sending to you some report of my progress. I write this in my high hotel bedroom, a beautiful summer day reigning outside, with the charming Nauheim town & country round-about, and round about them the great calm civilization of the new Germany, of which I confess that I like the feeling — tho Heaven knows that my acquaintance with it is so slight as to approach zero.

I came over, you may remember, to see whether I might not stop the downward tendency of my pectoral contents, so, after a month at Rye, where Henry[1] was not well, I went to Paris to see Moutier,[2] who found my radial blutdruck[3] only 150 (Pratt[4] had found it 170–80 3 or 4 years ago) and said he could do nothing for me, and that my angina was probably due to local cardiac vascular spasm which his methods couldn't relieve. He is just the reverse of a quack, but probably a "narrow specialist" who doubt-less generalizes his results too freely. He explains them as secondary results of hypertension being relieved. The excretories[5] then begin to excrete normally their poisons, and week by week the patient rejuvenesces, till after 6 months or so the arteries themselves may soften their walls. Hypertension is due to spasm, which his d'Ar-sonval currents[6] sometimes arrest in a single sitting, rarely taking 5, and this effect permanently or indefinitely continues. Groedel [7] here rather laughs at Moutier; but there is, I fancy, no question about some of his cases. Edgar Nichols has lately written me from Greece that since his 4 treatments he has gone on improving for six months, getting better all the time. Groedel says that *general* hypertension is always due to splanchnic sclerosis with spasm — this would well agree with all that Moutier says. Bergson has been treated by M. for *hypo*-tension, with what he considers bril-liant results. Mr. B. told Strong[8] that Moutier had enabled B. to write his evolution créatrice. Suspecting that Strong's invincible lethargy & lack of animal spirits might be low-tension symptoms, I took him to Moutier who found only 90 mm. Strong writes me that "3 treatments have bro't my pressure up to normal, where it has remained. But the effect, so far, on my power of work has been nil" — less than a fortnight after the change.

Groedel here is the next great man to Schott.[9] I like him very much. He has given me an admirably definite diagnosis (confirmed by radiograph in fact) of mitral insufficiency & aortic dilation. Thus are all my symptoms legitimately explained without the old reproach of "nervousness" thrown in my teeth. Both conditions are "moderate", (though the aorta in the cardiogram looks immense) and I am unquestionably more *sensitive* than most subjects. Blood pressure only 155; anginoid pain (so magically relieved by glonoin) due to spasm of coronaries, and *possibly* not to be relieved. He finds theobromine (double saliglate of th. with sodium) the great alleviator of dyspnea etc. from lung stasis. I tell you all these things, thinking they may be of interest in your own practice. I take my 12th bath in an hour — I can't guess at the result — so far I keep *feeling* worse and worse, tho my bathing is of the most limited sort. Enough! enough! of my pathology. I expect no answer! don't waste your precious time! To turn to pleasanter subjects, Fanny Morse[10] wrote me the other day a delightful letter about your whole family, and said in particular that you had had quite an "ovation" at the medical meeting at Washington,[11] which I much rejoiced to hear. If we live long enough we get appreciated; but then we mustn't take advantage of it to live *too* long! I was taken to a meeting of the Acad. des Sc. Morales, and feel now like a real "Membre de l'Institute." I had two delightful lunches at Bergson's — it is a pleasure to associate with a *really first* class mind. Europe is beautiful indeed; but I am so inactive that I can profit little by it, and should rather be at Chocorua.[12] Terraces and benches to sit on and take in views, are not like pine trees overhead & mother earth to lie on. My reading has almost stopped — when I say that the Paris N. Y. Herald forms a daily part of it, you'll pity the low ebb. I hope that yours can still go on in spite of all the calls of practice. I think of Marian[13] and ces demoiselles enjoying the water at Cotuit just now, and I hope you get there weekly. Passage home is taken for August 12th. Alice is still with Henry in England, but I hope for them here in 10 days. My love to *all* your sippschaft[14] whom I wont individually name! Heaven bless, you, dear Jim.

Yours ever
W. J.

---

[1] James's brother, the novelist, Henry James (1843–1916).

[2] Alexandre Moutier (d. 1916), a Paris physician, was well known for his clinical application of d'Arsonval currents, especially to hypertension. See A. Moutier, *Traitement de l'artério-sclérose par la d'Arsonvalisation* (Versailles, 1904).

[3] Radial blood pressure.

[4] Possibly Joseph Hersey Pratt (1872–1942), an instructor at Harvard Medical School.

[5] James's text is unclear. "Excretories," a Jamesian neologism, is the most likely reading.

⁶ High frequency alternating current produced by a forerunner of today's diathermy apparatus, invented by Jacques Arsène d'Arsonval (1851–1940), French biophysicist. The apparatus produced intermittent trains of heavily dampened oscillations of high voltage but low amperage.

⁷ Franz Maximilian Groedel (1881–1951), German cardiovascular specialist.

⁸ Charles Augustus Strong (1862–1940), professor of psychology, Columbia University, 1903–1910, author of *Why the Mind Has a Body* (1903). He had retired and was living in Paris.

⁹ Theodor Schott (1852–1920), German cardiovascular specialist. See Schott, *Zur Pathologie und Therapie der Angina pectoris* (Herzkrampf) (Berlin: E. Grosser, 1888).

¹⁰ Frances Morse (1850–1928), close friend of James and a cousin of Putnam.

¹¹ On May 3, 1910, Putnam delivered his first major address on psychoanalysis, "Personal Experience with Freud's Psychoanalytic Method" to the American Neurological Association. See *Journal of Nervous and Mental Disease*, 37 (November 1910), 657–674; Ad Psa, 31–53.

¹² James's New Hampshire farm.

¹³ Putnam's wife, Marian Cabot Putnam (1852–1932).

¹⁴ Kindred.

9

Putnam to James

[June 25, 1910]

106 Marlborough Street
VI. 25.10

Dear William¹

It is delightful to hear from you. You manage to put your whole self, voice and face and all, into your lines, to a remarkable degree. I was much interested in your accounts of Moutier and of the Nauheim doctor.²

What they both say harmonizes very well with the views given by Huchard,³ of whose address I spoke to you. He makes much use of thiobromine (as diuretic) and believes that the high tension is a physiological rather than an anatomical phenomenon, primarily at least. May the baths do you great service and may you come back in good season to enjoy something of your lovely Chocorua or, if it so happens, of Keene Valley.

I write this at Cotuit, with the voices of my children and their friends in my ears. It is a pleasant life and a lovely summer's day but all these luxuries and signs of health make one feel queer, in view of the fact that there are so many who are wholly ignorant of them. I wish you could bring home a clear philosophy and a justified religion. The 'necessary pre-suppositions' on which Miss

Blow[4] counts so much, and which taken together with an equally
'necessary' self-activity seem to lead to such momentous conclusions, give the most comforting assurances of anything I know; but
is there a flaw in them? If so, I cannot see it. And yet, to feel 'sure'!
What a luxury of luxuries, and one that, fortunately, the poor can
have as well as the rich. Continued VI.28. What terribly solemn
stuff this sounds; but I feel myself impelled to keep on for just a
few lines more. Why is not the argument a sound one that your
friend Schiller[5] makes and why, if sound, must it not be of fundamental importance? We must assume a primary activity somewhere, and if somewhere then everywhere. We see growth and
'progress' (?) and think we trace the birth of consciousness and
love and sense of freedom. But even mankind as a whole is finite
and self-activity is infinite. Our success cannot then measure the
possibilities of success or its actuality. Somewhere, somehow, there
must be a being wiser and better than ourselves, coeval with self-
activity having self-activity, not as a cause but as an attribute. Such
a being may be called a 'model' for mankind in the sense that we
have in our conscious life a 'freedom' of the same *quality* with
his. The responsibility, the suffering, the successes which we witness are our individual (*independent*) possessions, but as we see
our better qualities gradually prevail so the existence of such
an assumed being, whose body is the universe, is a warrant that
the conceivably *best* qualities are not in essential disharmony with
the whole scheme. And may we not regard the necessarily assumed
existence of such a being as a warrant that our existence is in some
sense *worth while?* I have been so much impressed with the
symbolism of dreams as pointing to the symbolism of all practical
life, that it seems but a short step to the metaphysics, expressed
so well by Bowne,[6] i.e. to the conclusion that everything finite is
symbolic only, but that there is an imperishable reality, above
storms and battles; something really desirable and permanent and
that our existences are not mere fleeting shows. 1 am just reading
Freud's "Der Witz" [7] and marvel at his keenness and tireless readiness to penetrate and penetrate. My longing to get all that metaphysics has to offer is indeed an indirect expression of a sort of
hope and belief that his terribly searching psycho-genetic explanations correspond only to one pole of human life, and that there
is another pole in which he takes no interest. My 'ovation' in

Washington to which you refer (as reported by F. R M.) was of course a Freudian victory alone, if victory it was.[8] I do think that as much interest was manifest as one could fairly look for. Of course there was much opposition also. Dr. Walton brought down the house by saying that he would rather have an ounce of Muldoon than a pound of Freud but I countered on him by joking him about his book "Why Worry?" and saying that it seemed cynical to ask 'why worry', without ever inquiring "Why *do* you worry"? [9] For certainly no *adequate* inquiry of that sort can be made except à la Freud. Since then there has been another contest of similar sort, this time at Toronto,[10] in which I also took part. You will doubtless smile at my above-stated metaphysics and say that nothing can be decided in that way. But I cannot see why the necessary presuppositions of all thinking are not binding; a *really eternal* universe capable of improvement and evolution to the extent of being able to produce even our consciousness, and yet still *entirely* in the making, that is, not containing anywhere evidence of the perfection (perfection in some sense) towards which we strive seems to me dreadfully absurd. Either eternity has no metaphysical meaning or else surely its meaning is that *in some sense* everything that could be actually is. In other words, the element of time, and with it the evolution that requires time must be eliminable from the scheme of the universe as a whole. Yet time, in the sense of evolution, pluralism, pragmatism, of course has its rights too.

And so some sort of absolute must be assumed, and likewise a progress towards it. And if we prize 'morals', or love then the universe must have a moral pole and individual effort must be of value. Of course, I don't believe in Royce's[11] *all containing* absolute. I am not a monist to that extent. But for all that I am not going to be forced into believing that everything is in flux; that there is no permeation of intelligence and feeling except such as Loeb would imagine as distilled from purely earthly crucibles. The alternative is surely between a gross [unthinkable?] materialism and a truly personalistic universe with love and hope in it from the start. And if 'in it' then an essential part of its eternal structure.

Best love to Alice

Ever affectionately,
J. J. P.

[1] In the upper left corner, Putnam wrote: "Send me back this perhaps absurd flight of fancy rather than destroy. Perhaps it may serve me as a suggestion for something less crude."

[2] See preceding letter.

[3] Henri Huchard (1844–1910), French specialist in cardiovascular diseases.

[4] Susan Blow (1843–1916), American educator. See Introduction.

[5] F. C. S. Schiller (1864–1937), philosopher, fellow of Corpus Christi College, Oxford, 1897–1926; professor of philosophy, University of Southern California, 1929–1936.

[6] Borden Barker Bowne (1847–1910), professor of philosophy at Boston University, author of *Personalism* (Boston: Houghton Mifflin and Co., 1908).

[7] *Der Witz und seine Beziehung zum Unbewussten* [Jokes and Their Relation to the Unconscious] (Leipzig and Vienna: F. Deuticke, 1905); SE, VIII.

[8] Frances Rollins Morse. For the mixed reception of Putnam's paper on psychoanalysis, see *Journal of Nervous and Mental Disease*, 37 (October 1910), 630–639.

[9] George Lincoln Walton (1854–1941), Boston neurologist. *Why Worry?* (Philadelphia: J. B. Lippincott, Co., 1908).

[10] Putnam addressed the Canadian Medical Association, June 1, 1910, "On the Etiology and Treatment of the Psychoneuroses," *Boston Medical and Surgical Journal*, 162 (July 21, 1910), 75–82; Ad Psa, 54–78.

[11] Josiah Royce (1855–1916), professor of philosophy at Harvard.

II

Freud–Putnam Correspondence

Letters 10–98

Sigmund Freud, 1909–1916

Freud's respect for Putnam's "unprejudiced perceptiveness" and Putnam's appreciation of Freud's integrity and greatness created the basis of their long correspondence. They wrote in a frank and affectionate vein that also characterized the letters Freud exchanged with the Swiss pastor Oscar Pfister.

Two elements in the psychoanalytic movement that sometimes have received less attention than they deserve emerge clearly from these letters. As Freud indicated time and again, psychoanalysis was open, experimental, and unformalized. Psychoanalysts were concerned with far more than therapy and theory. They were deeply interested in the reform of custom. Freud wrote that they wished to change "social factors so that men and women shall no longer be forced into hopeless situations." He observed to Ernest Jones that he hoped Jones would not deny to Putnam that "our sympathies side with individual freedom and that we find no improvement in the strictness of American chastity." [1] This reformist aspect of Freud was especially prominent from 1908 through about 1913, and was still present, although muted, in later years.

Certain themes recur — problems of psychoanalytic theory, the interpretation of dreams and symptoms, the role of philosophy and ethics and their relation to therapy. There also are unusually frank discussions of personal problems in Putnam's letter of September 30, 1911, and Freud's reply of October 5.

The correspondence falls into fairly distinct chronological groups. The first, from 1909 through 1911, discussed Putnam's new interest in psychoanalysis, aspects of theory and technique, and Freud's appreciation of Putnam's first eloquent papers defending

[1] Jones, *The Life and Work of Sigmund Freud*, 3 vols., II (New York: Basic Books, 1955), 103.

the psychoanalytic "cause." Freud carefully described his views of sublimation on May 14, 1911, a theme that especially interested Putnam. From June 16, 1910, through May 1911, the letters touch on Freud's request that Putnam found an American branch of the International Psychoanalytic Association, a topic taken up in detail by Ernest Jones. Beginning on August 20, 1912, Freud informed Putnam of the growing splits within the psychoanalytic movement and on June 19, 1914, frankly described his feelings about the final break with the Swiss. After 1912 Putnam's disagreements with Freud became more insistent, especially regarding the role of therapy. Putnam outlined his position in a popular book, *Human Motives*,[2] which Freud discussed in a notable letter on ethics of July 8, 1915. The correspondence ended six months before America entered the Great War.

10

Putnam to Freud

[November 17, 1909]

106 Marlboro St.   Boston
XI . 17 . 09.

Dear Professor.

Your visit to America was of deep significance to me, and I now work and read with constantly growing interest on your lines. In general 1 find myself in complete agreement with your ideas, except in some details, but I am looking forward to the day when I may venture to form an opinion of my own, with greater confidence.

I send you a few photographs of the Adirondacks, as a reminder of your three days' stay, and will try to get others showing our camp and camp-fire and perhaps some of the persons whom you met.

A quantity of questions have come to my mind which I should like to ask you if it were possible.

One is, just what you mean by the "Geld-complex" [1] as brought out by the Psychoanalyse. I have carefully noted what you say on that point in the paper on *Analerotik*,[2] which I have just read

2 Boston: Little, Brown and Co., 1915.

with much interest, but wish that I knew more fully to what you refer. I dwell on this because your reference to it shows me that in my own 'Analysen' I have not as yet learned to go deep enough to find all that can be found. In spite of this deficiency I can truly say that I do succeed in obtaining insights into my patients' minds and thoughts, of a far deeper sort than I have ever got before, and that I think you have thrown new and important light on the great subject of character-formation. Some of your conclusions I cannot as yet verify but there is so much that I can verify that I am in no mood for hostile criticism.

It still appears to me that — from the point of view of treatment — the psychoanalytic method needs to be supplemented by methods which seek to hold up before the patient some goal toward which he may strive. Thus, I am now treating a lady of much intelligence — a school-teacher — who is a great sufferer from morbid self-consciousness and blushing. I am making good headway and tracing out the origin of these symptoms, but find that I have also to meet the difficulty that she has lost all interest in life and living. The current theories of the universe do not bring her any satisfaction, her work bores her, and she wishes only to 'get out.'

I feel that it ought to be possible for us to work up ways of dealing systematically with such a state of mind as this. Perhaps you would say and perhaps it is true, that a complete Psychoanalyse accomplishes this result by discovering the causes for the state of general discouragement but if that is so I should like to see that side of the matter developed more fully. I have read your papers on the sexual ideas (or lack of them) characteristic of young children [Zur sexuellen Aufklärung der K.^{r}]^{3} and agree heartily with what you say. This is a subject which is being canvassed here a great deal just now and I should like your permission to translate the article, if on consultation it seems best to do so. I have almost finished a careful reading of the Sammlung Kl. Schr.^{n} II,^{4} and shall read, the 'Drei Abhandl.^{n} üb. Sexualtheorie' ^{5} as soon as I receive it.

I have also read a portion of Dr. Brill's translation of selected papers^{6} but wish it was expressed in better, more fluent and more impressive English. It is very conscientiously done but it is very hard for any foreigner to learn another language so well that he can use it adequately for literary work. Carl Schurz accomplished this and a few other men, of real literary skill, have done the same, but to translate really well is a rare talent. However, anyone who is looking for information and is willing to study hard to get it [as he would have to do in any case] will find himself greatly interested in the book.

I have recently had a letter from Dr. Ferencsi and was glad to learn that he enjoyed his visit to America. Let me thank you also for your card, sent to us on leaving for your home.

Be assured that I shall pay respectful attention to everything that you write, even if I cannot at once agree with all you say, and believe that I shall enjoy, and shall incline to accept your views much the more for having had the pleasure of making your acquaintance.

Yours very truly,

James J. Putnam

[1] Money complex.

[2] Freud, "Charakter und Analerotik" [Character and Anal Eroticism], *Psychiatrisch-neurologische Wochenschrift*, 9 (March 1908), 465–467; SE, IX, 167–175.

[3] "Zur sexuellen Aufklärung der Kinder" [The Sexual Enlightenment of Children], *Soziale Medizin und Hygiene*, 2 (June 1907), 360–367; SE, IX, 129–139.

[4] Freud, *Sammlung kleiner Schriften zur Neurosenlehre* [Collected Short Papers on the Theory of Neurosis], II (Leipzig and Vienna: F. Deuticke, 1909). Both essays referred to above were republished in this edition.

[5] Freud, *Drei Abhandlungen zur Sexualtheorie* [Three Essays on the Theory of Sexuality], 2nd ed. (Leipzig and Vienna: F. Deuticke, 1910); SE, VII, 123–245. Putnam wrote an introduction for Freud, *Three Contributions to the Theory of Sex*, trans. A. A. Brill, Nervous and Mental Disease Monograph Series No. 7 (New York: Nervous and Mental Disease Publishing Co., 1910).

[6] Brill included selections from Breuer's and Freud's *Studien über Hysterie* [Studies in Hysteria] (1895) and the two editions of the *Sammlung kleiner Schriften zur Neurosenlehre*. See Freud, *Selected Papers on Hysteria and Other Psychoneuroses*, trans. A. A. Brill, Nervous and Mental Disease Monograph Series No. 4 (New York: Nervous and Mental Disease Publishing Co., 1909).

11

Putnam to Freud

[December 3, 1909]

106 Marlborough Street

My dear Professor

I have just finished the Samml. Kl. Schr.[n] [1] and wish to say again how true and how important I find it all. I have ordered the 'Drei Abh.'[n][2] etc. and shall lose no time before I have carefully read all your writings and Dr. Jung's.

I send you by this mail the photographs of which I spoke, and shall endeavor to send others later.

I have written one half of my paper for Dr. Prince's Journal, giving my personal impressions of your work but think it may be better to wait for the publication of the second half before I send this to you.[3]

With kind regards,
James J. Putnam

XII . 3 . 09.

I believe I am gradually, though slowly, getting hold of the technique of Psycho-analysis. To carry it out thoroughly is evidently difficult I think — the real Ps. anal.[s] begins where the primary 'confessional' ends.

[1] Freud, *Sammlung kleiner Schriften zur Neurosenlehre.*

[2] Freud, *Drei Abhandlungen zur Sexualtheorie,* 2nd ed., 1910.

[3] "Personal Impressions of Sigmund Freud and His Work, with Special Reference to His Recent Lectures at Clark University," published in two parts, *Journal of Abnormal Psychology,* 4 (December 1909–January 1910), 293–310, and (February–March 1910), 372–379; Ad Psa, 1–30; also in James S. Van Teslaar, ed., *An Outline of Psychoanalysis* (New York: The Modern Library, 1925).

12
Freud to Putnam

[December 5, 1909]

5 Dec 09
Vienna, IX, Berggasse, 19.

Dear Dr. Putnam

Permit me to continue in German.[1] Our stay at your home was perhaps the most interesting part of our American experience, and the exchange of ideas with you, in spite of its brief duration, particularly strengthened my hopes that there might be a future for psychoanalysis in your country.

Although you are a decade older than I am, I found in you a high degree of general open-mindedness and unprejudiced perceptiveness to which I really am not accustomed in Europe. These qualities, which I value, lay the foundation for our relationship. It is not at all important that you agree with me in every particular. My work demands from the reader only this: that he seek to undergo the experiences on which it is based. Up to now I have not been disappointed in my hope that whoever does this will arrive at the same conclusions on all essential points. I neither demand nor expect that the reader accept everything I say without himself having first gone down and explored the sources of my observations. Actually most people demonstrate that they do not intend to accept anything new; they either approve or condemn what I advance in accordance with what they believe already. I know that you are free of such habits of mind, and therefore I assume that gradually you yourself will become convinced even of what may at the moment still appear inconceivable.

You are quite right in finding that our explanations are unsystematic and full of gaps. Actually our body of knowledge still is incomplete and as a whole is only in the process of becoming; there is ample room left for the contributions of others.

By the term "money complex," we mean the individual's attitude towards money: the intrinsic value he attributes to it; his tendency to attach to it a variety of unconscious complexes.[2] The attitude towards money should be especially revealing in the United States, where anal eroticism has undergone quite interesting transformations. By the way, the inter-relations between the money complex and anal eroticism only recently have been established.[3] With us, people are just as dishonest and as repressed in their attitude towards money as they are towards sexual matters, and thus they justify the analogy of money to sexuality.

I shall be quite satisfied by any use to which you put my writings. Dr. Brill[4] has the exclusive right to translate them. He surely will not object to relinquishing it to you in certain instances should you so desire.

I surmised that his translations were conscientious rather than beautiful. However, he cannot be looked on as a foreigner, for I believe that he crossed the ocean so early in life that one can consider English as his native tongue.

I believe that your complaint that we are not able to compensate our neurotic patients for giving up their illness is quite justified. But it seems to me that this is not the fault of therapy but rather of social institutions. What would you have us do when a woman complains about her thwarted life, when, with youth gone, she notices that she has been deprived of the joy of loving for merely conventional reasons? She is quite right, and we stand helpless before her, for we cannot make her young again. But the recognition of our therapeutic limitations reinforces our determination to change other social factors so that men and women shall no longer be forced into hopeless situations.

Out of our therapeutic impotence must come the prophylaxis of the neuroses. The more energetically one attacks the sexual problem in such cases, the more one is able to palliate. Where the conditions are not so hopeless sublimation creates new goals as soon as the repressions are lifted.

The *Drei Abhandlungen zur Sexualtheorie* is out of print; the second edition will not be available until February.

I look forward to the promised photographs of the Adirondacks and immodestly ask you for your recently published article on psychoanalysis, of which you spoke when we left and of whose appearance I have been told.[5]

In addition, please let me know briefly as soon as the six numbers of *Sammlung kleiner Schriften* have reached you. They were ordered quite some time ago, but the publisher asserts that such packages to America are often lost, (the same package to Stanley Hall did arrive). Please give my greetings to your brother as well as to the kind ladies of your family.

With best wishes,
Most sincerely,
Freud

[1] The salutation and first sentence are in English.

[2] Literally, "his ability to handle the stuff unhampered by unconscious complexes." See German text of the Freud letter.

[3] See Freud, "Charakter und Analerotik."

[4] Abraham Arden Brill (1874–1948), then a struggling young psychiatrist and psychoanalyst in New York, received the translation rights from Freud in 1908 during a year spent with Jung and Bleuler at the Burghölzli. Brill emigrated from Austria-Hungary to the United States at the age of fifteen.

[5] Putnam, "Personal Impressions of Sigmund Freud."

13
Freud to Putnam

[January 28, 1910]

28. J. 1910
Vienna, IX, Berggasse 19.

Dear Dr. Putnam

You surely will understand when I tell you that it has been a long time since I have begun reading anything with such intense anticipation as I brought to your first article in the *Journal of Abnormal Psychology*[1] in which my name has so honorable a place.

What I read did not surprise me in view of our correspondence. But it has given me pleasure and satisfaction. I hope your words will make a strong impression in America and will secure for psychoanalysis the lasting interest of your countrymen. I found your words on page 307, beginning with "All this is wrong", particularly fine.[2] This does credit not only to your qualities as a physician and a scientist but as a man. Probably my attitude toward religion is very different from yours. However, I do feel that all honest men share the same faith. I owe you special thanks for the seriousness with which you came to my aid in the matter of sexuality; that, too, should really be a matter of course among doctors, but unfortunately it is not. There is only one point on which I do not understand you: how you can accept Morton Prince's view of the unconscious.[3] I will never understand why it isn't an obvious prejudice to call the "suppressed mental states" of hysterics "conscious", when the most superficial investigation shows that they know nothing about them (and that this by itself is the distinguishing characteristic and the entire meaning of the Unconscious). This problem has nothing whatever to do with "awareness." Conscious mental processes announce themselves in consciousness as soon as they are become active; the processes we study become active and yet are not present in consciousness. Isn't this distinction sufficiently important to warrant an appropriate designation?

Naturally I am very curious to see the continuation of your article.[4] It gives me the opportunity to learn the proper English translations for my terminology. Don't expect anything from me in the near future. I must earn enough money for the coming year and for vacation expenses; in Austria as well as elsewhere, that means hard work. You will receive the second edition of the Sexualtheorie[5] in three to five weeks.

With many thanks
Yours,
Freud

[1] "Personal Impressions of Sigmund Freud."

[2] "All this is wrong. A fool's paradise is a poor paradise. If our spiritual life is good for anything it can afford to see the truth. No investigation is wrong if it is earnest. Knowledge knows nothing as essentially and invariably dirty. It is a piece of narrow intolerance, cruel in its outcome, to raise the cry of 'introspection', in order to prevent an unfortunate invalid, whose every moment is already spent in introspection of the worst sort, forced on him by the bigotry, however well meant, of social conventions, from searching, even to the death, the causes of his misery and learning to substitute the freedom, liberality, tolerance, and purity that comes from knowledge for the tyranny of ignorance and prejudice."

[3] The letter in which Putnam expresses this view is missing. Prince used "co-conscious" and "subconscious" as equivalent terms to describe the "dissociated ideas" of French psychopathology. These elements of consciousness were active but independent of the ego centers; the subject might or might not be aware of them. At the International Congress of Psychology in 1909 Prince urged that the term subconscious be dropped in favor of co-conscious. "Dormant ideas," which were not active and thus had no "psychic aspects," were to be considered "physiological brain dispositions." See Morton Prince, Hugo Münsterberg et al., "A Symposium on the Subconscious," *Journal of Abnormal Psychology*, 2 (April–May 1907), 22–43, and *ibid.*, (June–July 1907), 56–80; published as *Subconscious Phenomena* (Boston: Richard G. Badger, 1910); and *Journal of Mental Science*, 56 (January 1910), 187.

[4] See n. 1.

[5] Freud, *Drei Abhandlungen zur Sexualtheorie,* 1910.

14
Putnam to Freud
[February 15, 1910]

Dear Professor.

Thank you for your kind note. I become more interested in the psychoanalytic methods, day by day, and more expert also, though I recognize a strong tendency to try to hasten matters by lecturing to the patients, instead of drawing them out. I notice that you say that does no good and it certainly does not do much except that sometimes it may be made the basis of an earnest talk, I find.

I have been thinking carefully over what you say with reference to my remarks about Dr. Prince's view that the "suppressed mental states" may be called a form of consciousness.[1] It seems to me that there is not much real difference between us all, but a misunderstanding and perhaps misuse, of terms. Of course, it is absurd — strictly speaking — to say that a hysterical patient is 'conscious' of thoughts of which, *by agreement*, he is *not* conscious. On the other hand, there is a real difficulty in finding suitable words to express the complex conditions which are present. Münsterberg[2] would say that there is no 'Unbewusstes'[3] but that everything which is not, at a given moment, in consciousness [i.e. of which we are not consciously aware] is a *physiological brain-event*, not a 'psychological' or 'mental' process. This, I do not accept and I place myself squarely on the ground occupied by Bergson, who is, I believe, the keenest psychologist alive — up to a certain point at least. He shows, and I agree with him, that memories [without which no thinking can occur] are not brain-residua but a possession of the mind, having, as such, a real existence independent of physical laws. I should be content to adopt the term 'unconscious,' as you use it, to cover a large number of mental processes which we are engaged in studying, were it not that the word [unbewusst] is too *negative* to be fully satisfactory. It does not take stand sufficiently against the position of Münsterberg and it does not offer a satisfactory basis for further classification. It is true that the supplementary term "Vorbewusst"[4] helps out and seems to make unnecessary Morton Prince's word "co-conscious."[5] It should not, however, be forgotten that there is some real value in recognizing the relationship between the mental states of animals [even the vital powers of plants in so far as they secure a certain degree of *choice*] and the mental processes of man, and for this the term 'consciousness' has at least historical rights. Bergson says, for example, that there is no reason for denying 'conscience' [French] to an animal without a brain than power of digestion to an animal without a stomach. What we, in English, *commonly* call 'consciousness' contains always an element of 'self-consciousness,' i.e., consciousness or recognition of our *processes* of thought as well as of the objects of which we think. But this fact is usually overlooked and thus the word 'conscious' is almost universally used, with us, for mental processes in general [including das Unbewusstes] and also for those processes of which we are 'self-consciously' aware. I do not see any way out of this confusion except by clarifying our real psychological knowledge and conceptions, and the day for this is still far off though it approaches nearer.

You speak of my religion as probably different from yours. I do not know how this may be, but until recently I have had no religion at all, properly speaking, and was ready to let 'natural science' be the arbiter of everything. Within the past few years I have changed in this respect and I hope, some time, to have the chance of studying these matters over with you at some length. It may be quite true, as you say, that we get the *formal* explanation of our religious conceptions [idea of God, etc.] through 'projection' of our anthropomorphic ideas, but this does not rule out the view that we can obtain a knowledge of the existence of a form of consciousness and personality higher than ours, and a knowledge of the nature of this consciousness and of its relation to ourselves, only through philosophy and metaphysics. Psychologic observation of ourselves teaches us much, but it teaches *nothing* with regard to the essential nature of the universe or of ourselves. It is usually considered by men of science [so-called] that there is no positive conclusion to be drawn from philosophy. This, I believe, is a serious mistake. The symbolism which you found in dreams exists also in all life. The real thing to study, if one would be truly fundamental, is the mind, in all its aspects, and this cannot be done fully if we confine ourselves to pure psychology *as usually studied*. It is from this standpoint alone that I feel inclined to criticize your teaching. I feel that since you urge us to be completely truthful and completely thorough, you should urge us also to take in all the sources of knowledge and all motives and inducements for progress. Our psychopathic patients need, I think, something more than simply to learn to know themselves. If there are reasons why they should adopt higher views of their obligations [as based on the belief that this is a morally conceived universe, and that 'free-will' has a real meaning, then these reasons ought to be made known to them. I could refer you to books where these arguments are set forth with all the convincing logic and *reference to experience* that you have shown adherence to in your own work, but they have to be carefully studied in order to be appreciated. But perhaps you have done this and concluded that there is nothing for you there.

The second part of my paper goes to you today.[6] I am aware of its defects and if I were to write it again, even today, I should change it and add to it in various ways. In particular, I should say more of your views on character-formation and on the community and social aspects of these investigations.

I owe you an apology for sending you so long a letter.

With kind regards,

James J. Putnam

Feb. 15. 1910.

[1] See Freud to Putnam, January 28, 1910.

[2] Hugo Münsterberg (1863–1916), professor of psychology at Harvard.

[3] Unconscious (noun).

[4] Foreconscious.

[5] See preceding letter and Morton Prince, "The Psychological Principles and Field of Psychotherapy," in *Psychotherapeutics* (Boston: Richard G. Badger, 1909), pp. 24–26, and Prince, "Experiments to Determine Co-Conscious (Subconscious) Ideation," *Journal of Abnormal Psychology,* 3 (April–May 1908), 33–42.

[6] "Personal Impressions of Sigmund Freud."

15

Freud to Putnam

[March 10, 1910]

10. 3. 10

Vienna,, IX, Berggasse 19.

Dear Dr. Putnam

Many thanks for your letter and for the second article.[1] "You gave us a very good character; we shall take pains to deserve it." [2]

Your comments on the terminological misunderstandings involved in discussions of the unconscious relieved me greatly. Those who study the same facts cannot possibly come to dissimilar conclusions. Philosophy is a different matter; philosophers talk about the unconscious although they know nothing about it; this gives them the right to question its existence. But how can one analyze a single dream and still deny that it exists.

I make bold to say that from the very beginning I have agreed with Bergson's logical view of the matter.[3] I have made it mine. The confusion is less troublesome if one abandons the old meaning of consciousness, and sticks to this fact: The conscious consists of what one knows; the unconscious, of what one does not know but which nevertheless is actively at work. The fact that the word "unconscious" is merely negative really doesn't matter at all. Terminology does not have to fit perfectly; all we can do as knowledge progresses, is to pour new wine into the old wine skins.

It would be a great delight to me to discuss religion with you since you are both tolerant and enlightened. Perhaps we shall have occasion to do so at the next Congress, since we cannot expect you at this one; yet I am afraid that it may be only a pious wish-fulfillment. "Just God" and "kindly Nature" [4] are only the noblest sublimations of our parental complexes, and our infantile helplessness is the ultimate root of religion.

What we see around us gives us little evidence for the existence of an ethical order in the world. But this is not a logical consequence of psychoanalysis; one may or may not graft religion onto it; as a matter of principle I should not like to have psychoanalysis placed at the service of any specific doctrine. The second edition of *Die Sexualtheorie*,[5] (unchanged) shall be forwarded to you shortly.

Best wishes, and thank you for all your efforts on behalf of our cause.

Yours,
Freud

[1] See preceding letter.
[2] The words enclosed in quotation marks are in English.
[3] See preceding letter.
[4] The words in quotation marks are in English.
[5] Freud, *Drei Abhandlungen zur Sexualtheorie,* 2nd ed., 1910.

16
Putnam to Freud
[April 14, 1910]

106 Marlborough Street

Dear Dr. Freud

Your last letter and also the postal-card from Nuremberg[1] gave me great pleasure. I have also received, and carefully read, the Drei Abhandlungen Zur Sexual-theorie. It is a fine work.

The new Congress seems to have been a great success. Dr. Ferenczi sent me an account of it[2] which I shall read at the meeting of our new Society, which meets in Washington next month.[3] I am doing all that I can through addresses at different places, to help on the cause, and am sure that the interest in the psychoanalytic method and its results is on the increase.

I hope to talk over with you at length, some day, the subject of philosophy in relation to its bearing on religion and on our work. I accept all that you say as regards the significance of the *Vater-complex*,[4] etc., as giving the practical conception of God, but I still think we are in a position to say more about the nature of mind itself than this empirical, inductive reasoning gives us. I believe that there are certain philosophic *"necessary presuppositions"* [5] which require us to go further, and to entertain certain views about the meaning and destiny of man and the universe that can be made to form a valuable supplement to our psychotherapeutic work as represented by psychoanalysis.

I enclose a bird's eye view of our settlement.[6] It shows a part of the buildings only and unfortunately not that in which you slept. It was taken by Harold Bowditch.[7]

With kind regards from your friend,

James J. Putnam

IV. 14.

---

[1] Missing.

[2] Ferenczi had written Putnam about the organization of the International Psychoanalytic Association at the recent congress held in Nuremberg, March 30–31, 1910. See Ferenczi to Putnam, April 1, 1910.

[3] The American Psychopathological Association was founded May 2, 1910, in Washington, D.C. for physicians and psychologists interested in psychotherapy and psychopathology. See *Journal of Abnormal Psychology*, 5 (April–May 1910), 91.

[4] Father complex.
[5] See Putnam to William James, June 25, 1910.
[6] The Putnam camp at Keene Valley.
[7] Harold Bowditch (1883–1964), son of Henry Pickering Bowditch, who with Charles and James Putnam founded Putnam Camp at Keene Valley.

17

Putnam to Freud

[May 19, 1910]

106 Marlborough Street

Dear Professor

I have received the German edition of the Worcester lectures[1] [which I have already read in English] and am looking forward to reading them over carefully once more.

This morning I have been reading Dr. Jones' paper on your psychology, published in the Psychological Bulletin for April 1910.[2]

He is a fine, clear writer and also speaker, and his expositions of your views will do much good. We had a lively and interesting time at Washington, at the meeting of the Congress. Our new society, The American Psycho-pathological Assoc.[n], was duly founded, and several papers read, including one by Dr. Brill, another by Jones and another by myself.[3]

At the meeting of the American Neurological Association Dr. Hoch read an excellent paper on Dementia Praecox, with a good 'analysis', and I read on my personal experience with psychoanalysis.[4]

Both papers were listened to by relatively large audiences and provoked lively discussion.

Of course there was a good deal of criticism, of the usual sort, but it was universally recognized that a good impression had been made and much sympathetic interest aroused.[5]

Yours with kind regards.

James J. Putnam

V. 19.

On June 1st Dr. Jones and I both speak again, at Toronto, to be followed on the next day, by an adversary who is likely to make an animated opposition.[6]

He is a crazy-headed person.

¹ Freud, *Über Psychoanalyse* (Leipzig and Vienna: F. Deuticke, 1910); "The Origin and Development of Psychoanalysis," trans. Harry Woodburn Chase, *American Journal of Psychology*, 21 (April 1910), 181–218; SE, XI, 1–55.

² "Freud's Psychology," *Psychological Bulletin*, 7 (April 15, 1910), 109–128.

³ See preceding letter, n. 3, and A. A. Brill, "The Anxiety Neuroses," *Journal of Abnormal Psychology*, 5 (June–July 1910), 57–68; Jones, "The Art of Suggestion in Psychotherapy," *ibid.*, (December 1910-January 1911), 217–254; Putnam, "The Sex Symbolism in Dreams," unpublished.

⁴ August Hoch (1868–1919), Swiss-American psychiatrist, director of the Psychiatric Institute of the New York State Hospitals for the Insane, 1910–1917. See "On some of the Mental Mechanisms in Dementia Praecox," *Journal of Abnormal Psychology*, 5 (December 1910–January 1911), 255–273; also in Adolf Meyer et al., *Dementia Praecox, a Monograph* (Boston: Richard G. Badger, 1911). Putnam, "Personal Experience with Freud's Psychoanalytic Method." Read before the American Neurological Association, Washington, D.C., May 3, 1910. *Journal of Nervous and Mental Disease*, 37 (November, 1910), 657–674; Ad Psa, 31–53.

⁵ See the discussion of Putnam's paper, *Journal of Nervous and Mental Disease*, 37 (October 1910), 630–639.

⁶ Joseph Collins (1866–1950), a New York neurologist, who had attacked Putnam's speech before the American Neurological Association in May, was scheduled to discuss the psychoneuroses at the meeting of the Canadian Medical Association. See *Canadian Journal of Medicine and Surgery*, 27 (June 1910), 359 and Jones, *Sigmund Freud*, II, 115.

18

Freud to Putnam

[June 16, 1910]

16. 6. 10

Vienna, IX, Berggasse 19.

Dear Dr. Putnam

At last I am able to thank you — for your letters, your reports and the other things you have sent — with a small gift of my own. My essay, *Eine Kindheits-Erinnerung des Leonardo da Vinci*,¹ should have reached you by now. It contains much on which we do not think alike, and which I hope we shall be able to discuss in the exchange of ideas you have promised to have with me here in Europe. I would be greatly honored if I could persuade you to give me your opinion of this short study.

In addition, it has occurred to me — and I am writing this unofficially for I have no right to do so officially — that only you and only Boston could be the starting point for the formation of a psycho-analytic group to be joined by our friends in America, and which could then affiliate with the International Association that was planned in Nuremberg.[2] I understand that all important intellectual movements in America have originated in Boston. I also know that no one else is as highly regarded as you; because of your unimpeachable reputation for integrity, no one else could protect so well the beleaguered cause of psychoanalysis. Jung, the chairman of the International Association, will be glad to give you all the necessary information. Should you take this welcome step, it would give me one more occasion for which to thank you.

With best wishes,

Yours,

Freud

[1] [Leonardo da Vinci and a Memory of His Childhood], *Schriften zur angewandten Seelenkunde,* VII (Leipzig and Vienna: F. Deuticke, 1910); SE, XI, 57–137.

[2] The International Psychoanalytic Association was organized at Nuremberg, March 30–31, 1910. See Ferenczi to Putnam, April 1, 1910.

19
Putnam to Freud
[June 29, 1910]

Vienna IX, Berggasse 19, Austria;

June 29

Your letter of June 6 [1] reached me yesterday and was very welcome.

Your reprints arrived also by the same mail. I am reading them carefully and will reply very soon to letter.

Sincere regards from your friend

J. J. Putnam

[1] Putnam probably meant June 16, 1910.

20
Putnam to Freud
[Late July, 1910]

106 Marlborough Street

Dear Professor

I imagine that this note will find you off for Holland, to judge from what Dr. Jones has written me.[1]

I wish I was nearer either you or him or some reflecting source of light. However, reading does much, and the Jahrbuch[2] fills many gaps.

I have read the Leonardo very carefully and with the greatest pleasure. It seems to me that you establish your thesis very soundly and certainly you make an admirable contribution to the theory of character-formation as dependent on the early, infantile establishment of 'paths of least resistance.'

Of course I understand and appreciate that the religious conception of God is an idealized paternal complex. I believe that is true, but I still cling to the teachings of philosophy and metaphysics as adding something indispensable to such a genetic theory and conception. I find myself compelled to ask what is the fundamental nature of the universe, and compelled to answer that it is in some sense 'eternal,' and also that the mental life is the most real thing we know.

But if a scheme is *really* eternal it must *as a scheme* have already fulfilled its possibilities and be a perfect scheme. Otherwise it would have fulfilled its defects and have gone to pieces.

But if the universe is eternal and in some sense perfect, and if the 'mental' is the real, then the imperfection and evolution which we see around us must have some meaning compatible with the perfection of the general scheme. They must exist for a purpose, and I cannot imagine any better purpose than the elaboration of more and more desirable [and so 'viable'] forms of mental individuality. We don't know enough to say 'how' or 'why' exactly, but somehow the genetic scheme on which you are working, and which shows that men are elaborated forms of the lower and lowest organisms must harmonize with the principle of mental perfection and purpose as the real basis of the universe. All this may be very obscure and very absurd but it seems to me that some such reasoning is sound, and if sound then important. I believe there are two poles to an eternally existent universe; that we have something to work towards as well as something to work *out* of [Cf. a paper by Schiller in his essays on Humanism, on Aristotle's idea of energy in repose];[3] and that although the *form* in which we realize the higher mental qualities [love, etc.] is doubtless determined by evolution from below, yet there is an eternally existent form of these same qualities, which we can look at and aspire to as models of perfection.

I suppose all this sounds nonsense to you, but one must say what one thinks. I think there is a 'science' which works by certain presuppositions [laws of nature; assumption of causation, etc., i.e. by presuppositions which are arbitrary and conventional] and a 'philosophy' which works by certain other sorts of presuppositions [essential laws of thinking]. Why should we discard the latter, and why should we strive to silence our instinctive desire to know the essential nature of things, even though we may admit that the *form* which this desire takes [call it Grübeln[4] if you will] is dependent on infantile or childhood curiosity about fundamental facts in physiology.

I am — of course — getting more and more interested in Psychoanalyse, though I feel my deficiency in practice very much. I send you one more general address and will soon send another, but hope, some day, to be able to make some more specific contribution.

Dr. Jones and I will bring about the Branch Association meeting, but it seems to both of us that it would best take place in connection with the next meeting of our new American Psychopathological Assoc.[5]

I will, at any rate, communicate with Dr. Jung.

> Thank you for your letter.
> Sincerely,
> James J. Putnam

[1] See Jones to Putnam, July 18, 1910.

[2] The *Jahrbuch für psychoanalytische und psychopathologische Forschungen* [Yearbook for Psychoanalytic and Psychopathological Research] was published from 1909 to 1914.

[3] See F. C. S. Schiller, *Humanism: Philosophical Essays* (London: Macmillan and Co., Ltd., 1903), chap. xii, "Activity and Substance," pp. 204–227.

⁴ Speculation.

⁵ See Jones to Putnam, July 12, 1910, and Jones, *Sigmund Freud*, II, 87–88. The American Psychoanalytic Association was founded in Baltimore May 9, 1911. See *Zentralblatt*, 2 (1912), 236, 241–242, and *Journal of Abnormal Psychology*, 6 (October–November 1911), 328.

21
Putnam to Freud
[August 4, 1910]

August 4, 1910

Professor Sigmund Freud,
    Vienna, Austria.

Dear Professor:

I send you a copy of the Address before the Canadian Medical Association,¹ and also the Discussion of another paper, read before the American Neurological Association. I will send you a copy of this latter paper as soon as it comes out. The Discussion may entertain you, but I think it is fair to say that on the whole most of those present felt that the cause of psycho-analysis came out rather victorious.² The room was well filled and a good deal of interest was taken. The report of the Discussion here given is a very imperfect one, since it was drawn up by the reporter of the meeting, and I, at least, had no opportunity of revising my remarks. Let me say again that the paper here printed is not the one which was discussed.

Yours very sincerely,
James J. Putnam

¹ Putnam, "On the Etiology and Treatment of the Psychoneuroses." Read before the Canadian Medical Association, Toronto, June 1, 1910. *Boston Medical and Surgical Journal*, 163 (July 21, 1910), 75–82; Ad Psa, 54–78.

² Putnam, "Personal Experience with Freud's Psychoanalytic Method." For the discussion, see *Journal of Nervous and Mental Disease*, 37 (October 1910), 630–639; see also Putnam to William James, June 25, 1910.

22

Freud to Putnam

[August 18, 1910]

Noordwijk am Zee
Vienna, IX, Berggasse 19.
18 Aug. 10

Dear[1] Dr. Putnam

Thank you for your two letters and for sending the things you promised. In your first, your praise of the "Leonardo"[2] and your promise to found an American branch[3] pleased me very much. However, I was grieved that you should believe that I possibly could consider your idealistic views as nonsense because they differ from mine. I am not so intolerant as to wish to make a law out of a deficiency in my own make-up. I feel no need for a higher moral synthesis in the same way that I have no ear for music. But I do not consider myself a better man because of that. I console myself with this reflection: the idealistic truths which you are not willing to give up cannot be so certain if the basic principles of the science on which we do agree are so difficult to determine. But I respect you and your views. Although I am resigned to the fact that I am a God forsaken "incredulous Jew,"[4] I am not proud of it and I do not look down on others. I can only say with Faust, "There have to be odd fellows like that, too."

Dr. Jones who was my guest here in Holland for several days told me that he gave you the *Leonardo* to read. I hope that since then it has arrived from the publisher, for I asked him to send you all the subsequent volumes of the *Schriften zur angewandten Seelenkunde*.[5]

Soon a year will have passed, as I recall, since I enjoyed your hospitality and made friends who would be so important for the development of ΨA in America. Please give my sincerest greetings to your family.

Faithfully yours,
Freud

[1] In English.
[2] Putnam to Freud, [late July, 1910].
[3] Of the International Psychoanalytic Association.

23
Putnam to Freud
[September 1, 1910]

106 Marlborough Street
Sept. 1st.

Dear Professor

I write to thank you for your letter of August 18 and to say that I am sorry if I struck a foolish note in my careless remark about "nonsense." [1] In fact, if I should subject myself to a psychoanalysis, I should have to confess that I had a slight feeling of false shame, and was inclined to accuse *myself* of dealing in 'nonsense.' The best thing to do about that is perhaps to put my ideas to a further test, and that I intend, as soon as possible, to do. In general terms, I believe that psycho*genetic* knowledge and feeling, as based on a study of our own experiences of life, is not enough for a suitable 'Sublimation.'

I find that many of my patients, and I myself, need all the *motive* that can be secured, and I believe also that when one has taught himself to look into the matter in that way the strongest motive is that which comes from a recognition of our responsibility as self-conscious beings. Furthermore, I believe that if a psychoanalysis could be carried far enough it would be seen that we are constantly acting under instincts that are based on an unconscious recognition of the form and structure of the intellect. This scheme does not explain itself and could only be explained through an elaborate discussion and this I must try to give in print. I am sure that we have dwelt too exclusively on that portion of our mental life which is expressed only in our bodily life. But every student knows that our mental life transcends our bodily life (Cf. Bergson, for example) and I believe that we, as psychotherapeutists, are bound to act on that belief.

There is a self-active principle of life in the plant-world [Bergson's *poussée vitale*],[2] a still higher form of it in the animal world, a still higher form in man, and the highest and most thoroughly unified form is universe-al.

I write these things to you because I feel how much I owe you for mental stimulus in the study of the mind, and wish to express my acknowledgement.

Your Leonardo did not arrive but I ordered it and shall here-after receive regularly all the 'Schriften' as they come out. As I told you, I read it carefully and with the greatest interest and sympathy.

Sincerely yours,
James J. Putnam

[1] See Putnam to Freud, [late July, 1910].
[2] Life force.

24
Freud to Putnam
[September 29, 1910]

29 Sept. 10
Vienna, IX, Berggasse 19.

Dearest Dr. Putnam

Please forgive me if in this letter I cannot hold back an unac-customed enthusiasm. I have seldom been as proud or as satisfied with myself, as when I read your essay of July 21st, "On the Etiology and Treatment of the Psychoneuroses;" I did not read it until I returned from Italy today. You convince me that I have not lived and worked in vain, for men such as you will see to it that the ideas I have arrived at in so much pain and anguish will not be lost to humanity. What more can one desire?

Your exposition of the most intricate causal relationships was masterly. Such clarity and truth must have their effect on those who heard you and who were open to new ideas. You express my convictions more clearly than I do, in the broad cultural context in which they belong, and have imbued them with the all-inclu-sive viewpoint of a friend of humanity. I ask your permission to translate this essay for our *Zentralblatt*.[1] I cannot imagine any more dignified and forceful reply to the attacks against which we here have to defend ourselves. However, permit me to omit the lines in which you praise me so highly:[2] because I am the translator, it would not be fitting to include them, and this is all the more the case since I am also the publisher of the Zentralblatt. I do not wish to comment at length about your letter of Sept. 1. It does you great credit. I only regret that my own thoughts do not reach such heights. I have tried to correct the bookseller's carelessness about sending you the Leonardo.

Yours very cordially,

Freud

[1] See Putnam, "On the Etiology and Treatment of the Psychoneuroses," trans. Freud, *Zentralblatt*, 1 (1911), 137–154.

[2] Putnam wrote: "Finally, we come to the third group of investigators, whom I have designated as *analysts, inductive reasoners and broad thinkers*. The foremost representative of this group, at the present day, is unquestionably Sigmund Freud, a remarkable personage, whose observations and whose method have opened for us avenues of inquiry into which men of the best minds are pressing forward in ever increasing number. No future student of human character and motives, will ever make studies deserving serious recognition without familiarizing himself with the researches of the school of thinkers and observers of which Freud was the leader and is still the central figure. Janet's work and that of men following similar lines (Morton Prince, Sidis, etc.) have made a revolution in the field of scientific psychology; Freud's work has extended this scientific revolution and has set on foot an equal revolution in character-study, educational psychology, race-psychology, child-study and folk-lore."

This paragraph was retained, and a complimentary footnote about Putnam was added. See *Boston Medical and Surgical Journal*, 163 (July 21, 1910), 78; Ad Psa, 64–65; and *Zentralblatt*, 1 (1911), 137, 144–145.

25

Putnam to Freud

[October 10, 1910]

Oct. 10, 1910

Prof. Dr. Sigmund Freud,
Vienna, Austria.

Dear Professor, —

Your letter touched me very much and gave me great pleasure.[1] If I can do any service to the cause in which we are both so much concerned I think it is likely to be mainly through putting some of these questions in a clearer light before the medical profession, as I tried to do in that paper,[2] rather than by working out special points, though for that matter I have had some experiences that have interested me greatly.

I should, of course, feel much honored to have the paper translated into German, but I suggest that it might be well to wait a little so that I can send you a copy of a paper or article which was read at the meeting of the Neurological Association in Washington last May,[3] that should appear now very shortly, and parts of which may interest you. Possibly there may be a few paragraphs in that which you might wish to add.

I am sending copies of the Toronto paper to Dr. Ferenczi and to Dr. Jung.[4]

With very kind regards, believe me

Sincerely yours,
James J. Putnam

[1] See preceding letter.
[2] "On the Etiology and Treatment of the Psychoneuroses."
[3] Putnam, "Personal Experience with Freud's Psychoanalytic Method."
[4] Ferenczi, Jung, and Freud had visited Putnam Camp in the Adirondacks in September 1909.

26
Putnam to Freud
[December 26, 1910]

106 Marlborough Street

Dear Professor

I write a line to send you a New Year's greeting and to express the great pleasure and interest with which I have read the papers by you which came out in the Zentralblatt,[1] and of which you kindly sent me the reprints.

I trust that the next year will go well with you, and find you strong and active.

You spoke in your last letter of perhaps publishing my article on the Etiology and Tr^t of the Psychon^{ses}. If you still think it worth while to do this, I have been thinking that perhaps I could make a few slight changes, to advantage.

Yours with kind regards
James J. Putnam

Dec. 26th

¹ See Freud's major articles, "Die zukünftigen Chancen der psychoanalytischen Therapie" [The Future Prospects of Psycho-Analytic Therapy], *Zentralblatt*, 1 (1910), 1–9; SE, XI, 141–151; and "Über 'wilde' Psychoanalyse" ['Wild' Psycho-Analysis], *Zentralblatt*, 1 (1910), 91–95; SE, XI, 219–227.

27
Freud to Putnam

[December 29, 1910]

29 Dec 10
Vienna, IX, Berggasse 19.

Dear Colleague

I do not want to let this eventful and troublesome year close before having thanked you for many things: for your valuable articles, for the inestimable aid which you have lent our cause, for allowing your name to be used in America as a protection against the possible misunderstandings and abuses to which I otherwise would have been subjected. From the bottom of my egotistical heart I wish you untroubled health and energy.

Your Toronto lecture already is in print and will grace the fourth number of the *Zentralblatt*.¹ (The third issue already has appeared.) Your Washington lecture, translated by Otto Rank, will be published in a later number.² For form's sake I ask you to share the modest fee with the translator; in the case of the first lecture, the translator is I, although I did not sign it. Two small reprints of mine from the *Jahrbuch* and the *Zentralblatt* will be sent to you in the near future.

Our cause is doing very well here; the opposition is at its height. I am a bit tired, but that may pass, and my successors, especially my splendid Jung, are very hopeful.

I saw Bleuler and Jung recently in Munich. We plan to have the Congress meet at the end of September, 1911 in Lugano.³ The date was decided upon in the hope of seeing our American friends there.

With hearty greetings, yours sincerely,

Freud

---

[1] Putnam, "On the Etiology and Treatment of the Psychoneuroses." Trans. by Freud as "Über Ätiologie und Behandlung der Psychoneurosen."

[2] Putnam, "Personal Experience with Freud's Psychoanalytic Method." Trans. by Otto Rank as "Persönliche Erfahrungen mit Freuds psychoanalytischer Methode," *Zentralblatt*, 1 (1911), 533–548.

[3] Eugen Bleuler (1856–1939), professor of psychiatry at the University of Zurich. Freud met Bleuler in Munich to discuss his resignation from the International Psychoanalytic Association. Freud wanted Bleuler to play in Europe the same protecting role for psychoanalysis that Putnam performed in America. See Franz Alexander and Sheldon T. Selesnick, "Freud-Bleuler Correspondence," *Archives of General Psychiatry*, XII (January 1965), 1–10. Bleuler attended as a visitor the third International Psychoanalytic Congress held in Weimar instead of Lugano, September 21–22, 1911.

28

Putnam to Freud

[January 20, 1911]

106 Marlborough Street

I. 20. 11

Dear Professor

It was very pleasant to receive your New Year's greeting,[1] I assure you, and I trust that you received my note which perhaps crossed yours, telling of the pleasure which I had from reading your last papers.

Your industry and your power of grasping and illuminating new subjects, as in the essay on the words of opposite meaning,[2] fills me with amazement. I found that essay exceedingly interesting, and have made a note of one point which may serve as a text for future elaboration from a standpoint of my own.

You do me much honor in proposing to have my two papers translated for the Zentralblatt, still more in translating one of them yourself.[3]

I am only afraid that your German readers will think them rather juvenile and amateurish.

Of course I will do whatever you think best about the Honorarium, and should be entirely content to give the whole amount to the translator.

I am sorry to hear you say you are not well. Take good care of yourself for you are an important person.

With very kind regards,
James J. Putnam

[1] See preceding letter.

[2] Freud, "Über den Gegensinn der Urworte" [The Antithetical Sense of Primal Words], *Jahrbuch*, 2 (1910), 179–184; SE, XI, 155 161.

[3] Putnam, "Über Ätiologie und Behandlung der Psychoneurosen" and "Persönliche Erfahrungen mit Freuds psychoanalytischer Methode."

29

Freud to Putnam

[January 22, 1911]

22 Jan 1911
Vienna, IX, Berggasse 19.

Dear Colleague

Our New Year's wishes crossed. May they both be fulfilled.

The printed version of your Toronto lecture is here before me and will appear in the January issue of the *Zentralblatt*.[1] Your letter arrived too late for any additions. Even in its present form it brings the reader very much that is good and new. Jung agrees with me. We have taken advantage of your permission to have the Washington lecture translated; and it will be published a few months from now.[2] Meanwhile, perhaps you will have read Bleuler's nice apologia for psychoanalysis in the new volume of the *Jahrbuch*.[3] We shall wait and see whether or not it will have a calming influence on those in Germany whose feelings have been aroused. We hope to have the pleasure of seeing you and some of your countrymen at our September Congress as members of the ΨA Association.[4] It may take place in Lugano. Jung will send you the details.

With sincere regards,
Faithfully yours,
Freud

[1] Putnam, "Über Ätiologie und Behandlung der Psychoneurosen."

[2] Putnam, "Persönliche Erfahrungen mit Freuds psychoanalytischer Methode."

[3] Eugen Bleuler, "Die Psychoanalyse Freuds. Verteidigung und kritische Bemerkungen" [The Psychoanalysis of Freud. Defense and Critical Remarks], *Jahrbuch*, 2 (1910), 623–730.
[4] The third International Psychoanalytic Congress was held in Weimar instead of Lugano on September 21–22, 1911.

30

Putnam to Freud

[January 26, 1911]

106 Marlborough Street

Dear Professor

Your suggestion of a meeting of the Congress 'towards the end of Sept.' [1] has tempted me so much that I have already made plans to take my wife and children and make a trip in Eastern Europe (Engl., France and Switzerland), bringing up at Lugano and sailing for home from Genoa.

Do you think I could count on getting away from Lugano by Sept. 26 or 27? I must sail from Genoa, *unbedingt*,[2] on Sept. 28.

With kindest greetings and hopes of a meeting in Sept., I am sincerely

your friend
James J. Putnam

I. 26. 11

[1] Although the previous two International Psychoanalytic Congresses had been held in the spring, the third was scheduled for the fall to accommodate the Americans. See Freud to Putnam, December 29, 1910.
[2] Without fail.

31

Putnam to Freud

[February 6, 1911]

February 6, 1911.

Dear Dr. Freud,

You must have been surprised to receive my cablegram yesterday and I will explain the reasons for my sending it.

The neurological department of the Medical School publishes, once a year, a volume of papers by the different members.[1] I ought to have laid aside for this purpose a number of reprints of the Toronto address, but failed to do so and had intended therefore, in order to make up for these, to put in the reprints of the German translation. Perhaps it is too late to do this and if so, pray do not feel concerned.

I have just received your kind note of January 22nd and a week before that received three reprints, two of which I have already read with great interest.

I now write, in some haste, mainly to say that the date of our sailing from Genoa has been postponed until October first so that I trust I shall not have to incommode you with reference to the meeting of the Congress and yet shall be able to attend it.

Yours with kind regards,
James J. Putnam

[1] The volume included nine articles by Putnam, eight of them on psychoanalysis, with both English and German versions of "On the Etiology and Treatment of the Psychoneuroses." See *Department of Neurology, Harvard Medical School,* V (Boston, Mass., 1912).

32

Freud to Putnam

[February 19, 1911]

19 Febr. 1911
Vienna, IX, Berggasse 19.

Dear Colleague

I am delighted that you are definitely planning to attend the Congress.[1] We hope that it will be rewarding and promising for the future.

Perhaps we can meet and talk in Zurich before the Congress because until then I shall be Jung's guest beginning some time in September. That would be a pleasure for both of us.

Your Toronto lecture has just appeared in the fourth number of the *Zentralblatt.*[2] I ordered 400 reprints from Bergmann[3] after receiving your essay, but they have not yet been delivered. I shall ask whether he has sent them directly to you. Your Washington lecture[4] which we consider equally valuable already has been translated by Rank and will be published in due course. The *Zentralblatt* is already over supplied.

I am now working on the third edition of the *Traumdeutung*, and would like to know whether you have published the lecture you gave in 1910 on "Sex Symbolism in Dreams";[5] I would like to refer to it in the new edition.

The next issue of the *Jahrbuch* will contain several articles on paranoia by Ferenczi and by me.[6] Something that looks like a more considerable synthesis is taking shape for the summer.[7] I may find time to work on it while I'm taking the cure in Karlsbad; at the moment I am too busy with the demands of earning a living and carrying on my daily practice.

I am glad that here, as in America, psychoanalytic work itself as well as interest in it is progressing so well. Jones is especially active and untiring. With sincere greetings and wishes for your well being.

Faithfully yours,
Freud

[1] The third International Psychoanalytic Congress, scheduled for September 21–22 in Lugano.

[2] "Über Ätiologie und Behandlung der Psychoneurosen."

[3] J. F. Bergmann, Freud's publisher in Wiesbaden.

[4] "Personal Experience with Freud's Psychoanalytic Method."

[5] Freud, *Die Traumdeutung* [The Interpretation of Dreams], 3rd ed. (Leipzig und Wien: F. Deuticke, 1911). "Sex Symbolism in Dreams" was not published, see Putnam to Freud [late March, 1911].

[6] See Ferenczi, "Über die Rolle der Homosexualität in der Pathogenese der Paranoia," *Jahrbuch,* 3 (1912), 101–119; trans. Ernest Jones, "On the Part Played by Homosexuality in the Pathogenesis of Paranoia," in Ferenczi, *Sex in Psychoanalysis* (Boston: Richard G. Badger, 1916), and Freud, "Psychoanalytische Bemerkungen über einen autobiographisch beschriebenen Fall von Paranoia (Dementia paranoides)," *Jahrbuch,* (1911), 9–68; trans. James and Alix Strachey "Psychoanalytic Notes on an Autobiographical Account of a Case of Paranoia (Dementia Paranoides)," SE, XII, 1–79, and Freud, "Nachtrag zu dem autobiographisch beschriebenen Fall von Paranoia (Dementia paranoides)" [Postscript to an Autobiographical Account of a Case of Paranoia (Dementia Paranoides)], *Jahrbuch,* 3 (1912), 588–590; SE, XII, 80–82. Freud's "considerable synthesis" probably was *Totem und Tabu* (1912–1913); SE, XIII, 1–161.

[7] The word "summer" is uncertain in the holograph.

33

Freud to Putnam

[February 27, 1911]

27. 2. 11
Vienna, IX, Berggasse 19.

Dear Colleague

I am now in a position to conduct our first business transaction — concerning the publication of your article in the *Zentralblatt*.[1] You will see how much Bergmann pays for work which I consider beyond price. Half of the fee goes to me as the translator. The other half will be sent to you through my bank. Of the 400 reprints made, I have kept forty to be distributed in Europe in the Zurich and Berlin branches of the Association;[2] I hope you will find this satisfactory.

Since I don't want to mix science with business, I remain,

Yours sincerely,
Freud

[1] Putnam, "Über Ätiologie und Behandlung der Psychoneurosen."
[2] Psychoanalytic societies were founded in Zurich in 1907 and in Berlin in 1908; the latter had four members in 1911, in addition to Karl Abraham. Both groups joined the International Association that was organized in 1910.

34

Putnam to Freud

[Late March, 1911]

106 Marlborough Street[1]

Dear Professor

It was a pleasure to receive your letter of II. 19. and to hear that you are likely to be at Zurich in September.[2]

It is uncertain just what time will be at my disposal, for I shall probably be the only man in a party of ladies and children anxious to see something of Switzerland and Italy, and I may be obliged to act as escort, especially after September 9, when my son[3] returns home to Boston. Between Sept. 1 and 9 I could probably be free and perhaps earlier. At any rate, we shall meet at Lugano and I shall have many questions to ask you.

I am greatly obliged to you for attending to my reprints and shall not allow myself to be disappointed if it turns out that my message arrived too late for the reprinting.

You kindly ask about my paper on sex-symbolism in dreams. It has never been printed but its value would not be great except for persons as unfamiliar with the subject as I was prior to two years ago. We all know, now, that the variety of sex dreams[4] is simply infinite and those which I gave were simply a few out of a possible multitude of variations on the same theme. One of the latest was an Entbindung[5]-dream, in which a young married woman, — desiring yet fearing childbirth — found herself in company with an apparently new-born baby and, in obedience to an impulse, kept lifting the clothes that covered it and looking "to see how far the labor had advanced." In the earlier editions of the *Traumdeutung* you did not take up the subject of sexual dreams much, and I thought wisely. Do you mean to go into it fully in the new edition? [6]

Dr. Stekel [7] has kindly asked me to contribute short clinical observations to the Zentralblatt and I mean to do so, though I fear that, in my ignorance, I shall send what may not be much worth reading.

Now I wish to ask your advice upon another matter and shall be grateful for a frank statement of disapproval if you feel inclined to give it.

You are aware of my interest in certain aspects of philosophy and psychology, but I have not expressed as strongly as I feel that there are points of view which, I think, can be shown to be of distinctly practical importance as well as of theoretical interest.

What I wish to ask you is whether you think it would be (A) suitable and (B) worth while, for me to read a paper at the Congress on these views?

That which I should try to show, stated in brief outline, would be something of the following sort:

As I study patients and try to relieve them of their symptoms, I find that I must also try to improve their moral characters and temperaments. They must be willing, must *wish* to 'sublimate' themselves; must be ready to make sacrifices and to follow their best ideals. *But why?* This question Ψan as such does not (as I understand it) claim to answer. It would be said 'Moral philosophy is not our affair.' But this I do not admit. If there *are* reasons for *effort* in the world, for use of the *will* I think we are bound to give them and to make them clear, and especially so if these motives can be arrived at by introspection; that is, by a still further use of the Ψan^c process.

I consider that no patient is really cured unless he becomes better and broader morally, and, conversely, I believe that a moral regeneration helps towards a removal of the symptoms.

Now I do not ask that we should simply say, 'Be moral.' I have a wider plan than this. I wish to show that [in accordance with the Hegelian and Froebelian philosophy, and the psychology (and philosophy) of Harris and Bergson and Judd, etc.] [8] the current psychoan.^s *implies* (at least) a narrow, and so an incorrect because incomplete, view of human life and motive.

It is too materialistic, too purely interested in the bare *description* of genetic processes. It corresponds to an accepted but erroneous conception of evolution, which leaves out human will [Judd, Bergson, etc.] and fails to recognize that mind, consciousness, reason, emotion, will, are not merely *products* of evolution but underlying *causes* of evolution.

I cannot go into the matter here at greater length and indeed there is enough material for a book, which I hope to write some day, but I should try to show that the causes for conduct alleged by Ψan. [the *instinctive* strivings and cravings of the Oedipus complex, the parental complex, etc.], real though these are, are actually supplemented by quasi-volitional efforts partly 'unconscious' and yet not because painful but for other reasons and that it is our duty to learn to recognize [as Froebel did] the ever-present signs of these immature efforts of the will [just as we learned to recognize other infantile complexes] and to foster them by every means within our power. *We already utilize the will but we do this blindly and grudgingly and without quite believing in its existence.* We ought to do it consciously and skilfully.

There are many men among us — the great majority I think — who, even if not avowedly materialistic are avowedly deterministic. Their symbol of evolution is a straight line ———→ which begins with 'matter' [that is, they know not and care not where] and ends

— nowhere in particular. "Motive" has no place in such a scheme.

My belief is [an absolutely demonstrable doctrine as I think] that visible evolution occupies, not a strait line but small segments of a great circle ⌒ and that civilization and life consist in learning to realize ⌣ the whole of the circle, as we can do completely as a matter of formal insight and partially in practice, partially even in this life.

The only *reality* is in the nature of *personal consciousness*. This is present — or to be studied — under two aspects, (a) that of its *form;* (b) that of its *contents*. Ψan in common with observational sciences studies only a portion of the *contents,* of consciousness, but in so doing it leaves out of consideration some very actual and practical influences in human life and *we want the whole of human life*.

Would it be perfectly useless and ridiculous to bring *some portion* of this subject, that portion especially which relates to *practical motives* and the strengthening of *character,* before the Congress?

I must sometime, in print, have the courage of my convictions and express just what I think. But perhaps the Congress is not the place to do this.

Yours sincerely
James J. Putnam

¹ Above the heading Putnam wrote, "I owe you an apology for a letter which has far outgrown my first intention. Leave it till next September if you like."

² Freud was to visit Jung at his new home at Küsnacht, Zurich, before the third International Psychoanalytic Congress.

³ James Jackson Putnam (1890–   ).

⁴ See Freud to Putnam, February 19, 1911.

⁵ Birth.

⁶ The third edition was published in 1911; SE, IV, V.

⁷ Wilhelm Stekel (1868–1940), Viennese psychoanalyst, editor of the *Zentralblatt*.

⁸ Friedrich Froebel (1782–1852), German founder of the Kindergarten movement; William Torrey Harris (1835–1909), American Hegelian and U.S. Commissioner of Education from 1889 to 1906; Charles Hubbard Judd (1873–1946), American psychologist.

35

Putnam to Freud

[March 27, 1911]

March 27, 1911.

Dear Dr. Freud:

I have received your two letters and the reprints and two postal orders from Bergmann, — for all of which accept my sincere thanks. Your complimentary foot-note[1] is hardly true, but must pass for such. Your translation is exceedingly interesting, and I thank you warmly for making it.

I should have written to you before this, but could not quite make up my mind to send the enclosed letter[2] which I had written before yours arrived. However, I think I will send it after all, although it does not say quite what I mean. In it I ask you for an answer, but really no answer is required. I must think the matter over and make my own decision.

Yours sincerely

James J. Putnam

[1] Freud combined the compliment with a remark about Putnam's age. According to Jones, *Sigmund Freud*, II, 58–59, Freud had been annoyed by Putnam's reference to him as "no longer a young man" in the article "Personal Impressions of Sigmund Freud." In the complimentary footnote Freud wrote: "J. Putnam ist nicht nur einer der hervorragendsten Nervenärzte Amerikas, sondern auch ein wegen seines tadellosen Charakters und seines hohen ethischen Standard allgemein hochgeachteter Mann. Obwohl längst über die Jahre der Jugend hinaus, hat er sich seit dem Vorjahre unbedenklich in die erste Reihe der Vorkämpfer für die Psychoanalyse gestellt" [J. Putnam is not only one of the most eminent neurologists in America but also a man everywhere respected for his unimpeachable character and high moral standards. Although he has left his youth far behind him, he took his open stand last year in the front rank of the champions of psychoanalysis], *Zentralblatt*, 1 (1911), 137; SE, XVII, 272.

[2] See preceding letter.

36
Freud to Putnam

[May 14, 1911]

14. 5. 11
Vienna, IX, Berggasse 19.

Dear Dr. Putnam

I really must apologize for two reasons. First, I added a note about your qualifications to the translation of your lectures, little knowing that the German version would be distributed in America.[1] It must have seemed very odd that someone as unknown as myself should vouch for you over there. It would have been entirely different had it been you who were introducing me to the American public.

Second, please forgive me for answering your detailed letter on sublimation as if you had not written the postscript. I do it because the issue interests me so deeply and because I think your interest in ΨA might diminish if you assume that we disagree in this regard.

You say that ΨA experience shows you that whenever you want your patients to achieve complete recovery, you must direct them toward sublimation, but that ΨA theory does not show you *why* you must do so. Here I must disagree. ΨA theory really does cover this. It teaches that a drive cannot be sublimated as long as it is repressed and that this is equally true for every component of a drive. Therefore one must remove the repression by overcoming the resistances before achieving partial or complete sublimation. This is the goal of ΨA therapy and the way in which it serves every form of higher development.

If we are not satisfied with saying, "Be moral and philosophical,"[2] it is because that is too cheap and has been said too often without being of any help. Our art consists in making it possible for people to be moral and to deal with their wishes philosophically. Sublimation, that is striving toward higher goals, is of course one of the best means of overcoming the urgency of our drives. But one can consider doing this only after ΨA work has lifted the repressions.

There are two reasons why we have said so little about sublimation. First, because it is irrelevant, and second because so many of the patients we really want to help are incapable of it. For the most part, these patients have inferior endowments and disproportionately strong drives. They would like to be better than they can be, yet this convulsive desire benefits neither themselves nor society. It is therefore more humane to establish this principle: "Be as moral as you can honestly be and do not strive for an ethical perfection for which you are not destined." Whoever is capable of sublimation will turn to it inevitably as soon as he is free of his neurosis. Those who are not capable of this at least will become more natural and more honest.

These comments of mine will show you how delighted we would all be if we could hear something about your views on the relation of ΨA to ethics at the Congress in Weimar.

With reference to your additional demands on ΨA, I should like to say that it is only a tool which he who uses it can do with as he wishes. Personally I sympathize with your demands, but I do not go along with you in your attempts to fulfill them. Moderation, that is, aiming for certainty, seems to me to be the next best thing. There has never been a lack of the most uplifting Weltanschauungen, but these were born of pious wishes, of illusion, just as were the proud scientific systems we abandoned when we had to give up anthropocentric notions. We still know too little about the human soul. Only when this knowledge is greater, will we learn what is practicable in the field of ethics, and what we can do in the way of education without doing harm.

Thank you heartily for your letter which has absorbed me intensely; I hope to see you in the fall.

Faithfully yours,
Freud

---

[1] See n. 1, preceding letter.
[2] The words in quotation marks are in English; see Putnam to Freud, [late March, 1911].

37
Putnam to Freud
[May 30, 1911]

V. 30. 11
106 Marlborough Street

Dear Dr. Freud

Since writing to you last I have re-read your interesting letter several times over, with great care.[1] Of course, I agree with practically everything which you say but I think there is, nevertheless, a slight but real difference of attitude between us which I am very desirous of talking over with you.

I assure you that I, too, regard the Ψ^sche Methode[2] as "an instrument" and realize that one may use it without reference to his general views.

Nevertheless, I think it is also true — as illustrated, for example, by the remarks in the last few pages of Abraham's Traum und Mythus[3] — that the prevailing tendency of thought among most writers on Ψ^ic subjects, represents 'Weltauschauungen' which are less helpful and less true than certain others.

I assure you that *nothing* will ever weaken my confidence in the value of the Ψ^ic method. I only want to see it develop on the best philosophic background.

Very sincerely
James J. Putnam

[1] Freud to Putnam, May 14, 1911.
[2] Psychoanalytic method.
[3] Karl Abraham, *Traum und Mythus: eine Studie zur Völkerpsychologie* (Leipzig: F. Deuticke, 1909). Translated by William A. White as *Dreams and Myths: A Study in Race Psychology*, Nervous and Mental Disease Monograph Series No. 15 (New York: Journal of Nervous and Mental Disease Publishing Co., 1913).

38
Putnam to Freud
[July 15. 1911]

Address, care of Brown, Shipley & Co.
London
VII. 15.

Dear Professor

My wife and myself, with our children, have been making a short trip in the Highlands of Scotland and are now leaving Edinborough for London.

I received your kind letter giving your itinerary for the summer but fear we can hardly meet before Weimar, though I shall try to see you at Bozen.[1] We also had planned to be in Venice early in September but if the cholera is there, as you say, we shall probably remain in Switzerland or the Tyrol. After the Congress however, if not before, I trust that we may be able to have some good talks.

Meantime, I shall send you a type-written copy of the paper read by me at Baltimore,[2] through which I trust you will see that what I am trying to do is to show that we have now gone so far in probing the secrets of the mind that we can hardly avoid going further and studying the mind itself, à la Hegel, etc.

Sincerely yours
James J. Putnam

[1] Freud's letter is missing. Bolzano, town in the Tyrol.
[2] "A Plea for the Study of Philosophic Methods in Preparation for Psychoanalytic Work." Read before the American Psychopathological Association, Baltimore, May 10, 1911. *Journal of Abnormal Psychology*, 6 (October–November 1911), 249–264.

39

Putnam to Freud

[August 24, 1911]

Hotel Kurhaus Honegg
Bürgenstock

Dear Professor

Ihre Postcarte habe ich mit grossen Freude erhalten.[1] Ich hoffe allerdings in Zurich wenigstens eine Woche zu verweilen und werde Ihnen dankbar sein wenn Sie mir kundgeben werden des wahrscheinlichen Datums Ihres dort Ankommens.

Ich erlaube mir diesmal auf Deutsch zu schreiben weil es bei mir jetzt viel darauf ankommt mich ins Deutsche einzudenken, um mit meinen geehrten Collegen verkehren zu können.

Achtungsvoll [2]
James J. Putnam

VIII. 24. '11

[1] Missing.

[2] "I was delighted to receive your postcard yesterday. I hope to sojourn in Zurich for at least a week, and would be grateful to you if you would announce to me the probable date of your arrival there.

"Permit me to write you in German at the moment because my problem is to accustom myself to expressing my thoughts in German so that I may be able to converse with my honored colleagues.

Sincerely yours,"

40

Putnam to Freud

[September 30, 1911]

Paris
IX. 30.

Dear Professor

I find myself constrained to write to you once more, but I hope that although it will not be the last time that I write, it will be the last time that I trouble you about my private affairs.

Just now, however, when I am started on a Selbst-analyse,[1] I want as much help as I can have, to enable me to do justice to my patients and to get the satisfaction out of life which everyone ought to get, without needless and hampering sense of apprehension and anxiety.

The first question that I have to ask is one that you may find it hard to answer: I ask however only for some general advice.

A few days ago, while we were at the Hague, on our way to Paris, one of my children, a girl of 16,[2] had [for the first time] an attack which I fear was nothing less than epileptic in character. It came early in the morning, while she was dressing and at a time when her menstruation was expected. It seems also that for the past year she has had frequent, though very slight, momentary 'jerkings' or 'shakings' of the arms or the whole body, without any alteration of consciousness whatever as she thinks.[3] You can imagine my anxiety on this account. Remembering however our conversation about the difficulty of distinguishing epilepsy from hysteria, I wish to ask you whether you would think it decidedly advisable to have an 'Analyse,' even though it would be difficult from several points of view, and though the usual signs of a marked hysterical tendency are absent, as is the case. Except for the physical symptoms to which I have referred she seems to be a 'normal' and healthy girl, though small in stature for her age.

My next question is with reference to a dream which I had the night before leaving Weimar. This was, as usual, a picture, but the symbolism seems to me fairly clear. It appears that [as in an earlier dream] I was driving, and [perhaps] in a similar wagon [□D] to the one I described to you as a 'dog-cart.' I was near the top of a hill [indicated in outline by the line A B]

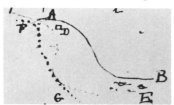

At first I was on the road indicated by the dotted line F.G., which wound down the hill in a generous curve. At once however I became aware of leaving this [safe?] road and driving across the grass, which was short, as if intending to make a 'short cut' in the general direction of E. At first all went well but very soon I became aware of two facts; first, that the hill was getting steep; next, that at E. it was marshy[4] [sumpfig] and that I could see several irregular spots or holes containing water, which reflected the blue of the [afternoon] sky [you may recall that I had another dream in which I saw a brilliant blue or yellowish Edelstein hanging from the neck of a young girl [my daughter had recently bought a bluish emerald pendant — this same daughter who has been taken sick]. I then tried to stop the horse but my pulling on the reins seemed to make no impression on him whatever. He plodded steadily on without seeming to notice my pull or perhaps the latter was like the efforts which patients with hysterical paralysis make, when they apparently use great effort but bring nothing to pass. Then I woke up.

My general interpretation is as follows: The horse stands for my Trieb[5] [sexual, mainly] which I would wish to regulate but cannot check. My 'driving alone' and leaving the safer road, yet feeling anxious on account of the steepness of the hill and the boggy ground below [in which I imagined I should get overturned] indicates my wish to be independent, yet points also to the fact that I am rather dependent on my brother and on my wife,[6] both of whom I associate in my mind with 'driving,' especially in the above mentioned 'dog-cart.' Possibly this feeling about my wife and my brother [dependence, yet 'protest,' and sometimes irrita-tion — really, at myself] may refer both to father and mother or homosexual vs. heterosexual. The holes containing water may have a sexual meaning, as I seemed to be going into them, yet dreading the fact.

I should say, in this connection, that my sexual relations with my wife have been rather infrequent for many years, of late years exceedingly infrequent, and that I have 'dreaded' them, — partly because I believed that many of my friends did not continue such relations at my age, but mainly because although the first effect was one of great relief from a very unpleasant state of tension [erythism, Angst,[7] etc.] yet for a number of days afterwards I always felt abgeschlagen,[8] sleepy, depressed, etc. At the time of the meeting at Weimar I had had no such relations for a good many months, but the 'tension' was I think coming on partly as a result of the fact that I was expecting to meet my wife after a two weeks absence, partly as a 'reaction' from the intellectual excitement of the congress. I did not sleep more than one or two hours that last night at Weimar and although I was not aware of any sexual excitement yet it may have been present 'in the unconscious.' It is certainly true that the sexual Trieb *has* always been like a horse that I could not satisfactorily drive or restrain, though I have never been, in any sense, a 'pervert,' and never experienced the Abgeschlagenheit[9] after sexual intercourse until a good many years after being first married.

My third question relates to the meaning of a 'Phantasie' of my youth,[10] one of the few that I remember. I used, namely, to long for a married life and home of my own and formed a picture in my mind, of myself sitting before an open fire in an otherwise unlighted room, with wife and young children [in my vision I think the *children* were more prominent] playing about and receiving the usual caresses and attentions — reading aloud, etc. In short this was one of the very common pictures of domestic happiness, I suppose, — perhaps idealized somewhat from personal memories, but possibly referring to a close feeling for my mother and father. Affection, readiness to be caressed, narcissism, 'protest,' autoerotism, homosexuality, heterosexuality — all played large parts in my early life, as also sense of Minderwertigkeit[11] ['too small sexual organs,' etc.] and desire for recognition as a means of escape from Minderwertigkeit. I think I have also tried, as I imagine many others have, to compensate for assumed internal lacks, by external aids — things that I could *buy*, influential friends, etc. I have always been fond of *trifling* means of Verschönerung,[12] of *little* successes, etc. of looking into shop windows though without any real intention of buying, as I am 'sparsam,' [13] even in essentials, though occasionally, as contrast or through 'protest,' extravagant, fond of courageous people, yet really timid; not at harmony with myself and — but *far less since married* — ill at ease with others.

One more brief question: When I told you my dream about Prof. James, with whom I had some conversation in a small auditorium, you said that the 'talking' by or with a dead person had some special symbolic meaning.[14] What was that?

I owe you an apology for writing at such length, but you can help me very much by even a few words, and I *must* get myself *free* and able to use my powers.

Sincerely yours
James J. Putnam

104 Marlboro St.
Boston, Massachusetts

[1] Self-analysis.

[2] Louisa Higginson Putnam (1895–1958).

[3] In the left margin of the first page of the letter Putnam wrote, *"I beg you not to mention these facts to any of our friends, while the diagnosis is so uncertain as it is."*

[4] "Boggy" was written above "marshy" in the text.

[5] Instinctual drive.

[6] Marian Cabot Putnam (1857–1932) and Charles Pickering Putnam (1844–1914).

[7] Anxiety.

[8] Exhausted.

[9] Exhaustion.

[10] "Adolescence" was written above "youth."

[11] Inferiority.

[12] Embellishment.

[13] Frugal.

[14] Possibly described during Putnam's six hours of analysis with Freud in Zurich before the Weimar Conference. Putnam's close friend, William James, died August 26, 1910.

41

Freud to Putnam

[October 5, 1911]

5 Okt 11
Vienna, IX, Berggasse 19.

Dear Colleague

You certainly describe yourself as a very bad character. But a far worse man would be uncovered were I to lay myself bare in an analysis as you have done. And you overlook the fact that your sincerity itself indicates greatness of soul. However, I was distressed to read that this would be the last time you would care to write about personal matters. I hope that will not be the case.

Let me hasten to answer your questions one by one, to the best of my ability.

(1) In regard to your daughter, as far as I can determine, the most probable diagnosis is nine to one in favor of hysteria rather than epilepsy. Consequently you can take your time and disregard the symptoms, if no others appear and the attack is not repeated. However, if it seems to be progressive, an analysis is surely indicated, and, I hope, would show you the advantage of this form of therapy in the case of someone dear to you. I shall of course keep the secret.

(2) As for your dream, all I can say is that I find your inter-

pretation entirely correct. I would only suggest this additional interpretation. The safe road that you followed might refer to the therapy you had used before; the new route which soon proves to be so disagreeable, is psychoanalysis, of which you seem to be very much afraid. You are much too frightened by your fantasies, and do not seem to wish to believe that they cannot possibly be transformed into reality. As soon as you give up that fear, you will learn more about your fantasies, find them interesting and experience relief. It strikes me, too, that you have used the letters ABDEFG in your drawing, but omitted C. (Charles).[1] Unfortunately I neglected to ask your wife's name.

(3) I can say least about your fantasy of a happy family life because you described the underlying motives so hastily and piled up everything disagreeable. I beg you not to attribute too much importance to Adler's concepts of organ inferiority, protest, and the desire to dominate because these are superficial, secondary and most often conscious.[2] They do not touch the real forces at work. On the whole I see that you are suffering from a too early and too strongly repressed sadism expressed in over-goodness and self-torture. Behind the fantasy of a happy family life, you would discover the normal repressed fantasies of rich sexual fulfillment. It is the influence of these fantasies which causes the sense of physical dissatisfaction with one's wife. These are symptoms of aging, which I am beginning to experience myself, as I told you in Zurich.[3]

I am always ready to talk with you by letter when distance makes personal communication impossible. I consider the understanding between us as one of the happy rewards of the Congress. I almost had forgotten your fourth question. I believe that communication with the dead, such as occurred in your dream about James,[4] can be interpreted to mean one's own death if the dream does not specifically stipulate, "I know that he is dead." It is interesting that you forgot this particular fact.

With best wishes,
Faithfully yours,
Freud

---

[1] Probably a reference to Charles Pickering Putnam (1844–1914), Putnam's older brother.
[2] Alfred Adler (1870–1937) resigned in July from the Vienna Psychoanalytic So-

ciety of which he was president. See Adler, "Der Aggressionstrieb im Leben und in der Neurose," *Fortschritte der Medizin,* no. 19 (July 1908), pp. 577–584; "Über neurotische Disposition," *Jahrbuch,* 1 (1909), 526–545.

[3] Putnam saw Freud in Zurich before the Weimar Congress and spent six hours in analysis with him.

[4] William James died August 26, 1910.

42

Putnam to Freud

[October 6, 1911]

On board R.M.S. "OCEANIC."
X. 6. 11

Dear Professor

As I wrote to you about my daughter, let me add that I see good reason to *hope* [and Janet[1] fully agrees with me] that her attack was primarily due to a rather severe infectious fever — possibly of the nature of poliomyelitis — by which she was attacked just a year ago.

The very slight 'jerkings,' without loss of consciousness, date apparently from a period about three months after that illness, which I think caused a localized encephalitis. This diagnosis — if it proves correct — seems to justify a better prognosis. I had a pleasant visit to Janet and found him friendly towards psycho-an. though of course he does not and cannot understand it and so misjudges it. He has made a real attempt to read your books but finds it well nigh impossible.

I am carefully reading the last ed[n] of the Traumdeutung[2] and hope to finish it tomorrow. *I read it in a new light.* I have had several short but interesting dreams and can understand them as never before, though still very imperfectly.

With renewed thanks
James J. Putnam

[1] Pierre Janet (1859–1947), French neurologist and psychopathologist.
[2] Freud, 3rd ed., 1911; SE, IV, V.

43
Putnam to Freud
[October 20, 1911]

X. 20. 11.

Thank you sincerely for your kind and very helpful letter. The dream-interpretation goes better, and I think I have had a 'baby-diapers' dream of comfortably lying in excretions (warm water and mud, turning into a bed — a long dream evidently taking place during waking). I have also recognized *Uebertragung*[1] towards yourself, and a 'revenge' in which I took you through a church (my philosophic ideas) and then made you (indignantly) confess that you had symptoms of depression (as I, *formerly*, and slightly of late) which Ψan. could not remove.

My daughter has had no further attack of unconsciousness, but the (very slight) shaking movements of the hand or hands, recur nearly every morning.

Very truly

James J. Putnam

I speak in New York, Nov. 14.[2]

---

[1] Transference.

[2] Putnam addressed the Harvey Society of New York November 14, 1911, "On Freud's Psycho-Analytic Method and Its Evolution," *Boston Medical and Surgical Journal,* 166 (January 25, 1912), 115–122; Ad Psa, 97–122.

44
Freud to Putnam
[November 5, 1911]

5 Nov. 11

Vienna, IX, Berggasse 19.

Dear Colleague

My heartiest thanks for the book about your grandfather[1] which arrived today. I shall read it with much interest. Surely it is not only a duty but a satisfaction to record the accomplishments of one's ancestors and then by one's own example disprove the idle gossip of those scientists who believe in the inevitable degeneration of civilized man. Your own English race offers many examples of the continuity of cultural achievement through several centuries and many generations.

I realize that it is quite impossible to make a definite judgment of your daughter's condition from a distance. Since the diagnosis is still uncertain, one is at a loss as to what treatment to suggest. That it is related to a poliomyelitis, as you wrote some time ago, seems to me particularly doubtful.[2]

I am glad to hear that our few attempts at analysis have not left you with a bad aftertaste. Self analysis is a never ending process that must be continued indefinitely. I notice in my own case how each renewed attempt at self analysis brings its own surprises.

The "politics" of the ΨA movement at the moment are relatively dormant. There is nothing new. You will be interested to learn that your lecture at Weimar[3] has impressed me deeply — although in a very strange way. I am trying to comprehend the psychogenesis of religion from an analytic point of view, and to use psychoanalysis to explain my own lack of a religious need. For this purpose I am studying Fraser, Andrew Lang, Tylor[4] and others, and I must soon read your late friend, William James. When I arrive at a final conclusion I hope that I will not have to offend the sincerely pious.

I hope I will have good news from you soon.

With best wishes,

Yours,

Freud

[1] Putnam, *A Memoir of Dr. James Jackson; with Sketches of His Father, Hon. Jonathan Jackson, and His Brothers, Robert, Henry, Charles, and Patrick Tracy Jackson; and Some Account of Their Ancestry* (Boston and New York: Houghton Mifflin, 1905).

[2] See Putnam to Freud, October 6, 1911.

[3] Putnam "Ueber die Bedeutung philosophischer Anschauungen und Ausbildung für die weitere Entwicklung der psychoanalytischen Bewegung" [The Role of Philosophical Views and Training in the Further Development of the Psychoanalytical Movement]. Read before the third Congress of the International Psychoanalytical Movement, Weimar, September 21–22, 1911. *Imago*, 1 (May 1912), 101–118; an earlier version is in Ad Psa, 79–96.

[4] Sir James George Fraser (1854–1941), British anthropologist; Andrew Lang (1844–1912), British folklorist, man of letters; Sir Edward Burnett Tylor (1832–1917), British anthropologist. See the bibliography in SE, XIII, 245–253.

45
Putnam to Freud
[November 14, 1911]

November 14, 1911.

Professor Sigmund Freud
Vienna, Austria.

Dear Professor:

I thought you might be interested in the two Ladder Dreams[1] which I enclose, and if you think them worthy of publication, perhaps you will be kind enough to send them to Dr. Stekel, who is welcome to deal with my German in any way he thinks best.

My daughter is doing well, we think. She has had no severe attack, and although the curious movements of the left hand continue, the mode and time of their occurrence make me feel more and more that they are in some sense of a hysterical nature.

I have just been delivering my address in New York.[2] I was pleased with the reception of it, and particularly that Dr. Dana,[3] who has hitherto been rather unfavorable, spoke very sympathetically in favor.

Yours sincerely,
James J. Putnam

[1] "Aus der Analyse zweier Treppenträume" [From the Analysis of Two Staircase Dreams], *Zentralblatt,* 2 (1912), 264–265; Ad Psa, 123–125.
[2] Putnam, "On Freud's Psycho-Analytic Method and Its Evolution."
[3] Charles Loomis Dana (1862–1936), professor of neurology at Cornell University Medical College.

46
Putnam to Freud
[November 20, 1911]

November 20, 1911.

Professor Sigmund Freud,
Vienna, Austria.

Dear Professor:

It is needless to say that your letter gave me great pleasure.[1] I wish, however, that instead of the books of which you speak, you would read certain ones *which I will send you*. There are, of course, others, and among them one on the 'Philosophy of Religion' by one of the remarkable Caird brothers, of Edinburgh, and another by Eucken, which no doubt you know. The best book of all is "Hegel's Logic" by Dr. W. T. Harris.[2] I hesitate, however, to recommend this, because I found it exceedingly hard reading.

I am just now trying to get my Weimar paper[3] into such form that it will be as convincing as one could expect within the space of a few pages.

My daughter continues to do well.

Yours sincerely,
James J. Putnam

[1] See Freud to Putnam, November 5, 1911.
[2] Edward Caird (1835–1908), Scottish philosopher, master of Balliol College, Oxford; John Caird (1820–1898), Scottish philosopher, professor of divinity, University of Glasgow; Rudolph Christoph Eucken (1846–1926), professor of philosophy at the University of Jena (1874–1920); William Torrey Harris, *Hegel's Logic: A Book on the Genesis of the Categories of the Mind. A Critical Exposition* (Chicago: S. C. Griggs and Co., 1895).
[3] Putnam, "Ueber die Bedeutung philosophischer Anschauungen."

47

Freud to Putnam

[December 25, 1911]

Weihnacht 1911
Vienna, IX, Berggasse 19.

Dear Dr. Putnam

I am using the first day of Christmas to thank you for the journals and the other things you sent. I will examine the books most carefully. That your daughter is getting on well probably confirms the diagnosis of a harmless hysteria. My study of the psychogenesis of religious feelings is progressing very slowly;[1] I have very little time and must do a lot of other things on the side. But I do not intend to give it up. All I need to achieve anything in that direction is a long life.

On the whole, doing this makes me feel like an elderly gentleman who contracts a second marriage late in life. L'Amour coute cher aux vieillards.[2] Our work in the psychoanalytic association progresses. We hope to publish the first number of the non-medical periodical in the spring.[3] With hearty greetings for the New Year of 1912,

Yours sincerely,

Freud

[1] See Freud to Putnam, November 5, 1911, and *Totem und Tabu: Über einige Übereinstimmungen im Seelenleben der Wilden und der Neurotiker* [Totem and Taboo: Some Points of Agreement between the Mental Lives of Savages and Neurotics], published in the first two volumes of *Imago*, in 1912 and 1913; SE, XIII, vii–162.

[2] Love is expensive for old men.

[3] *Imago, Zeitschrift für Anwendung der Psychoanalyse auf die Geisteswissenschaften*, herausgegeben von Professor S. Freud [*Imago:* Journal for the Application of Psychoanalysis to the Humanities and Social Sciences, edited by Professor S. Freud]. *Imago* was first published in March 1912.

48

Putnam to Freud

[March 2, 1912]

106 Marlborough Street

Dear Professor

Thank you for your two reprints from the Z.blatt, both of which I have read with great interest. I hope, some day, to make a comment on a point [ancestral experience] to which you refer in a foot-note.

Both the papers were helpful and it has occurred to me, in view of this fact, that it might *possibly* be worth while to have a 'question-page' in the Zentralbl. to which physicians in need of aid might send inquiries and statements of difficulties encountered. Perhaps, however, this privilege would be too often abused. Have you seen the notices in recent issues of the Amer. Jr. of Psychology?[1] They would interest you.

My own work goes better, I am glad to say. I have much to learn and various faults of method to correct, but I am getting gradually able to see many things which were formerly obscure.

I still feel very anxious about my daughter, and greatly fear that she has a mild form of epilepsy. She has lost consciousness three times, each time just before menstruation and each time in the morning, while dressing or after bathing, that is, while exerting herself and standing about, before taking food.

My hope is that she may gain with the improvement in her general health, towards which we are working. She is not strong and the digestion is not active.

Of course, if necessary, psychoan[s] should be used, but it would be difficult as there is no one here to whom I would entrust it and I do not like to undertake it myself.

Yours sincerely

James J. Putnam

III. 2. 09[2]

I have been re-reading a number of your older papers, with great profit.

---

[1] See Rudolph Acher, "Recent Freudian Literature," *American Journal of Psychology*, 22 (July 1911), 408–443, and Dr. James S. Van Teslaar, "Recent Literature on Psychoanalysis," *ibid.*, 23 (January 1912), 115–139.

[2] The date should be 1912.

49

Freud to Putnam

[March 28, 1912]

28. 3. 12

Vienna, IX. Berggasse 19

Dear Colleague

Each of your interpretations of ΨA pleases me better than the last. You make psychoanalysis seem so much nobler and more beautiful: in her Sunday clothes I scarcely recognize the servant who performs my household tasks. Your last communication gave me the same impression.

Imago came out today: we count on receiving contributions to it from you. I wonder whether the success of this new venture won't merely serve to antagonize experts in other fields. That will be the first result; I hope not the final one.

I am sorry you still have cause for anxiety about your little daughter. The differential diagnosis is so uncertain, a fact that you know better than I. The individual symptoms seem to imply hysteria, but one never really knows.

Whether we will hold a Congress or not is still undecided because of Jung's invitation to New York.[1] You will certainly see him there. Perhaps it is better that we meet only at long intervals; for then we will have more to say to each other. My studies in the psychology of religion have stopped at the psychology of primitive peoples. *Imago* will publish two articles of mine this year, "Taboo and Ambivalence," "Magic and the Power of Thought." An essay on the infantile re-enactment of totemism will probably be the final chapter of this work.[2]

With cordial greetings,
Freud

[1] At the invitation of Smith Ely Jelliffe (1866–1945), Jung lectured in September at Fordham University, New York. See Putnam to Ernest Jones, October 24, 1912. The Congress was not held.

[2] Freud, "Über einige Übereinstimmungen im Seelenleben der Wilden und der Neurotiker" [Some Points of Agreement between the Mental Lives of Savages and Neurotics], published in one volume in 1913 as *Totem und Tabu*; "Das Tabu und die Ambivalenz der Gefühlsregungen" [Taboo and Emotional Ambivalence], part II of *Totem und Tabu, Imago*, 1 (August 1912), 213–227, and (October 1912), 301–333, SE, XIII, 18–74; "Animismus, Magie und Allmacht der Gedanken" [Animism, Magic and the Omnipotence of Thoughts], part III of *Totem und Tabu, Imago*, 2 (February 1913), 1–21, SE, XIII, 75–99; and "Die infantile Wiederkehr des Totemismus" [The Return of Totemism in Childhood], part IV of *Totem und Tabu, Imago*, 2 (August 1913), 375–408, SE, XIII, 100–161.

50
Putnam to Freud
[April 1, 1912]

April 1, 1912.

Dr. Sigmund Freud,
    Vienna, Austria.

Dear Dr. Freud:

Thank you for your two last reprints — "Über neurotische Erkrankungstypen" and "Nachtrag zu dem autobiographisch beschriebenen Fall von Paranoia."[1] I have read them both carefully, and find the first especially useful.

I hope you received the copy of my Harvey paper, read in New

York.[2] The descriptions which one has to content one self with in such an address, delivered before physicians who are comparatively ignorant of the subject, must be extremely simple, and I fear you may be tired of hearing the arguments re-hashed over and over again in this way. In a few days I go to New York again, to read a paper before the Neurological section of the New York Academy of Medicine.[3]

I hope all goes well with you.

Yours sincerely,
James J. Putnam

[1] [Types of Onset of Neurosis], *Zentralblatt*, 2 (1912), 297–302; SE, XII, 227–238; [Postscript to an Autobiographical Account of a Case of Paranoia (Dementia Paranoides)]; SE, XII, 80–82.

[2] Putnam, "On Freud's Psycho-Analytic Method and Its Evolution."

[3] Putnam, "Comments on Sex Issues from the Freudian Standpoint." Read before the neurological section of the New York Academy of Medicine, April 4, 1912. *New York Medical Journal,* 95 (June 15, 1912), 1249–1254, and (June 22, 1912), 1306–1309; Ad Psa, 128–155.

51

Putnam to Freud

[April 6, 1912]

April 6, 1912.

Dr. Sigmund Freud,
  Vienna, Austria.

Dear Dr. Freud:

I have learned that the envelopes in which my pamphlets were sent out were too fragile, and that many of them broke. So I am sending you a duplicate pamphlet.

Yours very truly,
James J. Putnam

52
Putnam to Freud
[June 4, 1912]

106 Marlborough Street
VI. 4 1912

Dear Dr. Freud

I shall send you in a week or two the reprint of the paper on 'sex-issues,' which I read at New York on April 4th.[1] Of course, it is only a re-statement of known facts, but I put a good deal of thought into it and suspect that it will do good.

I felt very, very badly about Dr. Starr's[2] most undignified and discourteous and absurd attack, after my paper and several others. I went to the meeting determined to take all criticisms quietly and good-naturedly, and was so taken aback by what he said that I could not trust my words in answer.

Since then I have indulged in a great deal of esprit d'escalier[3] to no purpose, but have also had a talk with him personally and made him feel ashamed.

The meeting as a whole was a good one and so was the meeting of our Psychoanalytic Association, at Boston, on June 28.[4]

As for myself, my work is far from perfect and I suffer from certain complexes which I wish I could get rid of. Nevertheless, I make steady, if slow progress, and, whatever else I do *not* read, I *do* read everything of yours with great care. Have you any objection to my having a few of your shorter papers from the Zentralblatt translated and published by Dr. Jeliffe[5] in connection with the Monograph Series?

I think no one will do this if I do not and it should be done. I have a patient who is a good scholar and a thorough convert, and I would make myself responsible for the correctness of his work.

Please give my kind regards to Mrs. Jones, and to Dr. Jones if he is with you.

Sincerely, your friend
James J. Putnam

[1] "Comments on Sex Issues from the Freudian Standpoint."
[2] Moses Allen Starr (1854–1932), professor of neurology at Columbia University,

had attacked Freud's character after an address by Putnam before the section in neurology of the New York Academy of Medicine, April 4, 1912.

[3] Wit after the occasion.

[4] Putnam meant May 28. See *Zentralblatt*, 3 (1913), 102–103.

[5] Smith Ely Jelliffe, New York neurologist and psychoanalyst, inaugurated the Nervous and Mental Disease Monograph Series in 1907. The first volume was William Alanson White's *Outlines of Psychiatry,* which became one of the most popular American psychiatric texts.

53

Putnam to Freud

[June 19, 1912]

June 19, 1912.

Dr. Sigmund Freud,
Vienna, Austria.

Dear Dr. Freud:

I have just read twice over, with great care, and also great profit, your suggestions to budding psychoanalysts in the last number of the "Zentralblatt." [1] It is an admirable article, and only makes me long for an opportunity to talk over some of the points at greater length. I am not clear, for example, as to how much talking it is legitimate to do one's self, in the way of explanation or asking questions. In your Nüremberg address[2] you seem to say that we have now learned so much more about the structure of the different neuroses that we might give the patients the benefit of our knowledge, and so shorten the process of treatment. I judge, however, from this last article, that you still hold a very conservative position in this respect. It seems to me that many patients would utterly fail to get any adequate knowledge of dream symbolism without a great deal of help.

I am also in some doubt whether my own complexes are still so troublesome as to make it impossible for me to do real justice to my patients. I know most of these complexes, as it were, by name, but am well aware that I am still under their influence in some measure. So far as I can see, a psychoanalyst ought, theoretically, to have reached the millenium of perfection before he begins to work.

I trust that you will at least have gathered what I was vaguely striving for in the Weimar paper which came out in the last number of the "Imago." [3] I am sorry to say that there are several bad omissions and errors in the text, owing to the fact that I could not review the proof sheets. But I cannot help hoping, nevertheless, that you will find something to sympathize with in the ideas which I have attempted to convey. I will send you the last half of the New York paper in a few days. [4]

One thing which bothers me greatly, especially when beginning with a new patient, is the tendency which new patients sometimes show to go round and round in their descriptions of their symptoms and theories, without getting any deeper. Obviously the technical skill of an accomplished psychoanalyst enables him to break through this tendency without the use of too many words, and to bring the patients up against their own resistances. I wish you would sometime write one or two more papers in the "Zentralblatt," giving hints as to the best method of overcoming such difficulties as this.

Yours sincerely,
James J. Putnam

I am sorry that I used (in the Imago-paper) the expression 'Verdrängung' [5] with reference to the vagueness of outline which characterizes the feeling that people have about the action of their own minds.

I am tempted to write one more article on this and other points to make my meaning clearer.

---

[1] "Ratschläge für den Arzt bei der psychoanalytischen Behandlung" [Recommendations to Physicians Practicing Psychoanalysis], *Zentralblatt*, 2 (1912), 483–489; SE, XII, 109–120.

[2] "Die zukünftigen Chancen der psychoanalytischen Therapie," *Zentralblatt*, 1 (1910), 1–9; SE, XI, 141–151.

[3] "Ueber die Bedeutung philosophischer Anschauungen." *Imago*, I (May 1912), 101–118.

[4] "Comments on Sex Issues from the Freudian Standpoint."

[5] Repression. See p. 113 of *Imago*, 1 (May 1912).

54
Freud to Putnam

[June 25, 1912]

25. 6. 12
Vienna, IX, Berggasse 19.

Dear Colleague

I am sorry that you were upset by Dr. Allen Starr's remarks.[1] I was able to remain cool and untouched by them because I had never known Starr. Nor did the issue, no matter what its precise origin could have been, seem important enough. His information about my early years amused me mightily. Would that it had been true!

Your offer to have some of my shorter essays from the *Zentralblatt* translated delighted me, although I scarcely believe they deserve such a distinction. I wrote Dr. Brill last week and asked him to give you an answer directly because he has my formal promise to take charge of everything concerning translations into English.[2] I expect he will readily agree to your request.

Your article in *Imago*[3] has been highly praised and may prompt Dr. Ferenczi to make a reply which will present our less ambitious point of view.[4] I was truly delighted to hear from Jones that American interest in ΨA is not diminishing. Your name will enlist many partisans for us.

With friendly greetings,
Freud

[1] See Putnam to Freud, June 4, 1912.
[2] Putnam sent translations of a few short papers by Freud to Smith Ely Jelliffe.
[3] "Ueber die Bedeutung philosophischer Anschauungen."
[4] See Ferenczi, "Philosophie und Psychoanalyse. (Bemerkungen zu einem Aufsatze des H. Professors Dr. James J. Putnam von der Harvard Universität, Boston, U.S.A.)" [Philosophy and Psychoanalysis (Comments on a Paper of James J. Putnam of Harvard)], *Imago*, 1 (December 1912), 519–526; in Ferenczi, *Final Contributions to the Problems and Methods of Psycho-Analysis* (New York: Basic Books, 1955), pp. 326–334.

55

Freud to Putnam

[July 18, 1912]

Karlsbad
Vienna, IX, Berggasse 19
18. 7, 12

Dear Colleague

I received a letter from Dr. Brill today about the translations.[1] It seems clear that he has objections, is not satisfied with the publisher etc. He has done me an inestimable service in translating my writings, and I am sure you will understand why I do not feel ashamed in letting my loyalty prevail over my wishes. I therefore ask you to give up the project. I want very much to have each of my friends feel free to ask a favor from me. This time it is Brill's turn.

I am taking the cure here and am compelled to be inactive.[2] I hope that you, too, are having a holiday in camp or elsewhere and send you and yours my best greetings.

Faithfully,
Freud

[1] See Putnam to Freud, June 4, 1912, and Freud to Putnam, June 25, 1912.
[2] Freud was seeking relief for what he called his "American colitis." See Jones, *Sigmund Freud*, II, 90, 93.

56

Putnam to Freud

[August 1, 1912]

August 1, 1912.

Professor Dr. Sigmund Freud,
    Vienna, Austria.

Dear Professor:

Your note of July 18 is just received. I had already had some correspondence with Dr. Brill, and have withdrawn the paper which I had sent to Dr. Jelliffe.[1] I had also written Dr. Brill again, telling him this, and I think that all is clearly understood between us. You will of course understand that it was only through a misunderstanding of the situation that I did not communicate with Dr. Brill in the beginning. If he cares to use the translation which my friend has made, I shall place it at his service.

I wish to thank you also for your last letter, which I read and thought over very carefully. I shall be greatly interested to see Dr. Ferenczi's paper.[2] Although well aware that there are various weak points in my own argument, I believe that it contains some ideas of value, and sincerely hope that it will not be taken as implying an unfriendly attitude on my part towards psychoanalysis in its present form.

I have just been reading your "Bruchstuck einer Historieanalyse,"[3] even with greater pleasure and understanding than at first. I think it is difficult to appreciate all the bearings of the "Uebertragung"[4] doctrine, but succeed in appreciating them better as time goes on.

I shall shortly send Dr. Stekel two modest contributions.[5] With kind regards, and best wishes for a pleasant summer, I am,

Yours very truly,

James J. Putnam

[1] See Putnam to Freud, June 4, 1912, and Freud to Putnam, July 18, 1912.
[2] "Philosophie und Psychoanalyse."
[3] [Fragment of an Analysis of a Case of Hysteria], *Monatschrift für Psychiatrie und Neurologie*, 18 (1905), 285–309, 408–467; SE, VII, 7–122. Putnam misspelled "Hysterie-Analyse."
[4] Transference.
[5] "From the Analysis of Two Staircase Dreams"; and "A Characteristic Child's Dream" [Ein charakterischer Kindertraum], *Zentralblatt*, 2 (1912), 328–329; Ad Psa, 126–127.

57
Freud to Putnam

[August 20, 1912]

Karersee 20. Aug 12
Vienna, IX. Berggasse 19.

Dear Dr. Putnam

It was just three years ago yesterday that I started on the trip to America, a trip which among other good things, brought me

your acquaintance, and may I add, your friendship.[1] So I do not
wish to delay answering your letter which was forwarded to me
here at Karersee.[2] I am truly grateful to you for agreeing to give
up the translations you had planned and for not being sensitive
about the matter.[3] I know that your ideal is an ethical one and
that you live by it. Jones tells me that you really would like to
envisage analysts as perfect human beings, but we are far from
that. I continually have to calm down my own personal irritations
and must protect myself from those I arouse in others. After the
disgraceful defection of Adler, a gifted thinker but a malicious
paranoiac, I am now in trouble with our friend, Jung, who
apparently has not outgrown his own neurosis.[4] And yet I hope
that Jung will remain loyal to our cause in its entirety; nor has
my feeling for him been greatly diminished. Solely our personal
intimacy has suffered.

This does not argue, I believe, against the efficacy of psychoanalysis. Rather, it shows simply that we use it on other people's
personalities rather than on our own, and that, finally, we must
realize, as is quite natural, that our energies are limited and not
infinite.

I am spending the summer vacation in the most beautiful spot
of the Dolomites, and I wish you and yours the best possible
holiday at your camp or abroad.

Faithfully yours,
Freud

[1] Freud had traveled to the United States with Carl Jung and Sandor Ferenczi to
lecture at the 20th anniversary of the founding of Clark University in Worcester,
Massachusetts in September 1909.

[2] Lake in the Dolomites, fifteen miles northeast of Bolzano.

[3] See Putnam to Freud, June 4, 1912, and August 1, 1912; and Freud to Putnam,
July 18, 1912.

[4] Alfred Adler resigned from the Vienna Psychoanalytic Society, of which he was
president, in July 1911. Disagreements already had begun with Carl Jung, who
resigned the presidency of the International Psychoanalytic Association and left the
movement in 1914.

58
Putnam to Freud
[September 11, 1912]

St. Hubert's
Essex Cty
N.Y.

Dear Dr. Freud

Your last letter, with its pleasant reminder of the fact that it is just three years since your visit to America and to our camp, reached me a few days ago, and I am now writing to you from that peaceful retreat, just left in absolute quiet by the departure, for the morning or the day, of the various bands of walkers. My daughter, of whom I have written to you several times, is off among the rest, I am glad to say, for although she is by no means well, we feel that she is better and can be freely trusted to herself.[1]

Your visit of three years ago was a more significant event to me than you can easily imagine, for it helped to change radically the whole course of my life and thought. I only hope I am not wrong in thinking that the time will come when you will agree with me; first, that there is a metaphysics as well as a science of Ψan. [a metaphysics based on the work of such men as the Greeks and Hegel and Lotze and Froebel];[2] next, that there is a real place and need for the further personal development of the ps.an[sts] themselves, to which you refer. I *do* believe that we ought, logically, to become 'vollkommene Menschen' [3] and that without that we cannot lead our patients [those who want to go] to the real sublimation which is the only logical stopping place of a thorough Ψan[sis]. The unfortunate disturbances with Jung and Adler [I had not heard anything of the former and regret it very deeply] only make me feel this all the more.[4]

Fortunately, I believe that your profoundly philosophic spirit, which has carried you through so many trials and has enabled you to bear so many ungenerous and evil misconstructions, will make it possible for you to bear this last trial also.

I cannot believe that Jung, who if dogmatic and autocratic is also intelligent and fine-minded, can remain permanently alienated in any considerable respect, even personally.

Whatever happens, you have made a contribution of immense value to science and to medicine, and the number of those who appreciate this fact is rapidly increasing.

Also, you have a band of devoted followers in Vienna and they are doing splendid work.

I am reading your "Tabu" article with great interest, and propose to begin on Rank's Inzest-lehre as soon as I find time.⁵ I have also re-read the greater part of Stekel's Angstneurosen,⁶ and with better understanding than before.

As for myself, I am seriously preparing to write out, in book form, the evidence touched upon in the Weimar paper — the metaphysics and the sublimation-aspects of Ps.an.⁸·⁷

Troubles are sure to follow us, even into the erhabene Luft⁸ of the mountains, but I know how beautiful the Dolomiten are, from the glimpses that we had of them as we passed over the Brennerbahn, last summer. May they bring you health and vigor of mind and body and stimulate your imagination to new conquests!

Yours sincerely

James J. Putnam

Sept. 11, 1912

¹ See Putnam to Freud, September 30, 1911, and Freud to Putnam, October 5, 1911.

² Rudolph Hermann Lotze (1817–1881), German philosopher and psychologist.

³ Well-rounded human beings.

⁴ Wilhelm Stekel withdrew in November 1912. Difficulties between Freud and Jung grew serious early in 1912 and were exacerbated by Jung's lectures in America in September. See Jones, *Sigmund Freud*, II, 86 and chap. v.

⁵ "Das Tabu und die Ambivalenz der Gefühlsregungen," *Imago*, 1 (August 1912), 213–227; SE, XIII, 18–35; Otto Rank, *Das Inzest-Motiv in Dichtung und Sage: Grundzüge einer Psychologie des dichterischen Schaffens* [The Incest Motif in Poetry and Saga; Fundamentals of a Psychology of Poetic Creation] (Leipzig and Vienna: F. Deuticke, 1912).

⁶ *Nervöse Angstzustände und ihre Behandlung, mit einem Vorworte von Prof. Dr. Sigmund Freud* [Nervous Anxiety States and Their Treatment, Foreword by Professor Dr. Sigmund Freud], Berlin and Vienna: Urban and Schwarzenberg, 1908, and "Die Angstneurose der Kinder" [The Anxiety-Neuroses of Children], *Medizinische Klinik*, 14 (April 26, 1908), 621–623, and *ibid.*, (May 3, 1908), 659–662.

⁷ See Putnam, *Human Motives* (New York: Little, Brown and Co., 1915) and "Ueber die Bedeutung philosophischer Anschauungen."

⁸ Heavenly air.

59
Putnam to Freud
[November 21, 1912]

November 21, 1912.

Dr. Sigmund Freud,
  Vienna, Austria.

Dear Dr. Freud:

Your circular rather looks as if there had been a storm centre near Vienna.[1] I shall, of course, follow your fortunes, and will gladly do what little lies in my power to make your new enterprise successful. Please consider that my name is withdrawn from the "Zentralblatt," if that seems to you the proper step to take, and use the enclosed note to Dr. Stekel if you think it needed.

Yours sincerely,
James J. Putnam

[1] After the break with Wilhelm Stekel, Freud sent a circular to contributors of the *Zentralblatt* asking that they withdraw their support and join in establishing the new official *Internationale Zeitschrift für ärztliche Psychoanalyse* [International Journal for Medical Psychoanalysis], to be edited by Sandor Ferenczi, Ernest Jones, and Otto Rank. Stekel resigned from the Vienna Psychoanalytic Society in November, 1912, but continued to edit the *Zentralblatt* as his own journal until it ceased publication in 1914. See Jones, *Sigmund Freud*, II, 134–137.

60
Freud to Putnam
[November 28, 1912]

28.XI.12
Vienna, IX, Berggasse 19

Dear Colleague

The article you wrote me about on November 12 has not yet arrived.[1] However, I need not await its coming to know that it will be most interesting and that it will grace our journal. Our friend Ferenczi's reply does not overlook the significance of your views.

I hope you have no objection to having it appear in the new

Internat. Zeitsch. f. Aerztl. Psychoanalyse.[2] As you know, Stekel's treason forced me to give up the *Zentralblatt* to him. Almost all of our colleagues, however, have settled in the new home, and I hope that your agreement to its creation, which I requested in a circular letter, is on its way.

Last Sunday there was a meeting in Munich of Jung, Riklin, Seif, Abraham, Jones, myself and the Zurich secretary representing Maeder, which was most satisfactory.[3] We decided to make this new journal the official organ, replacing the *Zentralblatt*. Everybody was charming to me, including Jung. A talk between us swept away a number of unnecessary personal irritations. I hope for further successful cooperation. Theoretical differences need not interfere. However, I shall hardly be able to accept his modification of the libido theory since all my experience contradicts his position.

With cordial greetings, and I hope to hear that you are well,

Sincerely yours,

Freud

[1] Putnam's letter is missing. The article is apparently Putnam, "Bemerkungen über einen Krankheitsfall mit Griselda-Phantasien" [Remarks on a Case with Griselda Phantasies], *Zeitschrift*, 1 (March 1913), 205–218; Ad Psa, 175–193.

[2] Ferenczi, "Philosophie und Psychoanalyse," in Ferenczi, *Final Contributions*. See Putnam to Freud, November 21, 1912.

[3] Franz Riklin (1878–1938), secretary of the Association; Leonhard Seif (1866–1949), founder of the Munich Psychoanalytic Society; Karl Abraham (1877–1925), founder of the Berlin Psychoanalytic Society; Ernest Jones; Alphonse Maeder (1882–   ), Swiss psychiatrist, member of the original "Freud group" in Zurich. Riklin and Maeder later became followers of Jung.

61

Freud to Putnam

[December 3, 1912]

3. XII. 12

Vienna, IX, Berggasse 19.

Dear Colleague

Thank you very much for your willingness to join with us in our new publication. It is in fact not a new journal, but rather the former *Zentralblatt* which its editor's treason has forced us to issue under a new name. You will find all your familiar colleagues in the new *Zeitschrift für ärztliche ΨA*. I hope that you will contribute often. The article you wrote me about has not arrived.[1]

My colleagues, as is quite natural, sometimes provide as much trouble as the work itself. The loss of Stekel[2] is generally considered a great gain.

With best wishes,
Sincerely,
Freud

[1] Putnam, "Antwort auf die Erwiderung des Herrn Dr. Ferenczi" [A Rejoinder to Dr. Ferenczi's Reply], *Imago*, 1 (December 1912), 527–530.

[2] Beginning with the December issue, Stekel retained exclusive control of the *Zentralblatt,* until then the official journal of the International Psychoanalytic Association. A new official organ, the *Zeitschrift für ärztliche Psychoanalyse* began publication in January 1913.

62
Putnam to Freud
[December 19, 1912]

December 19, 1912.

Dr. Sigmund Freud,
  Vienna, Austria.

Dear Dr. Freud:

I was very glad to receive both of your letters, and especially glad to hear of the meeting in Munich.[1]

I shall want to be of what assistance I can in the new enterprise, and have several papers which are really under way, and which I will send you very soon.

It seems hard, after having done such an immense work in setting this great movement in motion, and giving it such a wonderful impetus, that you should be forced to contend with petty annoyances of the kind that you have had to meet. Looking at this matter psychologically, however, I suppose it may be considered that the defections are really in a measure an indication of the fact that the men who have been attracted to the enterprise have been men of a strong sense of personal initiative — which is, in itself, a good sign. Unfortunately, where the desire for personal distinction is so strong as to be a real hindrance to sublimation and general usefulness, it must be considered that the persons dominated by it are still, as you said on another occasion, "in der Neurose." [2]

This leads me to say that I have a strong desire to work up at greater length the subject of sublimation as related to psycho-analysis, and in connection with it to refer at some length to the work of Dante and of Emerson. It may be that this attempt will take a somewhat extended form, and that Dr. Van Teslaar (whose notices of the psychoanalytic literature you may have seen in the American Journal of Psychology)[3] will join with me in carrying it out.

Yours very sincerely,
James J. Putnam

[1] See Freud to Putnam, November 28, 1912, and Jones, *Sigmund Freud*, II, 145.
[2] Neurotic.
[3] James S. Van Teslaar (1886–?), was born in Romania and settled in Boston. He was secretary of the Massachusetts Mental Hygiene Society and edited *An Outline of Psychoanalysis* (New York: Modern Library, 1925), which contained Freud's Clark lectures and Putnam's "Personal Impressions of Sigmund Freud." Van Teslaar also translated several works of Wilhelm Stekel in the early 1920's. He claimed a medical degree from the University of California, but no record of this has been found. See *When I was a Boy in Roumania* (Boston: Lothrop, Lee and Shepard, 1917), p. 176, and University of California *Bulletin,* third ser. 15, no. 3, *Medical School, Directory of Graduates, 1864–1921* (Berkeley: University of California Press, 1921). See Dr. James S. Van Teslaar, "Recent Literature on Psychoanalysis."

63
Freud to Putnam

[January 1, 1913]

1. 1. 1913
Vienna, IX, Berggasse 19.

Dear Colleague

I am happy to begin the New Year by writing to you.

Thank you for indicating that you will give our new journal [1] your active support. I am equally grateful that your letter suggests that you have not lost faith in me in spite of the many personal attacks which I have undergone and will undergo for some time to come. I am sure you will believe that I have not been very shocked by them because I know too well that such developments are psychologically inevitable. I am not referring to Stekel, whose loss really was a gain, but rather to Jung, whom I overestimated greatly and in whom I had invested much personal feeling.[2] Differences in theory are unavoidable in the development of a science; even errors may contain elements of progress, as my own experience has taught me. But that such departures and theoretical innovations must be accompanied by so much injury to legitimate personal feelings surely does little credit to human nature.

Naturally I consider Jung's new views as regressive errors; but this need not constitute proof for other people. In this case, each person should judge the issue on the basis of his own experience and the merit of the arguments. For me it all seems like a 'déjà vu' experience. Everything which I encounter in the objections of these half-analysts I had already met in the objections of non-analysts. We look forward with great interest to your articles. Don't let our lack of understanding of philosophy interfere with the formulation of your ideas. We are not competent in these matters because we work in other fields; but nevertheless we listen to you attentively, and after us will come other, less limited analysts for whom your stimulus may prove fruitful.

With the best of wishes for yourself and your family in the coming year,

Yours faithfully,
Freud

[1] *Internationale Zeitschrift für ärztliche Psychoanalyse.* See Freud to Putnman, November 28, 1912.
[2] See Putnam to Freud, September 11, 1912, n. 4, and Putnam to Jones, October 24, 1912.

64

Putnam to Freud

[January 5, 1913]

106 Marlboro' St.
Boston

Dear Dr. Freud

I send an article — a Schriftchen[1] — to be used in any way that you desire. I only wish that it should *not* be published in the

Imago, because the patient whose history is here recorded takes and reads that journal.

I take the liberty of sending also another paper which I feel doubtful what to do with.² It was written as a reply to a review by Dr. Reik, of my Weimar address, which was published in the Zentralblatt for Oct. (or Sept.?).³

Properly speaking, this reply — which has taken on the form of an explanation of my ideas, and has grown to greater length than I intended, — should come out in the Zentrabl, and might still be offered there.

If, however, you choose to have it altered somewhat [leaving out all reference to Dr. Reik, for example] it *might be* published, some day, in the new journal.⁴ It seems to me very doubtful, however, whether you would care to have it there, and in that case it would be best to send it to Dr. Stekel ⁵ or back again to me.

With kind regards,

Yours very truly
James J. Putnam

Jan. 5. 1913

¹ Putnam, "Griselda-Phantasien."

² Putnam, "Psychoanalyse und Philosophie. Eine Erwiderung auf die Kritik von Dr. [Theodor] Reik" [Psychoanalysis and Philosophy (A Reply to the Criticism of Dr. Reik], *Zentralblatt,* 3 (1913), 265–269.

³ Theodor Reik, "Putnam, J. J.: 'Über die Bedeutung philosophischer Anschauungen und Ausbildung für die weitere Entwicklung der psychoanalytischen Bewegung' " [Putnam, J. J.: The Role of Philosophical Views and Training in the Further Development of the Psychoanalytical Movement], *Zentralblatt,* 3 (1913), 43–44.

⁴ *Internationale Zeitschrift für ärztliche Psychoanalyse.*

⁵ See Putnam to Freud, November 21, 1912, and Freud to Putnam, November 28, 1912.

65

Putnam to Freud

[January 9, 1913]

January 9, 1913.

Dr. Sigmund Freud,
 Vienna, Austria.

Dear Dr. Freud:

I send the paper of which I have spoken,¹ and will ask you to do with it what you like, except that for special reasons I do *not want* it published in the "Imago," since my patient reads it. If the article seems to you too long, please shorten it as much as you desire. The dreams can easily be left out, and the part which follows the dreams also, if it seems to you insignificant.

I am obviously pushing my philosophical ideas a little hard, but you will readily understand that I do this because it is absolutely the only way to bring them into notice; and as I read various articles, such as the "Recension" by Reik, which I have answered in the "Zentralblatt," and Jung's 'Libido' monograph,[2] I feel more and more convinced that the point of view in which I am interested has been too greatly overlooked.

Yours, with kind regards,

James J. Putnam

---

[1] Putnam, "Griselda-Phantasien."

[2] See Theodor Reik, "Putnam, J. J.: Uber die Bedeutung philosophischer Anschauungen;" and Putnam, "Psychoanalyse und Philosophie. Eine Erwiderung auf die Kritik von Dr. [Theodor] Reik." Carl Jung, *Wandlungen und Symbole der Libido. Beiträge zur Entwicklungsgeschichte des Denkens* [Changes and Symbols of the Libido. Contributions to the Developmental History of Thought] (Leipzig and Vienna: F. Deuticke, 1912); also part I, *Jahrbuch,* 3 (1912), 120–227; part II, *Jahrbuch,* 4 (1912), 162–464; authorized trans. of Beatrice Hinkle as *The Psychology of the Unconscious; a Study of the Transformations and Symbolisms of the Libido, a Contribution to the History of the Evolution of Thought* (New York: Moffat, Yard and Co., 1916, and Dodd, Mead and Co., 1925).

66
Putnam to Freud
[January 16, 1913]

106 Marlborough Street

Dear Dr. Freud

Your last, 'New Year's,' letter was welcome, as always, and it is very satisfactory to realize that you are full of energy and courage, and ready to begin new enterprises.

We ought all to help you at our best and I am sure that will be done.

If Dr. Stekel was only *a little* different, and a little less *personal* in his reactions, he would be admirable, for he certainly has much talent and much vigor and productiveness.[1] However, the facts must be accepted as they are.

I wish now to ask you whether you could find someone to make a few changes in or additions to the paper which I sent you, in consequence of some new facts which have come to my notice since I wrote it.² I shall be glad, of course, to pay for any translating or other work that must be done.

I have written the essential points on the next sheet.

With kindest regards and best wishes; I am yours truly

James J. Putnam

I. 16. 13.

I do not care at all to have all that I have written (with this) translated, but only the essential facts.

¹ See Putnam to Freud, November 21, 1912, and Freud to Putnam, November 28, 1912.

² Probably Putnam, "Griselda-Phantasien."

67

Freud to Putnam

January 21, 1913]

21. 1. 13
Vienna, IX, Berggasse 19.

Dear Colleague

I received your essay today, have read it and shall of course give it without any cuts to the *Internationale Zeitschrift,* whose first issue we expect to see one of these days.¹ Now when there is a definite need for a theoretical elaboration of the basic principles of ΨA, this exposition of your postulates will be of special interest.

The second essay you promised, the rejoinder to Dr. Reik's remarks, is missing.² Permit me to make this observation about its publication: the *Internationale Zeitschrift* considers itself the legitimate successor of the *Zentralblatt* because it has taken over the publisher and nine tenths of the contributors, and has left the *Zentralblatt* with only its name and its editor. The *Zeitschrift* claims the right to continue the series of articles, questions, etc., which were begun in the *Zentralblatt,* as you will notice when you see the first issue. We ask you to endorse this policy and to consider the *Zeitschrift* as the legitimate place for your reply to Reik's critique. We cannot maintain relations with what has become Dr. Stekel's personal publication.[3]

With thanks for your contribution, and best wishes,

Yours,
Freud

[1] Putnam, "Griselda-Phantasien."
[2] Putnam, "Psychoanalyse und Philosophie. Eine Erwiderung auf die Kritik von Dr. [Theodor] Reik."
[3] See Putnam to Freud, November 21, 1912.

68
Putnam to Freud
[Between January 21 and February 13, 1913]

106 Marlborough Street

Dear Professor

I have just received your letter of Jan. 21, and hasten to thank you for it, and also to express my regret that I did, after all, send my answer to Dr. Reik, to Dr. Stekel's journal. *I had not clearly understood the situation,* and thought that Dr. Stekel, and perhaps Reik also, would think it needlessly discourteous on my part if I should reply to the review of my paper in another periodical, even though I had withdrawn my support from the first.

I now see that it would have been better to send it to you, but you will understand my motives in not doing so.

With very kind regards — I am yours

James J. Putnam

I hope to ask you to publish, before long, a paper on a case recalling Fouqué's Märchen, Undine.[1]

[1] Baron Friedrich Heinrich Carl de la Motte Fouqué, *Undine, eine Erzahlung* (1811).

69

Putnam to Freud

[February 13, 1913]

February 13, 1913.

Dr. Sigmund Freud,
  Vienna, Austria.

Dear Dr. Freud:

I have received your postal card of February the 2d,[1] and shall, of course, be much pleased if you will make the insertions, provided you do not think I am demanding too much space.

I hope you understood my explanation of my reasons for sending the other paper to Dr. Stekel, instead of to your journal. I certainly intend to do my best to support your enterprise, and shall make that more clear as time goes on.

Yours sincerely,
James J. Putnam

[1] Missing.

70

Putnam to Freud

[February 24, 1913]

February 24, 1913

Dr. Sigmund Freud,
  Vienna, Austria.

Dear Dr. Freud:

I have received the first number of the journal, and have already read your article and Dr. Jones's, with great interest.[1] I only hope I am not too old myself to profit by your suggestions, which I think are admirable.

I enclose a copy of a letter I wrote recently to Dr. Stekel.[2] I did not suppose that it would really be possible for him to transfer the article, and indeed, I imagine it is already in print. But I wanted to make my position perfectly clear to him, and to you.

Yours truly,
James J. Putnam

¹ Freud, "Weitere Ratschläge zur Technik der Psychoanalyse: I. Zur Einleitung der Behandlung" [Further Recommendations on the Technique of Psycho-Analysis: I. On Beginning the Treatment], *Zeitschrift*, 1 (1913), 1–10; SE, XII, 121–134; Ernest Jones, "Die Beziehung zwischen Angstneurose und Angsthysterie" [The Relation between Anxiety Neurosis and Hysterical Anxiety], *Zeitschrift*, 1 (1913), 11–17.
² Putnam had withdrawn his support from the *Zentralblatt*.

71
Freud to Putnam
[March 11, 1913]

11. 3. 13
Vienna, IX, Berggasse 19.

Dear Dr. Putnam

Thank you very much for your promise to contribute to the new journal and also for informing me about your note to Dr. Stekel, which leaves no doubt as to your position.[1] Outwardly our movement may appear to have changed somewhat since we last met, because of the desertion of some and the desire to break away of others. However, nothing really harmful has happened; the movement is progressing and expanding satisfactorily. Naturally, unity within the ΨA movement is much more difficult to achieve than in other fields of science because the personal element plays such an important role. I do not know whether we shall have the pleasure of having you in Europe this September to take part in the Congress, which has been scheduled for the seventh and eighth of that month.[2] All of us would welcome your visit. Since you have not written for a long time about your daughter's condition, I assume that it has turned out to be an unimportant neurosis instead of the disease you feared it to be.

Whatever I manage to produce while I am carrying on my onerous practice is sent regularly to you. My next article, to be published in the fourth number of *Imago* this summer, should arouse your particular interest; however, it also may evoke doubts, even in you.[3]

With best wishes,
Sincerely,
Freud

¹ See preceding letter.

² The fourth Psychoanalytic Congress was scheduled to be held in Munich September 7–8, 1913. See *Zeitschrift,* 2 (1914), 405–407.

³ Freud, "Über einige Übereinstimmungen im Seelenleben der Wilden und der Neurotiker: II. Das Tabu und die Ambivalenz der Gefühlsregungen," *Imago,* 1 (October 1912), 301–333; SE, XIII, 35–74.

72
Putnam to Freud
[April 14, 1913]

106 Marlborough Street
Apr. 14th. 13

Dear Dr. Freud

Thank you for your letter of March 11, which I received a short time ago, and for the reprints of your valuable papers which I always read with great pleasure and profit.

Your practical advice is always sound and good but does not always save me from the disappointment of a failure where I had hoped for a success.

The causes — social, psychological and biological — that cause unexpected difficulties, seem to me very numerous, more so than I should have believed. Two or three patients have found their lives barren [öde, a fine word] after learning of tendencies which they felt obliged to give up after the treatment, and through which they had obtained much pleasure.

Some cool and callous patients do not suffer under the disillusionment but others seem to languish in their health while they improve in character.

The "Undine" [Baron Fouqué] ¹ of whom I wrote to you is of this sort. She had always been rich and wilful, — an "elemental" kind of person, without an adequate soul. I helped her to find a soul, but her health suffered in consequence and she became critical of the treatment though she admitted that it interested her.

If all the patients had a strong desire for sublimation, or any strong purpose in life, the treatment would be simpler. Of course, the difficulties created by the absence of these conditions may be among the very problems which we should fit ourselves to meet, but pure Ψa does not always seem enough to cover the ground.

I am sorry to say I shall not be able to get to Munich. My daughter, although better is not well and still requires great care and we have other causes for anxiety in addition.

The Zeitschrift seems to me excellent, both as regards appearance and contents.

With very kind regards and best wishes. I am yours sincerely

James J. Putnam

[1] A patient who reminded Putnam of the heroine of Baron Friedrich Heinrich Carl de la Motte Fouqué, *Undine*. See Putnam to Freud, [between January 21 and February 13, 1913].

73

Putnam to Freud

[August 6, 1913]

August 6, 1913.

Dr. Sigmund Freud,
  Vienna, Austria.

Dear Dr. Freud:

I beg to acknowledge the receipt of your two last papers, both of which I had read with great interest, and the reprints of which I like very much to keep.

I am just now reading Hitschmann's Schopenhauer paper,[1] and of course sympathize, in general, with his point of view. The only criticism I would make is that while the character of one's philosophy is undoubtedly modified by one's temperament, we can, nevertheless, utilize the partial view which a special temperament gives us to get a new glimmer of the truth that must lie as a background behind all the phenomena of life. All I contend for is that natural science does not and can not give us a true picture of this truth. Every method of inquiry, so far as I can see, is modified by our own personality; and the eternal question remains — to what do we owe our personality; and our capacity for having views at all? This is the question which insists on demanding some sort of an answer, yet which I admit we cannot wholly answer in a satisfactory way. The answer which best satisfies me must be one which best stimulates to sublimation, in the most complete sense of that term.

It is true that through psychoanalysis we find a certain basis for poetry and philosophy; or, in other words, poetry is only a partial and personal expression of the truth. Nevertheless, neither psychoanalysis alone, nor biology alone, in spite of their power to give a partial explanation of poetry and philosophy, can enable us to get on without poetry and philosophy in making our approaches toward the truth.

I remember reading in an essay by some English writer, I think Leslie Stephens,[2] that the search for truth was like jumping from one floating cake of ice to another in a limitless sea. This may be true, and the different modes which we adopt for arriving at the truth may be purely personal. Nevertheless, I still have the belief that some are less personal and more rational than others, and, at any rate, that no one set of men alone, but all of us must and do make this search.

Yours sincerely,
James J. Putnam

I wish I c^d join you in Sept. but it is impossible.[3] I send my best wishes and greetings, instead.

[1]Eduard Hitschmann, "Schopenhauer. Versuch einer Psychoanalyse des Philosophen" [Schopenhauer. An Attempted Psychoanalysis of the Philosopher], *Imago*, 2 (April 1913), 101–174. See Hitschmann, *Great Men; Psychoanalytic Studies*, ed. Sydney G. Margolin (New York: International Universities Press, 1956).
[2] Sir Leslie Stephen (1832–1904), philosopher, man of letters, author of *History of English Thought in the Eighteenth Century*, 2 vols. (London: Smith, Elder & Co., 1876).
[3] At the Psychoanalytic Congress.

74
Putnam to Freud
[October 22, 1913]

106 Marlborough Street
Oct. 22./13

Dear Professor

I have received your "Dritte Folge" and also your welcome postal card, for both of which I most sincerely thank you.[1]

I shall prize this collection of valuable essays very greatly and shall be glad, in looking at the title of either one of them, to be led on by the sight of all the rest, which I have read with so much pleasure.

I have had some accounts of the Munich congress, from Jones, and from Mensendieck, and wish I could have been present, even though the pleasure might have been a 'mixed' one.[2]

Would that I might have the chance of talking with you, not for a few minutes only but for a long enough time to reach conclusions.

That chance may never come but, at any rate, we shall remain friends and at least occasional correspondents.

Very sincerely
James J. Putnam

[1] *Sammlung kleiner Schriften zur Neurosenlehre* (III), *Dritte Folge* [Collected Short Papers on the Theory of Neurosis], 3rd ser. (Leipzig and Vienna: F. Deuticke, 1913). The postcard is missing.

[2] The last meeting between Freud and Jung occurred at the disagreeable Munich Congress, September 7, 1913. See Jones, *Sigmund Freud*, II, 102–103. Otto Mensendieck (1871–?), Swiss psychiatrist.

75
Freud to Putnam
[November 13, 1913]

Vienna, IX, Berggasse 19
13.11.13

My dear Colleague

Thank you for the various things you have sent. I shall reciprocate with my new book, Totem and Taboo.[1]

I, too, regretted that you were not present at the Congress in Munich.[2] Although I am aware that theoretically in some respects you tend to favor the other side, it would have been good if you could have been there to convince yourself of the nature of the differences that have arisen. Perhaps your very presence would have helped to mitigate the tone in which this conflict was expressed. That ΨA has not made the analysts themselves better, nobler or of stronger character remains a disappointment for me. Perhaps I was wrong to expect it.

With best wishes,

Yours,

Freud

[1] Leipzig and Vienna: Heller, 1913.

[2] This stormy Congress marked the last meeting between Freud and Jung.

76

Putnam to Freud

[November 29, 1913]

106 Marlborough Street

Dear Professor

I have again to thank you for both book (of excellent Totem and Tabu papers) and letter. I had read the greater part of the former, with pleasure and admiration, but shall read them through again now, connectedly. A new and interesting book has recently been published in England called Four Stages of Greek Religion which bears somewhat on the problems that you touch, although the author, Prof. Gilbert Murray, is not a psychoanalyst.[1]

I wish we might all meet again, in the near future, with the avowed purpose of dwelling on the *points of agreement* between us, instead of on the points of disagreement.

These (the former) would then be seen to be very numerous, and of far greater importance than the latter. Until then I suppose we must content ourselves by ascribing conscientious motives to all concerned. In one way it is a proof of the deep significance of this movement that it presents so many different aspects for study, and appeals in so many different modes to the minds of different sorts of men.

The principal lesson of Ψan, after all, is as to the absolute necessity of sincerity and frankness and thoroughgoingness. If we have philosophic tendencies we ought to search their underlying motives ["generic energy"] with complete honesty, as Hitschmann did in the case of Schopenhauer, etc. And so also with our religious tendencies; we ought to know how far they are based on superstition, how far on desires for expiation or propitiation, or for compromise, etc.

But if, after all that, we find that philosophic or religious tendencies continue to represent logical truths, then our ps.anᶜ studies will necessarily intensify this conviction. And so it results that the effect of ps.anᶜ work is to emphasize differences [even as regards our duties towards patients] among men who are all — or *may be* — sincere psychoanˢᵗˢ at heart.

Hitschmann makes his study of Schopenhauer and gains, or *seems* to gain, an increased contempt for the science of philosophy as such. Another person makes the same study and arrives at the conclusion that in spite of the defects in Sch.'s reasoning and the influence of his Unconscious, he expressed *partial* truths of considerable importance, and that if Sch.ʳ could have been thoroughly psychoanalyzed and made aware of his own neurosis and his consequent intellectual narrowness, he might have become; not merely an artist, not merely a healthy minded man and good citizen, but also the exponent of great truths.

The main question for me is; are there any logical arguments sufficiently strong to persuade us of such truths (Welt-anschauungen) as these, and do some patients carry the germs of a genuine belief in them, to such a degree that they ought to be given a chance to make these beliefs conscious and articulate, while under the influence of psychoanalytic criticism and stimulation to sincerity?

You and I might differ on these points, but I am sure we shall never differ in any way that will prevent us from working side by side, although in most respects it will always be as teacher on your part and learner on mine.

Very sincerely and sympathetically,

James J. Putnam

Nov 29.

---

[1] Gilbert Murray, *The Four Stages of Greek Religion* (New York: Columbia University Press, 1912). Murray (1866–1957), Regius Professor of Greek at Oxford from 1908 to 1936, translated Euripides and other Greek dramatists.

77

Putnam to Freud

[December 5, 1913]

106 Marlborough Street

Dear Dr. Freud

I trust that you did not misunderstand the note which I sent to you the other day.[1] I assure you that I did not intend it to be critical, but only explanatory. It was a great pleasure to see your handwriting again and I only wish I could be of some service in these uncomfortable times.

It is your keen power of observation and your insight into the practical workings of the mind, in health and in disease, that made possible the various Ausschweifungen[2] which have occurred, and this fact ought never to be forgotten.

Indeed, it will not be forgotten.

Sincerely your friend,
James J. Putnam

Dec. 5.

[1] See preceding letter.
[2] Aberrations.

78

Putnam to Freud

[December 21, 1913]

106 Marlborough Street

Dear Dr. Freud

I have just read your two last papers [Die Dispos. zur Zw[s] neurose and L'Intérêt de la Ps.Ans.] with great care.[1]

I think you present the doctrine of infantile fixation very impressively and convincingly, and find myself in complete sympathy with all your views, so far as they relate to the science or the practice of ps.a. I wish my ps.an^c training had been better. As it is I must be content to make as few mistakes as possible.

Sincerely your friend
James J. Putnam

Dec. 25.[1]

---

[1] "Die Disposition zur Zwangsneurose. Ein Beitrag zum Problem der Neurosenwahl" [The Disposition to Obsessional Neurosis. A Contribution to the Problem of the Choice of Neurosis], *Zentralblatt,* 1 (1913), 525–532; SE, XII, 311–326, and "Das Interesse an der Psychoanalyse" [The Claims of Psycho-Analysis to Scientific Interest], *Scientia,* 14 (1913), 240–250, 369–384; SE, XIII, 163–190.

79
Putnam to Freud
[December 25, 1913]

106 Marlborough Street
Dec. 25.[1]

Dear Professor

I feel that I almost ought to apologize for writing again so soon, but I have just received your letter of Dec. 11,[2] and am very anxious to offer certain explanations that it seems to make necessary; for I have an immense regard for your opinion and wish to reduce the differences between us to a minimum. I did not know the facts about Jung, nor — of course — do I know them now. I can, however, imagine some of them, for I have long since discovered that he is a person whose 'complexes' are stronger than he seems to know, himself, and the explanations of the situation which you offer appear to me reasonable and clear.

As for my own attitude with reference to Ψa, etc. etc., there are certain considerations which I wish to make perfectly understood:
1. I *desire* to practice this branch of medicine (Ψa). in accordance with the very best principles, and if I fail to do so it will be because I cannot rise to my own standards, on account of resistances which I realize to exist but find it hard to master. I believe heartily in your views on almost every point.
2. I assure you that I am greatly interested in what you say about the danger of obscuring scientific[3] truths by mixing in ethical and

aesthetical considerations, and I promise you that I shall be very careful not to err in that way if I can help it.

I also note carefully your statement that Ψa may, by unmasking a man's most vital tendencies, make him, at last, healthier [and honester?] yet viler? I can well believe that this might happen, for several patients have said to me, "I cannot help admitting the conclusions towards which the analysis points, but I feel that you are robbing me of all that makes life attractive."

3. I understand that the physician has no right to try to impose his own ethical or philosophical opinions on any patient, but must content himself with helping the patient to develop in his own way.

On this point my mind is perfectly clear, though I admit that I have not always been true to my own convictions in practice. Of course, the ethics of such persons as you speak of would be hypocrisy, if held at all, except in the sense of robber's ethics.[4]

4. There is, in fact, only one ethical consideration that seems to me especially significant in Ψc treatment, and, *unless I am wrong* (?), this can be developed without danger, though not with every patient. Thus, it comes out sometimes in the course of conversation that the patient feels [as one of "the more delicate torments of an unappeased aspiration"] that he owes a certain debt to his family, his state, his "team," etc; in short, that he acknowledges the calls of "loyalty," about which Prof. Royce has written so much of late.[5]

But what does such a patient feel as the further implications of this loyalty? To what other kinds of situations and communities does it apply? Where does he draw his line? *Is it possible* to draw any line between his family and some ideal community as regards loyal obligations of this sort? Does he actually feel that he is animated by a 'community-will' [à la Wundt[6] and others] in his conduct?

In short, if a patient *capable of such work* can be induced, by a strictly logical process of introspection, to arrive, through his own efforts, at some of the simpler yet vital truths of a — to him — sound philosophical psychology, I do not see how this can do him harm, or how aiding him to do this can injure the cause of legitimate Ψa, provided one does not try to impose one's own views. //Still, I am quite ready to be convinced that I am wrong.

5. I agree with you that one should not "listen to a physical inquiry into the future chances of the universe, when this inquiry was influenced by the desire to gain a proof for the rule of justice in the world."

But has one a right to argue from this premise that if one does believe that the world is ruled by justice, and has arrived at this belief through what seem to him thoroughly scientific and logical studies, he is therefore to be considered as incapable of conducting a truly scientific investigation? It is only a few weeks ago that I was talking with Prof. Richards[7] of Harvard, who is our formost chemist, and a man of greatest scientific accuracy, and I found that his *allgemeine Anschauungen*[8] coincided essentially with my own. In fact, logic and mathematics have been found recently to coincide in proving certain of these views, which have a distinct ethical bearing.

Suppose — what I believe — that a man cannot be strictly scientific, in the best sense, without [by inference, though perhaps unconsciously] admitting certain logical views such as, if followed further, would lead him to some such conclusions as I mentioned in the Weimar paper.[9] Is then every person who has gone thus further on this path, to be regarded as unfitted for ps.an[e] work? I assure you honestly that I believe the scientific value of my own work has increased of late, instead of diminishing, and that I am trying more conscientiously that[10] ever before, and with better results, to work out my "infantile fixations" and those of my patients.

———————

6. As regards Hitschmann, I may be quite wrong and I withdraw what I said of him.[11] Of course, in any case, I am an admirer of his work.

———————

Would you like a short paper pointing out the analogy between the literary style of the Old Testament and that of the dream, or has this already been done? Also, would you like an interesting Spermatozoa dream.

Please forgive this long letter.

Sincerely your friend,
James J. Putnam

[1] Above the heading Putnam wrote, "My best Christmas greetings."

[2] Missing.

[3] Ernest Jones noted in the margin of Putnam's holograph that Putnam first had written "ethical." This editor disagrees.

[4] This sentence was written in the margin.

[5] Josiah Royce regarded his later philosophical work as a development of the theme of loyalty. Putnam was among those who discussed with Royce *The Philosophy of Loyalty* (New York: The Macmillan Co., 1908) and *The Problem of Christianity* (New York: The Macmillan Co., 1913).

[6] Wilhelm Wundt (1832–1920), German psychologist. See Royce's discussion of Wundt in *The Problem of Christianity*, I, 64–65; II, 26–30, and Wundt, *Elemente der Völkerpsychologie: Grundlinien einer psychologischen Entwicklungsgeschichte der Menschheit* (Leipzig: A. Kröner, 1913), trans. by Edward Leroy Schaub, as *Elements of Folk Psychology: Outlines of a Psychological History of the Development of Mankind* (New York: The Macmillan Co., 1916).

[7] Theodore William Richards (1868–1928), professor of chemistry at Harvard, best known for his revision of atomic weights.

[8] General ways of thinking.

[9] Putnam's "Ueber die Bedeutung philosophischer Anschauungen."

[10] Putnam intended "than."

[11] Eduard Hitschmann (1871–1913), member of the Vienna Psychoanalytic Society. Putnam had criticized his treatment of Schopenhauer and philosophy; see Putnam to Freud, November 29, 1913.

80
Freud to Putnam

[March 30, 1914]

Vienna, IX, Berggasse 19
30.3.14

My dear Colleague

Today I received and read your article in the March number of the Am. J. of the Med. Sciences.[1] I like it exceedingly, perhaps best of all those excellent, eloquent and significant papers you have sent me. Possibly that is only because it was the last one; may it not remain the last for long. There is no part of it that concerns ΨA with which I could not identify myself. As you know, I comprehend very little of philosophy and with epistemology (with, not before), my interest ceases to function. I quite agree with you that ΨA treatment should find a place among the methods whose aim is to bring about the highest ethical and intellectual development of the individual. Our difference is of a purely practical nature. It is confined to the fact that I do not wish to entrust this further development to the psychoanalyst. I also do not believe that ΨA makes physical treatment unnecessary; but I have always found it impossible to combine ΨA with a somatic therapy. No matter how justified this may be in a given case such therapy immediately pushes the ΨA into the background. The reason for this is, I believe, the particularly great resistance which ΨA treatment meets. This resistance applies equally to the physician. Analysts themselves are far removed from the ideal which you demand of them. As soon as they are entrusted with the task of leading the patient toward sublimation, they hasten away from the arduous tasks of ΨA as quickly as they can so that they can take up the much more comfortable and satisfactory duties of the teacher and the paragon of virtue. This is just what the people in Zurich are now doing. Moreover, ΨA as a science itself is not even half complete; not to speak of the fact that it does not yet penetrate the individual deeply enough. "The great ethical element in ΨA work is truth and again truth and this should suffice for most people. Courage and truth are of what they are mostly deficient." [2]

Yours sincerely
Freud

[1] "On Some of the Broader Issues of the Psychoanalytic Movement." Modified from a paper of the same title read before the Association of American Physicians, Philadelphia, May 1913. *American Journal of the Medical Sciences*, 147, n. s. (March 1914), 389–406; Ad Psa, 194–222.

[2] The words in quotation marks are in English.

81

Putnam to Freud

[April 15, 1914]

April 15, 1914.[1]

Dr. Sigmund Freud,
  Vienna, Austria.

Dear Dr. Freud,-

I have read your letter very carefully, and assure you I have thought long and hard over what you say, both in this and in your previous letter.[2] I accept all your views, including those with reference to the limitations of the usefulness of the psychoanalytic method, except in one respect — which I will mention, and with regard to which I hope you will agree with me. I do not even care to place any emphasis on the metaphysical aspect of the subject. I admire immensely what you say about the importance of "the truth, the whole truth, and nothing but the truth and I realize that my own tendency to self-deception is strong and all pervading. How hard it is to get away from this Zug! [3]

The point to which I refer is this: — the individual is not to be thought of as existing alone, but should be considered as an integral part of the community in which he lives, and eventually of what must remain for him an ideal or idealized community. The great schism in every one's life is that involved in the instinctive attempt to set one's self up as having the right to stand alone. The interests of the community are implied in every one's motives and emotions, and sublimation consists in making these implicit interests explicit — i.e., in thinking out one's social obligations consciously and in the largest sense.

I feel sure that we should agree virtually as regards these propositions, and so far as I can see the only difference between us would concern the fact that I believe the community obligations and interests to be so deeply interwoven with the personal interests, and yet at the same time so deeply hidden, in many cases, that I believe they should be considered as forming a part of the repressed thoughts, in a psychoanalytic sense.

My "Ich-Trieb" and "Ich-Bewusstsein" [4] contain, I think, more of these social implications than yours do; and I find that one of the conflicts in some of my patients is the dim, and far too dim, recognition of these social bonds.

Of course, it is also true that in my belief the sense of these social bonds, as well as of a certain power which the individual gets by virtue of his belonging to the community, is something not derived from experience, but innate — i.e., a sort of endowment of the mind as such.

I imagine we should differ on this last point, and I cannot hope to bring you to my side concerning it. Perhaps I am mistaken in holding to my belief, but I hope not. If I understand you, you would believe that all this community and ideal community notion is something which is a projection from experienced relations between the infant and his entourage. Even if we do not agree about this, however, I think we might agree that the sense of loyalty, as has been so carefully worked out by Professor Royce,[5] is one of every man's best assets, and one which it makes him uncomfortable to feel himself lacking in, and therefore, a fit subject for psychoanalytical study.

In conversation with Mr. Royce, he has recently made the point, which seems to me a good one, that in so far as the psychoanalyst creates new social tensions, he should feel bound to deal with them in a suitable fashion. Otherwise, the patients might feel, as I once said, as Dante would have felt if Virgil had deserted him somewhere on the slopes of the Mount of Purgatory.

Yours very sincerely,
James J. Putnam

[1] Beside the letterhead, Putnam wrote, "I write this at my brother's house. He has been very sick for many weeks, but we hope and think that he will get well. He has been a very public spirited and useful man of great generosity and devotion." Charles Pickering Putnam was one of the nation's first specialists in pediatrics and a leader in social work in Boston. He was a founder of the city's Associated Charities in 1879 and a trustee of the Children's Institutions of Boston from 1902 to 1911.

[2] See preceding letter. Freud's "previous letter" is missing.

[3] Trait.

[4] Ego drive and ego consciousness.

[5] See *War and Insurance* (New York: The Macmillan Co., 1914) and *The Problem of Christianity*.

82

Freud to Putnam

[May 17, 1914]

Vienna, IX, Berggasse 19
17.5.14

Dear Colleague

After reading your last article in the Journal of Abnormal Psychology on the Interpretation of Dreams[1] I feel the urge to thank you once more. At the same time I ask myself why others cannot resolve these simple questions in the same way. You too hint that this can only be due to their motives, which is the way I also see it.

I do not share your great respect for Adler's theories.[2] They do not seem to me to be worth abandoning dream interpretation and the doctrine of the unconscious. It is their denial of these ideas that characterizes them rather than what they do assert, a large part of which we agree with. However, these points of agreement are not useful in treating the neuroses.

I am taking the liberty of sending you an article which you already may have read: its author does not publicly acknowledge having written it because in this exceptional instance, it does not deal with sexuality.[3]

Hoping that all continues to be well with you,

Yours very cordially,

Freud

[1] "Dream Interpretation and the Theory of Psychoanalysis," *Journal of Abnormal Psychology*, 9 (April–May 1914), 36–60. Ad Psa, 223–253.

[2] Alfred Adler, founded the school of Individual Psychology.

[3] Freud, "Der Moses des Michelangelo" appeared anonymously in *Imago*, 3 (February 1914), 15–36; SE, XIII, 209–236.

83
Putnam to Freud
[June 2, 1914]

106 Marlborough Street

June 2

Dear Dr. Freud

I thank you sincerely for your letter, and for what you say about Adler, which I have been thinking over carefully and shall take to heart.[1] I believe it is true and believe also that I am driven by my own complexes to overanxious attempts "to do justice," which are in reality attempts at conciliation.

Was die *sehr schöne* Moses Schrift betrifft, deren Styl mir als wohl bekannt vorkomt, und deren Bedeutsamkeit in mehr als eines Beziehung ich gerne anerkenne, brauche ich nur zu sagen dass sie nicht ohne wahren Genuss zu lesen ist.[2]

With kind regards and thanks, your friend

James J. Putnam

over[3]

I am sending you a reprint of my cousin Mr. Lee's notice of my brother, whose recent illness and death has been a serious affliction and whose loss I shall greatly feel.[4]

The group which you met at the Adirondacks four years ago, is thus broken into for the second time, this winter, by the death of very dear and very important members. The first was my daughter, then a gay and self-forgetting child of 12,[5] by whose friendly prattle at table I remember that you were amused; the second, my brother with whom you walked home from an excursion beyond the Ausable river. Without his energy and devotion the enterprise which has given great pleasure and brought much real "sublimation" to a large number of people in the course of the past thirty years, would never have come into existence.

I wish I could be with you at the Congress,[6] but it is impossible. I shall look at the reports of it with great eagerness and some anxiety.

[1] See preceding letter.

[2] "As for the fine essay on Moses, its style seems familiar to me. I note its significance in more than one respect most willingly and need only affirm that reading it is a real pleasure."

[3] Direction to overleaf.

[4] See "Charles Pickering Putnam," *Boston Medical and Surgical Journal*, 170 (May 7, 1914), 741–742, and Putnam to Freud, April 15, 1914, and June 2, 1914.

[5] Frances Cabot Putnam (1897–1913).

[6] The fifth International Psychoanalytic Congress was scheduled to take place in Dresden on September 20, but was not held because of the war which broke out in August. See *Zeitschrift*, 2 (1914), 482–483.

84

Freud to Putnam

[June 19, 1914]

19.6.14
Vienna, IX, Berggasse 19

Dear Friend and Colleague

I learned with great regret of your brother's death and thank you very much for sending me his obituary.[1] In reading it, I understood better why I had remembered so clearly his friendly kindness to me.

Thank you for the self-criticism you included in your discussion of Adler.[2] I take this opportunity to tell you that you will soon receive several copies of an article to be distributed among the members of the new Boston group, whose addresses we still lack.[3] As usual the hardest task falls to me: in this instance, I must protect myself against people who have called themselves my pupils for many years and who owe everything to my stimulus. Now I must accuse them and reject them. I am not a quarrelsome person, nor do I share the widespread opinion that a scientific quarrel brings about clarity and progress. However, I am not in favor of sloppy compromises, nor would I sacrifice anything for the sake of an unproductive reconciliation.

I hope that the Swiss and their following will desert the association after reading my polemic in the new *Jahrbuch*,[4] so that we can conduct our Congress in unity and with friendly feelings towards one another. It is possible that the schism may extend to America, where Jelliffe[5] is one of Jung's followers.

I learn with great regret that this year, too, you will not be coming to Europe. Nor do I expect to come to America in the near future: may I hope that this will not cause the slender thread of correspondence between us to break.

Very sincerely yours,
Freud

[1] For Joseph Lee's obituary see *Boston Medical and Surgical Journal,* 170 (May 7, 1914), 741–742.

[2] See Putnam to Freud, June 2, 1914.

[3] The Boston Psychoanalytic Society was founded in 1914 with Putnam as president and Isador Coriat as secretary. See *Journal of Abnormal Psychology,* 9 (April–May 1914), 71.

[4] "Zur Geschichte der psychoanalytischen Bewegung" [On the History of the Psychoanalytic Movement], *Jahrbuch,* VI (1914), 207–260; SE, XIV, 1–66.

[5] Smith Ely Jelliffe had published the opening of Jung's Fordham lectures as the lead article in the first issue of the *Psychoanalytic Review,* 1 (November 1913), 1–40, and the rest of the lectures in the subsequent issues of the *Review's* first two volumes. Jelliffe was in fact eclectic and regarded with distaste the "many and devious" European "currents and counter-currents." See "Glimpses of a Freudian Odyssey," *Psychoanalytic Quarterly,* 2 (April 1933), 327.

85
Putnam to Freud

[July 7, 1914]

106 Marlborough Street
July 7, 1914

Dear Dr. Freud

I think your historical sketch, with its characteristically honest statement of the present situation is *very fine* and impressive.[1] It is a model to all the rest of us in the way of clear thinking and intelligent expression.

Sincerely Yours
James J. Putnam

[1] "Zur Geschichte der psychoanalytischen Bewegung."

86
Putnam to Freud

[Early 1915]

106 Marlborough Street

Dear Professor

I know not whether letters from here will reach you, but there can be no harm in trying. I sent you one little note of greeting at Christmas time, and another earlier, in the autumn, and can assure you that I have thought of you very, very often.

I presume it would not be appropriate to talk of public matters, so I will speak only of our common and personal interests.

In the first place, I wish to thank you for referring two patients to me, Mr. X (the artist) and Mr. Y (an odd but interesting man with curious perversions).[1] Both of them have improved a good deal and indeed Mr. X is very nearly well, certainly much better. You may perhaps recall that he had a well marked Mutter-Complex, with Oedipus like dreams in some respects (incest-dreams) and a fear of death. His personal history in many ways was very interesting. Mr. Y is not likely to get just like other men, but he is a good fellow and good student of dramatics, and feels himself a good deal better off than when you saw him.

I believe that the interest in Ps.a is on the increase in America, though it is not likely that many persons will carry it out with real thoroughness, in practice.

Drs. Hoch, Clark, and McCurdy[2] came on here from New York about three weeks ago and some of us here (Drs. Coriat, Prince, Emerson, Van Teslaar, and a few others)[3] had two long sessions with them. The New York men have been making excellent studies in the depressions, as well as in paraphrenia, and have come to interesting conclusions.

We have also a small group that meets at my house every Friday afternoon, and although we are not geniuses, yet we do fair work, and, I think, keep our heads level.

As for myself, I have been writing a book — not a large one — intended to lay before intelligent "lay" readers, my views on ps.a., on the one hand, and Welt-anschauung on the other.[4] You know that I think this latter both important and also susceptible of scientific treatment, and while the space allowed to me does not permit of thorough treatment, I have tried to be clear and explicit.

Of course, I cannot expect you to agree with all I say, but I have taken pains to avoid putting ps.a in any light that could be considered objectionable.

In fact, I have said very little on the subject of therapeutics but have treated ps.a as one of the two modes of approach to the study of human nature and have followed Rank and Sachs carefully in what I say about art, poetry, etc.[5] I wish I might hope to persuade you to agree with me that one cannot estimate how much influence to attribute to repressions, etc., until one has formed some judgment as to the other influences at work.

I have used, in part, a diagram of this sort, the two figures being thought of as superposed, one above the other. This is intended to illustrate the fact that both of the two sets of influences to which I have referred exert their action throughout each person's life and in all his acts.

The book is to be called "Human Motives," and my thesis is that the real source of *all* motives is the unpicturable energy of which the mind represents a typical form. The mind (or what corresponds to it) makes and modifies the body, and not the body the mind, at least not directly.

I will not undertake to explain the whole argument in this letter but will only say that I feel as convinced of its truth and of its practical importance as I do of the truth and practical importance of your views, and that is saying a great deal. I have just re-read very carefully your "Zur Geschischte der ps.an. Bewegung" and have taken great care to endorse your statement that the ps.an^c doctrines make no claim to account altogether for the action of the mind, but only to indicate a certain qualification of motive and action due to repressions, etc.

Dr. Hoch told me that Dr. McCurdy and he are reading over again all your writings, systematically, and it has long been a plan of mine to do the same.[6] As soon as I get this book off my hands I shall go to work on this and other much neglected reading.

Meantime, I shall not let so long a time go by again without writing.

I have had a foolish feeling that no mail would reach you.

With sincere regards, believe me always your friend

James J. Putnam

[1] Names withheld.

[2] August Hoch was a member of the American Psychoanalytic Association. L. Pierce Clark (1870–1933), New York psychoanalyst and neurologist, a specialist in epilepsy and a consulting neurologist to the Manhattan State Hospital; John P. MacCurdy (1886–1947), lecturer in medical psychology at the Cornell University Medical School from 1913 to 1922 and, from 1923 on, lecturer in psychopathology at the University of Cambridge, England.

[3] Isador Coriat (1875–1943), Boston psychoanalyst, had worked under Adolf Meyer at the Worcester Insane Hospital, and became interested in psychoanalysis around 1911; Louville Eugene Emerson (1873–1939), a member of the American Psychoanalytic Association, was appointed psychologist in the Neurological Department of the Massachusetts General Hospital in 1911.

[4] *Human Motives.*

[5] Otto Rank and Hanns Sachs, *Die Bedeutung der Psychoanalyse für die Geisteswissenschaften* [The Significance of Psychoanalysis for the Social Sciences and the Humanities] (Wiesbaden: J. F. Bergmann, 1913). A translation by Charles Rockwell Payne, *The Significance of Psychoanalysis for the Mental Sciences,* was published in volumes two and three of the *Psychoanalytic Review* in 1915 and 1916 and as number 23 of the Nervous and Mental Disease Monograph Series (New York: Nervous and Mental Disease Publishing Co., 1915).

[6] MacCurdy and Hoch spent "hundreds of hours" together in 1913 and 1914 reading critically what Freud had written. See John P. MacCurdy, *Problems in Dynamic Psychology* (New York: The Macmillan Co., 1922), p. xi.

87
Putnam to Freud
[February 22, 1915]

Dear Friend.

Your postal[1] has just reached me, and I hasten to assure you that neither war nor differences in opinion can change the estimate which I formed long ago. I trust it may be the same with you, and feel sure of it. May we meet again before too long, on one side of the ocean or the other. My book is now practically finished and I shall send it to you in a few months.[2]
Read it carefully, if you have time, and try to put yourself leniently in my place.

Yours,
James J. Putnam,

II. 22/15.

[1] Missing.
[2] *Human Motives.*

88
Freud to Putnam
[March 9, 1915]

Vienna, IX, Berggasse 19
9.3.15

Dear Friend

Your handclasp across the wide ocean made me very glad. Let me assure you that even the postal disruptions of this war will not estrange us. I could reproach myself for not having answered your communications sooner in more detail; however, the idea that there is a censor paralyzes the desire to write.

From one of Jones's letters, which get through occasionally, I know that you are engaged in writing a book.[1] I regret to hear that I will not be able to read it until a few months have elapsed.

Naturally, the times are not propitious for creative work. At the beginning of the war I energetically forced myself to write an extensive case history, which is now awaiting publication in the yearbook.² Since then paralysis has set in; work is an effort for me; and I produce little. We are continuing our two periodicals. The first number of this year's *Internationale Zeitschrift* contains a technical article by me (on transference love) about which I should like to hear your opinion.³ For the next number of *Imago* I am to write a topical essay on the disappointment this war has brought, which gives me no pleasure whatsoever and probably will not please others either.⁴ My practice is reduced to a poor third, but the time thus gained is to no advantage.

Two of my sons are in the army, one of them already has been fighting for weeks in Galicia and is pleased with things as they are so far. The other probably will be sent from the training camp to the front in several weeks.⁵ A third son and both my sons-in-law have not yet been called up.⁶ The women of the family try as far as they are able to fulfill the tasks which these days bring them.

I remember Mr. X and Mr. Y⁷ very well. I am grateful to you for all the news concerning the interest in our science that you see around you. I note with satisfaction that mail is still going to and from America.

With sincere greetings,
Yours,
Freud

¹ *Human Motives.*

² Possibly "Mitteilung eines der psychoanalytischen Theorie widersprechenden Falles von Paranoia" [A Case of Paranoia Running Counter to the Psycho-Analytic Theory of the Disease], published in the *Zeitschrift,* 3 (1915), 321–329; SE, XIV, 261–272.

³ "Weitere Ratschläge zur Technik der Psychoanalyse: III. Bermerkungen über die Übertragungsliebe" [Further Recommendations on the Technique of Psychoanalysis: III. Observations on Transference-love], *Zeitschrift,* 3 (1915), 1–11; SE, XII, 157–171.

⁴ "Zeitgemässes über Krieg und Tod" [Thoughts for the Times on War and Death], *Imago,* 4 (1915), 1–21; SE, XIV, 273–302.

⁵ Martin and Ernst Freud. See Jones, *Sigmund Freud,* II, 180.

⁶ Oliver Freud, Robert Hollitcher, and Max Halberstadt.

⁷ Patients of Freud, names withheld. See Putnam to Freud, [early 1915].

89
Putnam to Freud
[April 5, 1915]

106 Marlborough Street
April 5/15

Dear Friend[1]

Your letter of March 9 reached me a few days ago, after —
evidently — a long passage, and was read with deep interest. If
the news is waited for, day by day, with thrilling interest, by us
here, how much must it mean for you, with your sons actually
engaged and all your interests so intimately involved! Would that
each person engaged might be 'analyzed,' as a part of his preparation for the war.

Meantime, I have read carefully your Narzicismus paper,[2] and
find it full of interest. You certainly pack a great deal of meaning
into your words, and one has to ponder over them; and that is
good.

My own ideas have gradually been defining themselves more
and more since the Weimar paper was written,[3] though on the
whole that covers most of the ground, if interpreted as I meant
it. I wish I had the chance to explain my view to you at length and
repeatedly, the more so that I fear the new book,[4] which is both
condensed and popular, will not give an adequate idea. Let me
attempt another condensed statement in the following terms:

1. I propose no abandonment of any of your views, or of any part
of the original ps.an[c] doctrines or of the therapeutic procedure.

The only modifications that I should suggest are as to secondary
conclusions — as with relation to the nature of "ideals," of "conscience" of "art," etc. etc.

2. I ask, as a preliminary consideration, What are the main sources
from which an individual derives his desires and motives? We
should all agree on two of these, namely, (a.) the repressed, infantile
desires, based on strong instincts, and (b.) the pressure of social
conventions. But what are these social convent[ns]?

Most scientific men would say that they are the results of previous repressions, etc; or, in other words, they are traceable eventually to infantile instincts.

But I believe that society really antedates the individual, in a logical sense, and that "society," in its turn, is the name for a conception which must be taken in an ideal sense. And I regard this opinion, not as an idle theory, of no practical bearing, but as extremely practical and I believe that the inferential recognition of it enters in to all our thoughts and acts, just as the infantile incest motive enters into them.

3. If this is true, we cannot afford to overlook the fact, or to keep ourselves consciously unaware of it, while at the same time we are *unconsc*^{ly} aware of it. This opinion is, I think, a natural outcome of psychoanalytic doctrine of the best sort.

4. If, now, you ask me why I affirm that this unconscious recognition of universal truths is present, I reply that it shows itself whenever a person (i.e. an intelligent person, free from resistances) is urged to give, one by one, the logical and necessary presuppositions or inferences without which his own thought is lacking in clearness, provided it is called upon to grasp such ideas as those above noted [the nature of "ideals etc.]

When I say "lacking in clearness," I mean, "unable to withstand a demand for modifications of certain sorts, when properly presented."

5. I am quite willing to agree that *as a matter of ps.an^c procedure*, i.e. for clinical and practical reasons, it may be unwise and unsuitable for us to endeavor to bring out these "necessary inferences and presuppositions," or that if we do so, and especially if we develop, or cause them to develop the special ethical conclusions which naturally flow from them, this should be done only under special precautions and with the recognition that special forms of self-deception and Uebertragung⁵ are liable to come into play. [I believe, for ex., that *a part* of my own interest in these matters is the desire to escape from seeing my own Complexes]. Nevertheless, in spite of the defense-reaction tendency, I feel sure that I cannot make myself blind to this sort of truth, without injury to my own best intelligence. *And we must all agree to make intelligence the final guide.* Feeling as I do, ought I cease calling myself a ps.anst?

Sincerely your friend

James J. Putnam

There are many evidences of this. Of course, the principle of 'motive' culminates in 'religion,' and this again is closely related

to the sense of responsibility based on recognition of our origin
and destiny as self-conscious beings. Formerly I cared nothing for
these matters, but I have learned through study of philosophy,
to care a great deal and to believe that they are important for
everyone as well as for myself.[6]

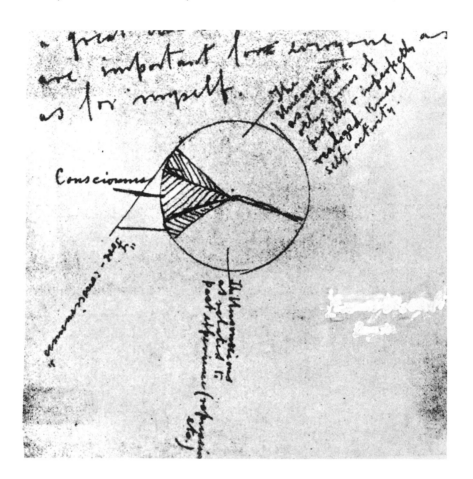

[1] Above the greeting, Putnam wrote, "Der Inhalt dieser Mittheilung is ausschlies-
slich freundschaftlischer und wissenschaftlicher Natur" [The contents of this communication are entirely of a friendly and scholarly nature].

[2] "Zur Einführung des Narzissmus" [On Narcissism: An Introduction], *Jahrbuch*,
6 (1914), 1–24; SE, XIV, 67–102.

[3] Putnam, "Ueber die Bedeutung philosophischer Anschauungen."

[4] *Human Motives*.

[5] Transference.

⁶ This paragraph is on a separate page attached to the letter of April 5, 1915, although not necessarily belonging to it.

90
Putnam to Freud
[May 19, 1915]

May 19, 1915

My dear Friend:

You will receive in a few days a copy of the little book of which I have several times spoken to you, and with which I hope you may find it possible to sympathize in some respects.¹

You will understand, I trust, that while I am entirely ready to admit that my motive in writing the book was one partly to be explained in accordance with psychoanalytic principles, yet it was inspired also, and I hope with good reason, by a wish to inquire what it is, after all, that makes men go ahead at all, whether in the direction that their libido points, or in that of sublimation. I cannot convince myself that life, with all that makes it admirable, is to be explained purely and simply through the study of conflicts; and I do not believe that we can study repressions adequately without having in our own minds an adequate idea of what there is in life over and above that which is repressed. I do not mean that we should make it an essential part, or perhaps any part, of our treatment to convince patients on a point such as this; but I do feel that we ought to have it clearly in our own minds. Friendship and love do not seem to me explicable on the basis of the conflicts of instincts, although I can readily believe that the force which underlies love and friendship makes itself felt on a lower plane as instinct.

I have been reading your last two papers (the "Weitere Ratschläge)² with great care and interest, and sympathize with them very heartily. Among the many sentences which I have marked as particularly noteworthy is the last sentence of the second article, in which you speak of the undoubted fact that psychoanalysis will always have a place in spite of the dangers that go with it, because the need for it is so great. This same great need I feel to exist not only with reference to the serious forms of the psychoneuroses, but also with reference to the life of the members of the community, in an ethical sense, where the need is quite equally great. I am well aware that psychoanalysis can never develop its entire capacity for usefulness as regards problems of an ethical sort, but I hope I am not wrong in thinking that the more intelligent members of the community may be led to take an interest in the principles under-lying it, and that it may thus indirectly come to play an important part in education, especially ethical education.

The recognition of this need has impressed itself the more clearly on my mind through my observation of psychoanalysts themselves. One hears it said — and I believe it to be true — that a psychoanalyst should himself have been analyzed. Not a day passes that I do not feel the need of this with regard to myself. But on the other hand a great many psychoanalysts have been analyzed, and yet they are far from being perfect persons from any point of view. If one inquires why this is so, why the analysis did not succeed in eradicating all the infantile tendencies which stood between them and the best sublimation of which they were capable, a part of the answer must be, I think, that those by whom the analysis was conducted had not themselves realized what the final goal was which these infantile fixations had prevented them (their temporary patients) from reaching.

There are two other points about which I should like to speak, because they came up in the course of our discussion at the meet-ing of the Psychoanalytic Association in New York about two weeks ago.[3] One of these has reference to your interpretation of the main element in repression. It was maintained by two promi-nent members of the society that you interpreted this element as a negative one, — that is, that you believed it was the desire to *escape from "Unlust,"* [4] rather than the *craving for* some more infantile form of *"Lust,"* [5] which contributes the main impulse to repression. I maintained, on the other hand, that I believed your real meaning to be that a craving of some sort was by implica-tion always the really active factor. In other words, it seems to me, — and as I have understood it seems to you, — that we have to reckon all the time with *positive,* rather than with *negative,* factors in the world. Our fears are desires in disguise, etc.

The other point has reference to *acts* (and experiences) vs. *tend-encies.* I have supposed your meaning to be that when we study experiences, whether in the form of "Traumata" or otherwise, the real thing that we wish to know about is in obedience to what tendency, or trend of character, or impulse, or instinct the experience assumed the form which it did assume. In other[6]

[1] *Human Motives.*

[2] "Weitere Ratschläge zur Technik der Psychoanalyse: II. Erinnern, Wiederholen und Durcharbeiten" [Further Recommendations on the Technique of Psychoanalysis: II. Remembering, Repeating and Working Through], *Zeitschrift,* 2 (1914), 485–491; SE, XII, 145–156; and "Weitere Ratschläge zur Technik der Psychoanalyse: III. Bermerkungen über die Übertragungsliebe."

[3] The American Psychoanalytic Association met in New York, May 5, 1915.

[4] Unpleasure.

[5] Pleasure.

[6] Remainder of letter missing.

91
Freud to Putnam
[June 7, 1915]

Vienna, IX, Berggasse 19
7.6.15

Dear Friend

What a very pleasant surprise!

I believed that there was no prospect that a letter from here could get across the ocean. Therefore, in deep resignation I had left your last friendly communication unanswered. I am now learning how illogical hope makes one! The fact that letters reach Vienna from America still does not prove that the reverse route is open.

Send me a card as proof that this letter has reached you. Then I shall have the courage to write to you in detail — a courage I still lack today — after receiving the book you have announced.[1] My chief impression, however, is that I am far more primitive, more modest and more unsublimated than my dear friend in Boston. I see his noble ambition, his profound curiosity. I compare them with my own way of restricting myself to what lies nearest, is most tangible, and yet is actually petty, and with my tendency to be satisfied with whatever is attainable. I believe that I do not lack appreciation of what you are striving for, but I am somewhat frightened by uncertainty. I am timid rather than courageous and gladly sacrifice much for the feeling that I am on solid ground.

The unworthiness of human beings, including the analysts, always has impressed me deeply, but why should analyzed men and women in fact be better. Analysis makes for integration but does not of itself make for goodness. I do not believe, as do Socrates and Putnam, that all vices originate in a sort of obscurity and ignorance. I feel that one puts too great a burden on analysis when one asks that it realize each of one's dearest ideals.

Do assure me about the fate of this letter. In my present isolation I shall be doubly glad to be able to answer you.

Ever your friend,
Freud

¹ *Human Motives.*

92
Freud to Putnam
[July 8, 1915]

Vienna, IX, Berggasse 19
8.7.15

Dear Friend

Your book, *Human Motives* has arrived at last long after it was announced. I have not yet finished it, but have read the parts on religion and psychoanalysis that were most significant to me, and I am following my impulse to write you something about it.

Surely you do not expect praise and commendation from me. It pleases me to think that the book will make an impression on your countrymen and will shake the deep rooted resistance of many of them.

On page 20 I found a passage which, I must admit, applies to me. "To accustom ourselves to the study of immaturity and childhood before . . . undesirable limitation of our vision" etc.¹

I recognize that that is my case. I certainly am incompetent to form a judgment on the other aspects of the subject. Probably I must have made use of this limitation in order to be able to observe what had been hidden from others. Let that justify my defense.

The limitation, in this case, proved rather useful. On the other hand, the fact that I have never been strongly impressed by arguments for the Reality of our Ideals is less significant. I cannot bridge the gap from the Ψ [2] Reality of our Ideals of Perfection to their concrete embodiment. This should not surprise you: you will know how little one can expect from argument. Let me add that I am in no way in awe of the Almighty. If we ever met one another, it is rather I who should reproach Him, than he me. I would ask him why he had not provided me with a better intellectual equipment; he could not accuse me of not having made the best use of my alleged freedom. As an aside, let me say that I know that every human being represents a piece of vital energy, but I really do not understand what energy has to do with freedom (i.e., the absence of causal determination).

You really should know that I always have been dissatisfied with my talents and am aware of the respects in which they are defective. But I consider myself a very moral human being, who can subscribe to the excellent maxim of Th. Vischer:[3] What is moral is always self-evident. I believe that in a sense of justice and consideration for one's fellow men, in discomfort at making others suffer or taking advantage of them, I can compete with the best men I have known. I have never done anything shameful or malicious, nor do I find in myself any temptation to do so. I am not proud of this. I interpret morality, such as we speak of it here, in the social, rather than the sexual sense. Sexual morality as society — and at its most extreme, American society — defines it, seems very despicable to me. I stand for a much freer sexual life. However, I have made little use of such freedom, except in so far as I was convinced of what was permissible for me in this area.

The public emphasis on ethical demands often makes a painful impression on me. What I have seen of religious-ethical conversion has not been inviting. Jung, for example, I found sympathetic so long as he lived blindly, as I did. Then came his religious-ethical crisis with higher morality, "rebirth," Bergson and at the very same time, lies, brutality and anti-semitic condescension towards me. It has not been the first or last experience to reinforce my disgust with saintly converts.[4]

But there is one point on which I can agree with you. When I ask myself why I always have striven honestly to be considerate of

others and if possible kind to them and why I did not give this up
when I noticed that one is harmed by such behavior and is victim-
ized because others are brutal and unreliable, I really have no
answer. It surely was not the sensible thing to do. Nor did I feel
any special ethical bent even in my youth. When I judge myself
to be better than others I feel no special satisfaction. Probably you
are the first person to whom I have boasted of this. You might
almost cite my case as a proof of your assertion that such ideal
impulses form an essential part of our nature. If only other people
exhibited more of this precious disposition! Privately, I'm convinced that if one had the means to study the sublimations of instinct as thoroughly as their repressions, one would come upon
quite natural psychological explanations, and you could do without your benevolent assumption. But as I said before, I know
nothing about this. Why I — as well as my six adult children —
are compelled to be thoroughly decent human beings, is quite
incomprehensible to me. Let me add the following consideration:
if knowledge of the human soul is still so incomplete that my
poor talents could succeed in making such important discoveries,
it seems likely that it is too early to decide for or against hypotheses
such as yours.

Permit me to correct an insignificant error that is without importance for world history. Actually, I was never Breuer's assistant.[5] I never saw that famous first case of his and learned of it
only from his reports many years later. This historical error is
certainly the only one which you have made. I can accept un-
reservedly everything else you have said about ΨA. At the moment
ΨA can accommodate itself to any number of different Weltanschauungen, but has it really said its last word? For me an all
embracing synthesis never has been the important issue. Certainty,
rather, always has been worth the sacrifice of everything else.

I send you cordial greetings, and I wish you lasting good health
and zest for work. As for myself, I am taking advantage of this
holiday to complete a volume of twelve psychological essays.[6]

Faithfully yours,

Freud

---

[1] Putnam had written: "The mature man is a more natural object of primary
study than the immature man or the child, because the traits that make him mature correspond to the traits with which we, as rational beings, enter on our task.

To accustom ourselves to the study of immaturity and childhood before proceeding to the study of maturity and manhood is often to habituate ourselves to an undesirable limitation of our vision with reference to the scope of the enterprise on which we enter" (pp. 19–20).

² Here Freud is using psi to mean psychical or psychological.

³ Friedrich Theodor Vischer (1807–1887), German philosopher, critic, and novelist.

⁴ The passage "What I have seen of religious-ethical conversion . . . saintly converts." was omitted from previously published versions of the letter.

⁵ Putnam had written that Freud was associated "as student and assistant" with Joseph Breuer, in *Human Motives*, p. 74. Breuer was a distinguished older physician and scientist in private practice. See Jones, *Sigmund Freud*, I, chap. xi. For a brief account of Breuer's famous case see, Freud, *Über Psychoanalyse* (1910) and "The Origin and Development of Psychoanalysis," *American Journal of Psychology*, 21 (April 1910), 181–186; SE, XI, 10–15.

⁶ Between March 15 and August, 1915, Freud completed a dozen metapsychological essays, including "Instincts and their Vicissitudes," "Repression," "The Unconscious," etc. The last seven were never published. See Jones, *Sigmund Freud*, II, 185–186; SE, XIV, 105–258.

93
Putnam to Freud

[August 13, 1915]

August 13, 1915.¹

Dear Friend:

Your letter of July the 7th² has given me much to think of and suggests much that I wish to say to you, in the hope that in the end we may be found to agree more nearly.

To begin with, I wish to express my very great regret in regard to my careless blunder in representing you as Breuer's assistant, etc., etc. Whenever the chance comes I shall take pains to correct the mistake and I sincerely apologize for having made it.

As regards the difference in our attitude, I believe that in the end it will not turn out to be so great as it now seems, and I hope to be able to make it clear that you believe in free will and in religion as much as I do, or more than I do. It cannot be that we differ radically in the workings of our minds or in our ability to see the truth. The main difference, as I conceive it, is one of "Widerstand." ³ You have overcome my "Widerstand" in matters of psa., and I wish if possible to overcome yours in regard to the doctrines which I consider so important. Or, again, if the doctrines themselves are not true, I wish to be convinced that that is so.

You say that "arguments" are of no great value; and this is true in so far as the use of arguments means the attempt on the part of one person to impose his own opinion on another. If, however, for the word "arguments" we substitute the term "analysis" — that is to say, the interpretation of one's thought and the discovery of opinions really held — the case is very different. Thus, if anything I say leads you to discover that you do at heart believe what I th⁴ you believe, and that you do actually recognize the importance of so believing, then the effort on my part will have been worth the making. I entirely agree with you that it was very fortunate that you did not concern yourself with "Weltanschauungen" during the long period when you were working over psa. as a pioneer. I would not urge you even now to abandon the exclusive attitude of the pioneer and the specialist were it not for two considerations: (1) the principles of psa. are now so well established that you can afford to consider them, no longer exclusively in themselves, but more in relation to other matters (as, in fact, you are doing); and (2) you do hold "Weltanschauungen" of a sort which, as I think, do not help your work but hamper it. For example, in your "Totem und Tabu," you describe the three modes of looking at the world under the heads animism, magic, and scientific reasoning; and you speak of the last as the best and the ultimate way. Again in your last letter you say that you believe each one of us represents a portion of the world energy but do not see that it has anything to do with the possession of freedom. That is, you again seem to assert a belief in a rigid determinism (as represented by the physical sciences as ruling the world). This is surely a "Weltanschauung" of a very serious sort, and one that is either literally true or literally not true. If it is true, then surely the world would have run down long ago, like a clock, and there would have been no evolution; for a lot of fixed, determinate, interdependent forces could never, without some outside aid, have made anything better than themselves, any more than a man could pull himself over a fence by his own boot straps.

I believe as thoroughly as you do that the greater part of our acts is *virtually* determined. I should be perfectly willing to admit that freedom characterizes only a millionth part of any act or thought. But this millionth part is, I believe, our most precious possession, and deserves our most careful study, all the more so from the fact that it is "verborgen"⁵ and that so many men are inclined to deny its existence, just as they deny the existence of the infantile complexes.

I am sure you do not believe, either as a scientist or as a man, that when you make some great sacrifice for the advancement of the truth (as you have done so often), or when you do some painful task in obedience to a sense of duty, you do not exert any power of free will or choice, or that you do not rearrange the forces of the world in a way that they never could have rearranged themselves. I feel sure that if anybody should threaten to take away that amount of freedom — be it never so small — which you feel yourself possessed of, you would resist the attempt with all your strength and with your life. In other words, you cherish this sense of freedom, however slight it is, and you cherish it as something which does not belong exclusively to yourself but which can be shared by other men and can constitute a bond among men in general.

To put this in another way, your feeling toward your sense of freedom and your love of truth is a "religion." You feel yourself bound by these; and that is all religion means. It is also a universal religion because all men feel themselves bound, in some measure, by these ties, although they may express them in different terms. In my opinion this bond is the very essence of the social bond, and is stronger than any single form of the social bond, like that proposed by Adler,⁶ and stronger even than the sex bond, though by no means exclusive of it.

I would claim further that if there is *any* spontaneity or freedom in the world (what we call *spontaneity* in simpler forms of life is fairly spoken of as *freedom* when one comes to deal with beings like men, who are able to see and estimate the significance of their acts) it must virtually be present everywhere in some measure. I say this in the same sense that one would say that a tree is virtually present in a seed from which the tree will spring. A scientific man might study the growth of the seed without seeing as yet any evidences of the tree, and might therefore readily deny the tree; but the fault would be in the narrowness of his conception.

I cannot agree that the existence of these feelings of recognition (like yours toward the truth) are of no practical significance. It is not only that sublimation could not go on were it not that the

end toward which sublimation moves was already virtually present; but voluntary sacrifice is necessary at every moment and for
every man in order that he may do his best. And strange as it may
seem, the voluntary sacrifices which excite our admiration the most
are those where the advantage to the individual is the least apparent.

You speak of referring these processes to a "psychological cause."
But how does that help the matter? Whence comes the impulse
that makes this psychological cause operative? If you call it the
"Libido," what is the mainspring of the "Libido?" This is a
question which I think we are bound to answer. If you call the
"Libido" a "Weltenergie," [7] and think in that way to avoid the
necessity of defining it still further, you are again brought face
to face with the question whether you mean it "Weltenergie" in
the sense of a purely physical force or of a force which is essentially
mental and analogous to voluntary effort. It surely cannot be both,
for no one has ever shown or has ever dreamed of showing that
the mental forces are really subject to any such law as that of
"the conservation of energy." And one cannot imagine two sets of
laws in the universe constantly interacting and yet having no
common origin or nature. If you turn again and say the mental
processes are only physical processes in disguise, then you have
the strange phenomenon to deal with of physical processes turning
on themselves and learning to appreciate and contemplate themselves. But this again proves them to be no longer physical laws.
In short, we can imagine a universe made on the principle of
spontaneity and personalism, and yet having so-called physical laws
operative within certain limits as one of their own forms of existence; but we cannot imagine the reverse.

It is well known, I believe, that none of these physical laws is
really a complete expression of the truth. They are only partial
expressions.

One more point, which seems to me of considerable importance.
You asked me, in the letter received before this last one,[8] on what
grounds I thought that psychoanalysts ought to be better than
other men; and following the same reasoning you have at different
times thought me rather excessive in thinking that psa. could be
used to any extent in the interests of ethics.

In answer to these questions or sentiments I would say that

when one is doing an analysis one does not hesitate to discuss everything that comes up — a man's character and civic attitude, etc., etc. If, then, such a person is a cheat, we try to learn to know it; and I see no point at which such an inquiry should stop except at the point of ideal perfection. You and others have many times made it clear to us that the effects of our repressions vary or mix themselves in with everything that happens to us through life. If this is so, a complete analysis would leave one, theoretically, a perfect person. Such an analysis done on a physician with the purpose of fitting him to deal with patients should surely make him a more perfect person in the ideal sense.

I would confidently maintain that the cause of the attitude of our Zurich friend [9] toward you was not that he had too much religion, but aver that it was too little or too false. In other words, he did not show this worship of the truth which is the basis of religion, and his failure to do this ought not to be laid at the door of religion itself, any more than the behavior of soldiers, as you yourself pointed out in your paper on the war, ought to be laid to the failure of sublimation. You said, very truly, that we ought not so much to feel disappointed at the apparent downfall of civilization in war, but ought, instead, to recognize that we had overrated the amount of civilization which had actually been present, and had mistaken a venture for a really interstitial penetration and observation.

I repeat that I consider you as a more religious man than myself because I think you are a more honest and courageous man. I would also say that the "Weltanschauungen" which I hold do not, I find, make me less inclined, but make me more inclined, to do good analytic work. This is very difficult, and very often I fail; but unless I greatly err, the difficulty does not lie in any such influence as that exerted by my beliefs in the nature of life and human obligations.

Still one more point seems to me of interest. This is that one may fairly demand a patient attention to those inferences of our logical thought from one who has done such incredibly great service in pointing out the inferences of our unconscious thinking. In both cases, of course, we are dealing with manifestations of the unconscious, and in both cases, if I am right, one proceeds from one point of vantage to another with the aid of inference.

It is true that in the psycho-analytic investigation one tries to reproduce actual experiences; whereas you might urge that in the process of leading the thought on from one presupposition to another this was not true. But I really think — and this is a point which I tried to make evident in my book[10] — that what we call experiences in analysis are really symbols or expressions of an energetic process, call it "Libido" or what you will; and that on the other hand we do discover what may fairly be called experiences through which it is possible to express to ourselves our relations to our ideals, and that, too, in a very practical form.

Yours very sincerely, as ever,

[1] Above the date of this typewritten letter is the note, "Dr. Freud Copy (not sent)."
[2] Putnam probably meant July 8, 1915.
[3] Resistance.
[4] Think.
[5] Hidden.
[6] See Putnam, "The Work of Alfred Adler, Considered with Especial Reference to That of Freud." Read before the New York Psychoanalytic Society, November 23, 1915. *Psychoanalytic Review*, 3 (April 1916), 121–140; Ad Psa, 312–339.
[7] Cosmic force.
[8] Freud to Putnam, June 7, 1915.
[9] Carl Jung.
[10] *Human Motives.*

94
Putnam to Freud

[September 15–October 3, 1915]

106 Marlborough Street
Sept. 15. 1915.

Dear Friend

Your kind letter has given me much to think about and I wrote a long reply which however — because it was so long — I have decided not to send. The main point of it was that we do not and cannot stand so far apart as one might think, — and for the simple reason that we are both attempting, by the use of our intelligences and our intuitions, to reach the truth, and there cannot be two sorts of logical process in the world. It is you that have helped to teach me to be "religious" and to believe in the reality of the unseen, and in "free will." — Even though our freedom accounts for only 1/1,000,000 of our acts and thoughts, that small fraction is the most valuable part of them.) For it is you that have taught me to believe in "truth" and "justice" as in things outside of us yet in us, and to make *voluntary* sacrifices for them, and that *is* re-ligion and the worship of the unseen.

You say that our (or your) tendency to show reasonableness etc. etc. might perhaps be explained as a psychological outgrowth of our repressed instincts, etc. But supposing that is true; what then? How are our instincts to be explained, and our libido? Whence do they come? If, *as forces,* they transcend any given or particular manifestation of their power, — bringing about, now this, now that result, — then they are forces which can interlock with our own volition and of which we can get the best idea by studying them under the form of introspection, which Ps.a has taught us how to do. You say you have no leaning toward philosophic reasoning of this sort and no capacity for it, and that in your work you have purposely kept yourself in a "scientific" attitude and free from general philosophic conclusions.

But have you not shown that you have ten times my capacity for *every sort* of reasoning that you think it best to use; and is it not a case of "resistance," partly conscious, partly unconscious? You cannot really believe that "science" (i.e. "natural science," so-called) has the last word about the psychology of intellect and emotion — unless indeed it be science as interpreted by thought and feeling. For the less, while it may seem to *precede* the greater, cannot really create it.

One word more: you said in the letter before the last that you did not think me justified in claiming that ps.an^sts. ought to be better men than others, and you have several times said that Ps.a. should not be looked to, in the degree that I have sought to use it, as a means of promoting ethics. Now of course I realize that Ps a. owes its success to *clinical studies on neurotic patients.*

But when we have to deal with such patients does it not often happen that matters come up for discussion which are practically questions of ethics (or "Sublimation"), and do we not then, at least, feel obliged to conclude that ethics and the higher reaches of sub-limation and character are fit subjects for ps.an^e investigation? Is it not to be believed that if our Zurich friend ¹ would really open his mind and allow himself to be analyzed to the very depths, he would probably come out of it to advantage. Is it not, in short, at least *logically* true that all imperfection implies an undue preponderance of immaturity?

Of course, the issue is a practical one, and that I entirely admit.

If I felt the ability to make the same fine scientific analyses that you make, I should probably devote myself to that sort of work, and it would be none the less good, I believe, for the fact that a philosophic background lay behind it. My much admired Hegel became very practical under certain influences and wrote papers, as you know, on politics and statecraft. But he never ceased to feel that his main life-work lay in bringing home to people's minds the great mental laws that underlay science and politics and aesthetics, etc.

————————

Last evening I re-read a portion of your paper on the war,[2] and again admired the vigor of your thought and style.

I had a letter from Jones only a few days ago, in which he said he was very busy and that he was about to read a paper before the Sociological Assoc.[n] on 'outlets for the emotional needs of women.'[3] I am sure it will be interesting and opportune, for the poor women of the next generation are likely to have a hard time of it. He also told me about Rank and Sachs,[4] to whom, if you have a chance I wish you would remember me warmly.

I trust that all goes well with your own sons.

Very sincerely your friend
James J. Putnam

Oct. 3[d] (my 69th birthday).

[1] Carl Jung.

[2] "Zeitgemässes über Krieg und Tod."

[3] Jones's letter is missing. *The Sociological Review,* journal of the Sociological Society (London), lists only Jones's "The War and Individual Psychology," 7 (July 1915), 167–180. The Society held a number of informal symposia, however, whose proceedings were not published.

[4] Otto Rank and Hanns Sachs, both members of the Vienna Psychoanalytic Society and Freud's closest assistants, remained in Vienna until they were called up for service in June and August of 1915. Sachs was released after 12 days. See Jones, *Sigmund Freud,* II, 181.

95
Putnam to Freud

[October 6, 1915]

106 Marlborough Street
October 6, 1915.

Dear Professor:

I wish just to add to my letter my sincere regret at having made in my book the careless blunder about your relation to Dr. Breuer.[1] I shall take the first opportunity to set the matter straight.

Yours sincerely, as ever,
James J. Putnam

Professor Dr. Sigmund Freud,
Berggasse 19, Vienna IX, Austria.

[1] See Freud to Putnam, July 8, 1915.

96
Putnam to Freud

[January 3, 1916]

106 Marlborough Street
Jan. 3rd

Dear Friend

Communication between us is difficult and it would not surprise me if my last letters had not reached you.

At any rate, I must send a line of greeting for the New Year, to assure you that I have you constantly and warmly in my mind, and rate Ps a higher than ever.

I have just been spending a lot of time over Adler, and the fact that his writers[1] have served as a handle, or tool, for some men here to use for striking at Ps a.

I read a paper on this subject in New York and have written it out, at perhaps too great length, for the Psychoanalytic Review.[2]

I am aware that one does better to put one's efforts into more constructive work, but that comes hard to me.

I hope and trust that all goes well with you and with your sons and family (!!); also that you were interested in Prof. Holt's book called The Freudian Wish[3] which he tells me he has sent to you.
  With best regards,

Yours sincerely
James J. Putnam

[1] Putnam intended "writings."
[2] "The Work of Alfred Adler, Considered with Especial Reference to That of Freud."
[3] Edwin B. Holt, *The Freudian Wish and Its Place in Ethics* (New York: Henry Holt and Co., 1915).

97
Freud to Putnam
[January 26, 1916]

Vienna, IX, Berggasse 19
26. Jan 16

Dear Friend
  Communication is really difficult nowdays. Judging by the example of Prof. Holt's book,[1] which did not arrive, I may have suffered the loss of many a letter from you which would have delighted me had it come. To have your assurance that your feeling for me is still a friendly one and that you continue to be actively interested in our science pleases me all the more. Surely I shall be able to read your essay on Adler[2] some day. I deeply feel the loneliness which surrounds me. My best assistants Rank, Abraham and Ferenczi are far away and so occupied that we seldom hear from one another.[3] The war has greatly magnified all distances. With the co-workers who are still here, within calling distance, I continue to keep the two periodicals going. Six issues of the *Internationale Zeitschrift* appeared in 1915, and three numbers of *Imago*. I do not know whether any of them reached you. I have not sent off any of my reprints in recent months. This is not a propitious time for physical well being, nor does it matter. Two of my sons both of them well until now, are at the front, and both have distinguished themselves. They are both officers — while my son-in-law from Hamburg is serving as an artillery man in

Flanders.[4] We have armed ourselves with patience; our hopes for an early end of the war proved to be mistaken.

I am writing down the lectures which I am giving at the moment on the "Introduction to ΨA." [5] They are to be published by Hugo Heller in Vienna.[6] They will contain nothing new for the initiated. You know what my wishes are for you — a long Otium cum dignitate et studio[7] and added to this, the well being of your family. Do remember me from time to time.

Yours very cordially,
Freud

P. S. I have written this letter in a script unusual for me in order that you may not need the help of E. Jones or rather Loo J.[8]

---

[1] Edwin B. Holt, *The Freudian Wish.* However, on July 27, 1916, Freud wrote to Lou Andreas-Salomé that he would forward the book along with "Putnam in the Psychoanalytic Review," probably his article on Alfred Adler. See n. 2 below and *The Letters of Sigmund Freud,* Selected and Edited by Ernst Freud (New York: McGraw-Hill, 1964), pp. 313–314.

[2] "The Work of Alfred Adler, Considered with Especial Reference to That of Freud."

[3] All three were serving in the armed forces.

[4] Martin (1887–1967), and Ernst Freud (1892–1970) and Max Halberstadt (1882–1940). See Jones, *Sigmund Freud,* II, 180.

[5] *Vorlesungen zur Einführung in die Psychoanalyse* [Introductory Lectures on Psycho-Analysis], Leipzig and Vienna: Heller, 1917; SE XV, xvi. They were delivered at the University of Vienna during the winter terms 1915–1916 and 1916–1917.

[6] Hugo Heller (1870–1923), a member of the Vienna Psychoanalytic Society, and publisher of *Imago.*

[7] Dignified and scholarly leisure.

[8] Loe Jones, with whom Ernest Jones lived for seven years, had helped him to decipher Freud's German script. See Jones to Putnam, October 17, 1910, and Jones, *Free Associations* (New York: Basic Books, 1959) pp. 139–140.

98
Freud to Putnam

[October 1, 1916]

Vienna, IX, Berggasse 19
1 Oct. 16

Prof. J. J. Putnam
106 Marlborough Street,
Boston, Mass., U.S.A.

Dear Friend

I deeply regret not having heard from you for such a long time. I wanted to send you the first volume of my "lectures" [1] but learned that the post office will not accept it at this time. Let us hope for better times! My best wishes and greetings

Yours,
Freud

[1] The first volume of Freud's *Vorlesungen zur Einführung in die Psychoanalyse: Die Fehlleistungen* [Parapraxes] was published by Hugo Heller before the end of July 1916, although the exact date is uncertain. See SE, XV, 1–79.

III

Jones–Putnam Correspondence

Letters 99–157

Ernest Jones, 1909–1917

Putnam regarded Jones as a brilliant, disciplined, and tireless young crusader, an opinion in which Jones doubtless would have concurred. Perhaps more than any other single individual, Jones was responsible over the years for guiding the psychoanalytic movement. Imbued with visions of the paladins of Charlemagne, in 1912 Jones organized the secret "Committee" whose mission was to protect Freud and champion orthodoxy. Ferenczi, Abraham, Rank, Sachs, and Jones each received a Greek intaglio from Freud as a sign of membership. No American was included in this secret directorate.

Jones insisted uncompromisingly that psychoanalysis was Freud's theory and technique alone, uncontaminated by other varieties of psychological analysis or by the errors of those who differed with Freud and left the movement. Jones developed a clear sense of the function of personal contacts and of the need for organized groups whose purpose was not only to protect rigor of method and theory but to work through clinical and personal problems.

Ambitious and curious, Jones mastered the new literature of medical psychology as it appeared. He was much in demand as a speaker, probably for his provocativeness as well as for his lucidity. From 1909 through 1911 he made repeated "raids" over the Canadian border from Toronto on behalf of psychoanalysis, chiefly in the mid-West. Regularly he rode the train for eight hours each way to attend the meetings of the Detroit Neurological Society. He spoke to the Chicago Society, probably on the initiative of Hugh T. Patrick, a leading local authority, who had been impressed by Putnam's speech to the American Neurological Association in 1911. Jones was among the distinguished guests, including Eugen Bleuler, who spoke at the dedication in 1913 of the new

Phipps Psychiatric Clinic that Adolf Meyer directed at The Johns Hopkins University in Baltimore.

In 1910 Putnam broached the possibility of a position for Jones at Harvard and sounded out Hugo Münsterberg, head of the University's psychological laboratory. Münsterberg wrote to Putnam, March 23, 1910, praising Jones's combination of "medical experience and full neurological knowledge with psychological interest. Among the younger men I hardly know anyone who seems to fill the bill so well as Dr. Jones. The only objection which troubles me is his inclination to put more emphasis on sexual factors than would be desirable in a course which is not intended for medical students and which is open to undergraduates. It might too easily degenerate into a sensational course by the loafers on account of its piquancy. But I trust that Jones would see that himself and would 'repress' his ideas of sexual explanation." Nothing came of Putnam's informal suggestion, which had it succeeded, would have altered the history of the psychoanalytic movement.

Jones met more opposition to Freud's sexual theories in Canada than Putnam encountered in Boston. These theories exacerbated the danger all psychotherapists faced of charges of unprofessional conduct and even blackmail by patients. Jones described such an episode to Putnam in letters of January 13 and 23, 1910, and February 5, 1911. The matter must have been settled to the satisfaction of the University, for Jones remained on the faculty until November 13, 1913, when he resigned to live permanently in London. Beginning in the summer of 1912 he had been spending larger amounts of time in Europe, partly because of the poor health of Loe, a young Dutch woman with whom Jones lived for seven years, introducing her to family and friends as his wife. After her psychoanalysis with Freud in 1913, she and Jones separated, and each married someone else. At Freud's suggestion, Jones was the first psychoanalyst to undergo a didactic analysis. He spent one hour twice a day with Sandor Ferenczi in Budapest during the summer and autumn of 1913.

Jones's correspondence with Putnam falls largely within the years 1909 through 1911 and includes the only contemporary account yet available of the founding of the American Psychoanalytic Association, which was undertaken at the request of Freud and

Ferenczi. Few of Putnam's letters for this period have survived and none of Jones's after 1912.

In retrospect, Jones observed characteristically that A. A. Brill's support of psychoanalysis in America was more "completely whole-hearted and based on a much better understanding of it"[1] than Putnam's. In his autobiography, Jones also concluded:

Putnam "was much more than his philosophy. For one thing, he was the only man I have ever known, in a vast experience of scientific discussions, to admit publicly that he had been mistaken. He had a superb integrity of soul, and no personal interest ever even weighed with him in the balance against his devotion to his ideals."[2]

99
Jones to Putnam
[June 1, 1909]

June 1.
407 Brunswick Avenue,
Toronto

Dear Dr. Putnam.

Your letter arrived this morning.[1] The two men in London I should most recommend for such a case as you mention are Harry Campbell, 23, Wimpole St. W, and Purves Stewart, 94, Harley St. W. As to Holland I think I know all the neurologists there, and would say Winckler Professor of Neurology, Amsterdam, Rosenstein, Hague, and Jelgersma, Leyden in this order.[2] I enclose a couple of my cards, which if you think fit might serve as an introduction.

It was most good of you to put me up for the Amer. Neur. Assoc. I thank you very much. I hope to attend it next year. Isn't it good news about Prince being made President?[3] It is a triumph for the Boston school in her fight against materialism.

---

[1] Jones, "Reminiscent Notes on the Early History of Psychoanalysis in English-speaking Countries," *International Journal of Psychoanalysis*, 16 (parts I and II, 1945), 9.

[2] Jones, *Free Associations* (New York: Basic Books, 1959), p. 189.

I am glad the Kleine Hans⁴ interested you, even before you came to the end of the article which is of course of most general value. What a problem it is to make such unpalatable facts clean. If only we were all imbued with the aesthetic passion for truth and progress, however hateful, that Keats so wonderfully depicts in his Hyperion! The coming generation must adapt itself — or suffer the consequences.

I believe that the complex Freud studies in this case are throughout representative of the normal, and would quite subscribe to a sentence from a letter I had last week from Jung; *"es ist ja recht eigentlich die erste Psychologie des Kindes."* ⁵ Such matters *have* to be taken into account if we ever wish to understand the later reactions and character formation of the individual.

Yours very sincerely

Ernest Jones

¹ Putnam's letter is missing.

² Harry Campbell (d. 1938), physician at the West End Hospital for Nervous Diseases, London, editor of the *Medical Press and Circular* from 1919 to 1933; Sir James Purvis Stewart (1869–1949), Lecturer on Nervous Diseases at the Westminster Hospital Medical School, London, author of *The Diagnosis of Nervous Diseases* (10th ed., 1948); Cornelis Winkler (1855–1941), professor of neurology and psychiatry, University of Utrecht; P.H. Rosenstein (d. 1943), neurologist practicing at The Hague, M.D., University of Leyden, 1898; Gegrandus Jelgersma (1859–1942), professor of psychiatry, University of Leyden. As Rector, Jelgersma invited Freud to lecture in the autumn of 1914, and he discussed Freud's theory of dreams at the 339th anniversary of the founding of the University.

³ Morton Prince became president-elect of the American Neurological Association in 1909 and served as president for the year 1910.

⁴ Freud, "Analyse der Phobie eines fünfjährigen Knaben" [Analysis of a Phobia in a Five-year-old Boy], *Jahrbuch,* 1 (1909), 1–109; SE, X, 5–147.

⁵ "This is indeed the first true insight into the psychology of the child."

100

Jones to Putnam

[November 19, 1909]

Nov. 19/09.

407 Brunswick Avenue,

Toronto.

Dear Dr. Putnam.

My primary object in writing to you is a business one. The Canadian Medical Association meets in Toronto next June, and proposes to arrange a symposium on the Neuroses and Psycho-neuroses. The Committee of the Medical Section, who is arranging this, has commissioned me to invite you to read an address on the subject. Dr. Adolf Meyer[1] is also invited, and possibly some other American neurologist will be. If you could see your way to entertaining the suggestion favourably we should all be delighted, and I need hardly say that I in particular should be very happy and that I should consider it a great honour to be allowed to extend to you all the hospitality in my power.

Materialism (views of intestinal toxaemia, etc.) is even more rampant here than anywhere in the States, and it is a great opportunity to strike a blow at it.

I have here an unanswered letter of yours dated July 19.[2] I got it only on my return in the middle of September, and I am afraid that by now most of it has answered itself. I can only reply in the positive as to your question of the *possibility* of an obstinate priapism being a conversion.

I got this week a long and rather bitter letter from Dr. Prince on the subject of Freud's work. From various indications that are easy to read between the lines it is pretty plain that his resistance springs from personal grounds. It is indeed hard for a man to have to confess that he has devoted his life mainly to elucidation of the psycho-neuroses, and has overlooked so many important secrets of them. He is but following the way of all flesh in striving to resist, reject and minimise the work that would show him he must begin all over again. It is the old story of the attitude taken by leading authorities whenever a revolutionary discovery is made. Still the true greatness of a man then has the opportunity of being put to the test, and the noble man is the one who under those circumstances can acknowledge and deal with these unconscious personal prejudices, and sink personal questions in the general onward march of the army of society towards the goals of truth and progress.

I am afraid that he, Sidis[3] and others are using their great influence powerfully in the effort to crush the tender plant of psychoanalysis in America, and I am sorry for it. The other attitude, of readiness to listen to the new, is so stimulating an example than[4] one greatly regrets its rarity.

These remarks about Prince are of course for your ears only, and I only make them in the hope that you might be able to make some general suggestions about him.

Pierce[5] has asked me to read a short paper at the Amer. Psychol. Assoc. next month. I have accepted with pleasure, and am thinking of taking as a subject Freud's Dream Theory. It would of course be impossible even to outline it in the time, but it may serve the purpose of arousing some interest in it. Prince warned me that if I chose a Freud subject I would be opposed, but I feel it is my duty to do what little I can regardless of that.

My practice has much increased of late, and I have had some very satisfactory results in even old-standing cases. It is a great joy to watch these chronic sufferers revive day by day and take up life again with a new zest.

I have recently had letters from Freud and Jung. They greatly enjoyed their stay with you, but it was a pity that Freud was feeling so unwell.[6]

With kindest regards, and with keen hopes of receiving a favourable reply to our invitation

I am

Yours cordially

Ernest Jones

[1] Adolf Meyer (1866–1950), professor of psychiatry at The Johns Hopkins University, 1910–1941, director of the Psychiatric Institute of the New York State Hospitals for the Insane, Ward's Island, New York, 1902–1910.

[2] Missing.

[3] Boris Sidis (1867–1923), psychopathologist, had received a PhD in psychology under William James and a medical degree from Harvard. He practiced in Brookline from 1904, and in 1909 opened the Sidis Institute at Portsmouth, N.H.

[4] That.

[5] Arthur Henry Pierce (1867–1914), professor of psychology at Smith College, secretary of the American Psychological Association. Putnam spoke on "Freud's and Bergson's Theories of the Unconscious," and Jones on "Freud's Theory of Dreams" at the eighteenth annual meeting of the American Psychological Association, Cambridge, Mass., December 29. See abstracts, *Psychological Bulletin*, 7 (February 15, 1910), 44–46.

[6] Freud, Jung, and Ferenczi had visited Putnam Camp at Keene Valley in the Adirondacks for three days in September, and Freud had suffered from a mild attack of appendicitis. See Jones, *The Life and Work of Sigmund Freud*, II (New York: Basic Books, 1955), 59.

101
Putnam to Jones
[November 22, 1909]

Dear Dr. Jones, —

I have read your letter with much interest and accept your kind
invitation to read a paper at the Toronto meeting, although I
suppose it will imply giving up the meeting of the Neurological
Association.[1] I also thank you very much for your kind offer of
hospitality. The subject of which you speak is unquestionably the
important one for me.

I am very glad to hear that you are to attend the meeting of the
Psychological Association.[2] I hope to see a good deal of you and
you will, I trust, dine with me. If it were not that every room
will probably be occupied, I should ask you to stay with me while
you are here.

I also am to read a short paper at this meeting and have chosen
as a subject, A Comparison od [3] Bergson' and Freud's Theories of
the Unconscious Mental Life.[4] I am very glad that you are to read
on Dreams.[5] It is a great subject and although I have not found
it possible to verify all that Freud says, yet with regard to this,
as with regard to his observations in other directions, I have been
able to confirm so much that I am ready to believe that the rest
will come.

The visit of Freud and Jung to the Adirondacks was on the
whole satisfactory. They were curiously unlike most of the other
persons gathered there, but I believe they found the experience
an interesting one. I will tell you sometime something of their
comments.

Yours sincerely

Nov. 22, 1909.

P.S. The best answer I can make now to the remaining portion of
your letter is to say that I am just writing two papers, of an introductory nature, on Freud matters to be published in Dr. Prince's
journal.[6]

---

[1] Putnam read "On the Etiology and Treatment of the Psychoneuroses," before
the Canadian Medical Association at Toronto, June 1, 1910. See *Boston Medical and
Surgical Journal,* 163 (July 21, 1910), 75–82; Ad Psa, 54–78. Putnam also attended

the American Neurological Association meetings in Washington, D.C., May 2–4, 1910.

² The American Psychological Association held its eighteenth annual meeting in Cambridge, Mass., December 29–31, 1909. The afternoon of December 29 was devoted to Freud and abnormal psychology.

³ Putnam intended "of."

⁴ See the abstract of Putnam, "Freud's and Bergson's Theories of the Unconscious," pp. 44–45.

⁵ See Jones, "Freud's Theory of Dreams," *American Journal of Psychology*, 21 (April 1910), 283–308; PPsa, eds. 1–5.

⁶ Putnam, "Personal Impressions of Sigmund Freud and His Work, with Special Reference to His Recent Lectures at Clark University," *Journal of Abnormal Psychology*, 4 (December 1909–January 1910), 293–310, and (February–March 1910), 372–379; Ad Psa, 1–30; in James S. Van Teslaar, ed., *An Outline of Psychoanalysis* (New York: The Modern Library, 1925).

102
Jones to Putnam
[November 25, 1909]

Nov. 25/09
407 Brunswick Avenue,
Toronto.

Dear Dr. Putnam.

It is very good indeed of you to promise to come to Toronto, and we shall all, I am sure appreciate your paper. I do not think the meeting will clash with the Amer. Neurol. Assoc., for I fancy it is later. Meyer can't come, as he will be in Europe at that time, so we shall try to get August Hoch instead.¹

Many thanks for your kind invitation as concerns Boston. I hear that Dr. Prince is reading a paper on Dreams, as I am doing, so that our three papers will have much in common.² It ought at all events to act in stimulating a little more interest among psychologists in our practical problems. By the way, if you wish to discuss with me beforehand any special points in relation to Freud's views on the Unconscious, you know I should be most happy to do so.

I shall be most interested to read your forthcoming papers in Dr. Prince's Journal, and shall eagerly look forward to them.³

I am busy at present writing two long reviews, one for Jung's Jahrbuch on the subject of the English and American literature on psycho-pathology, the other for the Psychol. Bulletin on Freud's work.[4]

Yours very sincerely

Ernest Jones

[1] August Hoch (1868–1919), succeeded Meyer in 1910 as director of the Psychiatric Institute of the New York State Hospitals for the Insane on Ward's Island and as professor of psychiatry at the Cornell University Medical School. He edited the *Psychiatric Bulletin*.

[2] All three spoke before the eighteenth annual meeting of the American Psychological Association December 29, in Cambridge, Mass., at a session devoted to abnormal psychology, with special emphasis on Freud's work. See Morton Prince, "The Mechanism and Interpretation of Dreams," *Journal of Abnormal Psychology*, 5 (October–November 1910), 139–195; Jones, "Freud's Theory of Dreams"; Putnam, "Freud's and Bergson's Theories of the Unconscious" (abstract), pp. 44–45.

[3] "Personal Impressions of Sigmund Freud."

[4] The *Jahrbuch für psychoanalytische und psychopathologische Forschungen* began publication after the Salzburg Psychoanalytic Congress in 1909 under the direction of Eugen Bleuler and Freud. It was edited by Carl Jung for the next five years. Jones's reviews were "Review of the Recent English and American Literature on Clinical Psychology and Psychopathology" [Bericht über die neurere englische und amerikanische Literatur zur klinischen Psychologie und Psychopathologie], trans. W. Stockmayer, *Jahrbuch*, 2 (1910), 316–346; this review appeared in *Archives of Neurology and Psychiatry*, 5 (1911), 120–147; "Freud's Psychology," *Psychological Bulletin*, 7 (April 15, 1910), 109–128; PPsa, eds. 1–5.

103

Jones to Putnam

[January 13, 1910]

Jan. 13.

407 Brunswick Avenue,

Toronto.

Dear Dr. Putnam.

My psycho-analytic experience with stammering is but slight. I have made one complete psycho-analysis in an adult a recently acquired case (male hysteria) and two incomplete ones in young boys. I have had however a very extensive clinical experience of it, as I was deputed by the London County Council to enquire into it in the schools, and have full notes of over 100 cases. I think the clinical features, together with my slight psycho-analytic experience of it, justify me in forming a general opinion of it by analogy with allied neuroses. I fully accept all that Stekel [1] says of it, that it is an Angsthysterie,[2] always of sexual origin, and allied in mechanism to a Versprechen[3] and accompanying embarrassment. I see every reason to believe that it should be possible completely to eradicate it by psycho-analysis, with this addendum. In long standing cases it comes to resemble tics in that the affective basis sinks from expression and a direct habit is set up. One has therefore to combine the attempt to resuscitate the old affective tone, before getting to the root of this, with other exercises of the ordinary (Gutzmann)[4] kind. I might also add that I don't think the aetiology is always the same, e.g. fear of betraying a secret. The greater incidence in boys (3:1) and other features make me assimilate it often to psychical sexual impotence. I should much like the opportunity of making a few full analyses of it, and will be very interested to hear the result of yours.

I have just got the second number of the Jahrbuch, and like Ferenczi's article very much.[5] I haven't yet read the others.

Yours very sincerely

Ernest Jones

[1] Wilhelm Stekel, *Nervöse Angstzustande und ihre Behandlung, mit einem Vorworte von Prof. Dr. Sigmund Freud* [Neurotic Anxiety States and Their Treatment, Introduction by Prof. Dr. Sigmund Freud], Berlin and Vienna: Urban & Schwarzenberg, 1908, pp. 231–234.

[2] Anxiety hysteria.

[3] Slip of the tongue.

[4] See Albert Theodor Karl Gutzmann, *Das Stottern und seine gründliche Beseitigung durch ein methodisch geordnetes und praktisch erprobtes Verfahren. Eine Anleitung für Eltern und Lehrer, sowie zum Gebrauch für Erwachsene* [Stuttering and Its Radical Elimination by Means of a Methodical, Practical and Proven Treatment: An Introduction for Parents and Teachers with Exercises for Adults], Berlin: Edwin Staude, 1895, 1906.

[5] Ferenczi, "Introjektion und Übertragung" [Introjection and Transference], *Jahrbuch,* 1 (1909), 422–457; in Ferenczi, *Sex in Psychoanalysis,* trans. Ernest Jones (Boston: Richard G. Badger, 1916), pp. 30–79 and (New York: Basic Books, 1950), pp. 35–93.

104
Jones to Putnam
[January 16, 1910]

Jan. 16/1910.
407 Brunswick Avenue,
Toronto

Dear Dr. Putnam.

I enclose a letter from Dr. Hattie,[1] which shows that we can't expect much from him. Will you please send it back sometime.

I have just heard that the Freud Congress in Nuremberg takes place at Easter, March 28.[2] Can you get off then? I doubt if I can, as the session will be still on.

You spoke to me about over-sensitiveness etc., in children. Curiously Adler deals with it in the second number of the Jahrbuch in a very interesting article.[3] How did you like Stekel's article?[4] Some of his interpretations are wonderfully quick sighted. There is no doubt that dream analysis is the centre of our practical therapeutic work, strange as it may appear to an outsider.

Do you see the American Journal of Psychology? You should look up the January number, P. 168, where there is a review of Freud, evidently written by Stanley Hall.[5] My Hamlet article is in the same number, and of course I shall send you a reprint as soon as they arrive.[6] I was wondering if I might ask you to review or abstract it for the Journal of Abn. Psych.[7] I know how busy you are, but there is no one else who could do it, and I think it is an article that is likely to arouse general interest if people hear of it.

Yours very cordially
Ernest Jones.

[1] William Harop Hattie, M.D. (1870–1932), Canadian psychiatrist, served as medical superintendent, Nova Scotia Hospital for the Insane, Halifax, from 1908 to 1913. He also was to participate in the symposium on the neuroses, to be held June 1, before the Canadian Medical Association.

[2] The second International Psychoanalytic Congress was held in Nuremberg, March 30–31, 1910.

[3] Alfred Adler, "Über neurotische Dispositionen: Zugleich ein Beitrag zur Ätiologie und zur Frage der Neurosenwahl" [On Neurotic Tendencies: A Contribution to Etiology and to the Problem of Choice of Neurosis], Jahrbuch, 1 (1909), 526–545.

[4] Wilhelm Stekel, "Beiträge zur Traumdeutung" [Contributions to Dream Interpretation], Jahrbuch, 1 (1909), 458–512.

⁵ "Psychological Literature," *American Journal of Psychology*, 21 (January 1910), 168–170.
⁶ "The Oedipus Complex as an Explanation of Hamlet's Mystery: A Study in Motive," *American Journal of Psychology*, 21 (January 1910), 72–113.
⁷ For Putnam's review see *Journal of Abnormal Psychology*, 5 (June–July 1910), 114–115.

105
Jones to Putnam
[February 12, 1910]

Feb. 12/10.
407 Brunswick Avenue,
Toronto

Dear Dr. Putnam.

I apologize for the delay in answering your letter,¹ but I was daily expecting to hear from August Hoch, to whom I wrote a fortnight ago. I have not yet heard from him, and have written to Macfie Campbell to find out if he has turned up.² As soon as I hear I will let you know. With regard to your Toronto paper I think you kindly agreed to take up the Aetiology *and Treatment* of the Psychoneuroses. If you deal with the principles of psychoneurosis and conversion, and especially tackle the vexed sexual question, I shall feel freer to refer to the *specific* aetiology of the individual neuroses, only however briefly mentioning it. I shall stick more to the question of classification, and the psychopathological basis for this.³ Don't you think it might be worth while for us to interchange our papers beforehand?

I am deeply obliged to you for kindly promising to review my Hamlet article.⁴ I sent you a reprint this week, and hope it may interest you, though of course there is nothing new in it.

Neither Brill nor I can get to Nuremberg, so that we must postpone making an American contingent until perhaps next year.

I have just read Gross' Über psychopathische Minderwertigkeiten (Braumüller);⁵ it is remarkably original and interesting and well worth your attention.

With kind regards

Yours very cordially
Ernest Jones

¹ Putnam's letter is missing.

² Charles Macfie Campbell (1876–1943) psychiatrist at the Psychiatric Institute of the New York State Hospitals, professor of psychiatry, The Johns Hopkins University, 1914–1920, and from 1920, director of the Boston Psychopathic Hospital and professor of psychiatry at Harvard Medical School.

³ Putnam, "On the Etiology and Treatment of the Psychoneuroses"; and Jones, "A Modern Conception of the Psychoneuroses," *Interstate Medical Journal,* 17 (August 1910), 567–575; PPsa, eds. 1–3, 417–428. Both papers were read before the Canadian Medical Association, Toronto, June 1, 1910.

⁴ "The Oedipus Complex as an Explanation of Hamlet's Mystery." For Putnam's review see *Journal of Abnormal Psychology,* 5 (June–July, 1910), 114–115.

⁵ Otto Gross, [Concerning Psychopathic Inferiorities], Vienna and Leipzig: Braumüller, 1909.

106
Jones to Putnam
[April 9, 1910]

April 9/10.
407 Brunswick Avenue,
Toronto

Dear Dr. Putnam.

Many thanks for your abstract. I wish I were getting on with my article as rapidly as you seem to be with yours. By the way I notice you say "there are several psycho-analytic methods," one of which is Freud's. Surely this refers to several methods of making a psychological analysis, for one must give Freud the exclusive priority to at least the name "psycho-analysis," if only to avoid confusion. For instance Prince often writes of having made psycho-analyses of his patients,¹ which only causes misapprehension in the minds of his readers, for how are they to know that he has never spent five minutes making a psycho-analysis a procedure they naturally associate with the method legitimately known as Freud's? I can foresee all sorts of amateur claims and confusions in the future if we relax strictness in this. It sounds very presumptuous of me to say so, but do you think your note should stand in view of this consideration?

I quite agree with you as to the need for something to supplement the Ψ–A. method, though I feel it will have to be something of a non-medical nature. I find ΨA quite adequate to solve all internal conflicts, and cure the resulting troubles; where its effect is limited is in the case of external conflicts, though even here I think it enables the patient to face these and, by understanding, to gain some control over his reactions to external situations far better than any therapeutic measure. The next step we need is a *social* one, but that is a big subject — relation of parents to children, sex questions etc.

By the way you don't forget you have aetiology as well as therapeutics to deal with, do you? ²

With many thanks

Yours very cordially

Ernest Jones

¹ See Prince, "The Psychological Principles and Field of Psychotherapy" in Frederic H. Gerrish et al., *Psychotherapeutics* (Boston: Richard G. Badger, 1909), pp. 40–41.

² Putnam read "On the Etiology and Treatment of the Psychoneuroses" in Toronto.

107

Jones to Putnam

[June 19, 1910]

June 19/10.

407 Brunswick Avenue,

Toronto

Dear Dr. Putnam.

I am extremely sorry but I can't find your last letter any where.¹ I know you asked me several questions in it, of which I can only recall two. Possibly the ones I have "forgotten" may explain my "misplacing" the letter.

As to stammering, I think the services of a speech teacher are very useful for speech defects (stammeln), but not for stammering (Stottern) for he is too likely to introduce wrong psychological attitudes. The exercises are of no very great value, rather a faute de mieux. There are several books by Gutzmann; those by Albert are better than those by the older Gutzmann.² I think the most useful practical books on the subject are by Denhardt, and A. Liebmann; Sikorski's is the best historically.³

I enclose copies of my association tests. They have, you will see, a number of interpolated critical words, but they are faulty in two chief respects. (1) there are too many substantives. (2) the order I find by experience to be not carefully enough selected, in that some words usually produce responses which are apt by perseveration to influence subsequent reactions. I am getting out a better series when I have time. Jung's are not suitable in English, for linguistic reasons.[4]

Have you read Freud's Leonardo book yet?[5] It has a very dainty analysis, with all sorts of suggestive remarks in it. What a lot there is to learn!

Yours very sincerely,
Ernest Jones

[1] Missing.

[2] See, for example, Albert Theodor Karl Gutzmann, *Das Stottern und seine gründliche Beseitigung durch ein methodisch geordnetes, und praktisch erprobtes Verfahren. Eine Anleitung für Eltern und Lehrer, sowie zum Gebrauch für Erwachsene;* Hermann Albert Karl Gutzmann (1865–1922), *Die Sprachstörungen als Gegenstand des klinischen Unterrichts* (Leipzig: G. Thieme, 1905) and "Über das Stottern" in A. Gutzmann, *Das Stottern und seine gründliche Beseitigung* (Berlin, 1910), I, 128–150.

[3] Rudolf Denhardt, *Das Stottern. Eine Psychose* [Stuttering: A Psychosis], Leipzig: E. Keil's Nachfolger, 1890; Albert Liebmann, *Vorlesungen über Sprachstörungen* [Lectures on Speech Defects], *Die Pathologie und Therapie des Stotterns und Stammelns* [The Pathology and Treatment of Stuttering and Stammering], Berlin: O. Coblentz, 1898; Ivan Aleksandrovich Sikorski, *Über das Stottern* [On Stuttering], Berlin: A. Hirschwald, 1891. Ger. trans. Dr. V. Hinze.

[4] Like many analysts who had been influenced by Carl Jung at the Burghölzli Clinic in Zurich, Jones used word association tests as a preliminary method of uncovering his patient's complexes. See Carl Jung, "The Association Method," delivered at the celebration of the twentieth anniversary of the opening of Clark University, September 1909, trans. A. A. Brill, *American Journal of Psychology,* 21 (April 1910), 219–269; and *Diagnostische Assoziationsstudien: Beiträge zur experimentellen Psychopathologie* (Leipzig: J. A. Barth, 1906, 1910–1911, 1915); *Studies in Word-Association: Experiments in the Diagnosis of Psychopathological Conditions Carried Out at the Psychiatric Clinic of the University of Zurich under the Direction of C. G. Jung,* trans. M. D. Eder (New York: Moffat, Yard, 1919).

[5] *Eine Kindheitserinnerung des Leonardo da Vinci* [Leonardo da Vinci and a Memory of His Childhood], *Schriften zur angewandten Seelenkunde,* VII (Leipzig and Vienna: F. Deuticke, 1910); SE, XI, 57–137.

108
Jones to Putnam
[June, 27, 1910]

June 27.
407 Brunswick Avenue,
Toronto.

Dear Dr. Putnam.

Freud's Leonardo da Vinci is the last number of the Schriften z. ang. Seelen Kunde.¹ Don't you take them regularly?

I am very fond of Der Witz² and think it shows Freud at his best. The clearness of the first part and the extraordinary way he generalises such a mass of apparently disparate facts, picking out the essential, is very striking. The second part has a number of very profound thoughts. The book is over neglected. It is a good one to recommend to psychologists.

Would you mind letting me know when Adler's paper came out.³ I don't think I have seen it.

Many thanks for your test words, which I am going to try. They strike me as very good, except that the variation in syllabic length is rather great.

My Father had to go home suddenly soon after you were here. My sister went later, and got to London last Saturday. On the same day to my great surprise I had a cable saying she was going to marry Trotter in a week's time.⁴ It was quite unexpected, but it will be an excellent match. You see the Old Country is not always slow.

My wife sends her kind regards, in which I heartily join.

Yours sincerely,
Ernest Jones.

P.S. Where have you been reading — any abstracts of mine?

¹ Freud edited this series of twenty monographs on applied psychology for the educated public between 1907 and 1925.

² Freud, *Der Witz und seine Beziehung zum Unbewussten* [Jokes and Their Relation to the Unconscious], Leipzig and Vienna: F. Deuticke, 1905; SE, VIII.

³ Alfred Adler, "Der psychische Hermaphroditismus im Leben und im der Neurose (Zur Dynamik und Therapie der Neurosen)" [Psychological Hermaphroditism in Life and in Neurosis (On the Dynamics and Therapy of the Neuroses)], *Fortschritte der Medizin,* 28 (April 21, 1910), 486–493.

⁴ Jones's sister Elizabeth married his friend the British surgeon Wilfred Trotter (1872–1939). See Jones, *Free Associations,* p. 181.

109
Jones to Putnam
[July 1, 1910]

July 1.
407 Brunswick Avenue,
Toronto.

Dear Dr. Putnam.

Many thanks for sending me Adler's article.[1] I want to read it yet again before returning it, but shall not keep it long. I wish these Vienna people were better at sending reprints. I used to take the Fortsche. der Med., for its neurological abstracts are especially well done, but have dropped it lately; one must draw the line somewhere.

I have not had enough experience to confirm all Adler's remarks, and one or two of them strike me as very doubtful, especially his acceptance of laryngeal symptoms as feminine. It is however an exceedingly suggestive and important line of thought, and I fully agree with the great significance of mental hermaphrodism in children. I suffered badly from it myself, in ways too numerous to write. I will only mention one half-sublimated effect, which may interest you. I can trace my excessive interest in hemiplegia* [2] and allochiria, on which subjects most of my work has been done, only a tithe of which is published,[3] to the same source i.e. which is it, right or left, male or female? I say half-sublimated, for the best test that it was not fully so is the fact that there was a distinct Zwang[4] about it, irritation at being interrupted, passionate ardour, etc. There are obviously grades in success of sublimation, a point that deserves special study; it would suit your genius, and I humbly recommend it to you.

I will send your kind message to my father.

Yours very cordially
Ernest Jones

[1] "Der psychische Hermaphroditismus."
[2] On the left margin Jones wrote, " * I think you have my earlier papers on this subject."
[3] Hemiplegia, paralysis of one side of the body. Allochiria, a transference of sides in the localization of sensation. See, for example, Jones, "The Precise Diagnostic Value of Allochiria," *Brain*, 30 (1907), 490–532, "Allochiria," *Lancet* (September

21, 1907), pp. 830–837, "The Significance of Phrictopathic Sensation," *Journal of Nervous and Mental Disease,* 35 (July 1908), 427–437.
    4 Compulsion.

110
Jones to Putnam
[July 12, 1910]

> July 12/10.
> 407 Brunswick Avenue,
> Toronto

Dear Dr. Putnam.

I am sending the "Leonardo" by even post. I had two copies, one ordered and one sent by Freud, but I have presented the other to a friend in England, so I will ask you kindly to return this one — quite at your leisure.

I do not think there are any analyses published of alcoholism. There have been several casual references to it, which I cannot place; the fullest account, however, is in Abraham's paper in the Zeitschrift für Sexualwissenschaft, 1908.¹ (I have no copy I could send you, but the whole journal is worth buying. It only ran one year, being then incorporated in Sexual Probleme.) Probably you have read it.

I cannot suggest anything about Laocoon. It is worth working out. Have you read Lessing's Laocoon? ² What did you think of my remark about my interest in hemiplegia, etc.? ³

As to the branch society I agree that the A. Pp. A. fills the bill at present.⁴ We are too few to make it worth while to organise a new society. On the other hand it would please Freud if we simply got up a *formal* branch of the Internat. ΨA Verein, and it might strengthen their hands a little. We could hold a short meeting once a year just before the A. Pp. A., and in a couple of years should be large enough to hold more definite meetings. It might also be of service in co-ordinating our work a little, and exchanging experiences and views. On the whole, therefore, I am in favour of forming a branch. Jung is in charge of the whole matter, and perhaps you could get details of it from him.⁵

> Yours very sincerely
> Ernest Jones

P.S. When do you take your holidays?

[1] Karl Abraham, "Die psychologischen Beziehungen zwischen Sexualität und Alkoholismus" [The Psychological Relations between Sexuality and Alcoholism], *Zeitschrift für Sexualwissenschaft*, 8 (1908), 449–458; *International Journal of Psychoanalysis*, 7 (1926), 2–10; in Karl Abraham, *Selected Papers of Karl Abraham, M.D.*, trans. Douglas Bryan and Alix Strachey (London: The Hogarth Press and the Institute for Psycho-Analysis, 1927, 1942, 1950; and New York: Basic Books, 1953), pp. 80–89.

[2] Gotthold Ephraim Lessing (1729–1781), *Laokoon: oder über die Grenzen der Mahlerey und Poesie . . . mit beyläufigen erlauterungen verschiedener punkte der alten kunstgeschichte* [Laocoon, An Essay upon the Limits of Painting and Poetry in the History of Ancient Art], Berlin: C. F. Voss, 1766.

[3] See preceding letter.

[4] The American Psychopathological Association was founded by Ernest Jones and Morton Prince May 2, 1910, for physicians and psychologists interested in psychotherapy and psychopathology.

[5] Jung was elected president of the International Psychoanalytic Association at the Nuremberg Congress, held March 30–31, 1910.

111
Jones to Putnam
[July 18, 1910]

July 18/10.
407 Brunswick Avenue,
Toronto.

Dear Dr. Putnam.

I have just decided to cross this year after all, and leave tomorrow by the Lusitania — to return end of August. I shall probably see Freud in Holland where I am to stay with some relatives.[1] I shall read a paper[2] at the Internat. Congress of Med. Psychol. in Brussels (by invitation from Forel).[3] It will be a pleasant relaxation.

Yes, certainly, I have plenty of evidence about my self-analysis of rt. and lt., which I didn't give in my letter.[4] Your argument that on the contrary my interest "might be like that of Dana[5] and others" does not, I am afraid, much impress me, for I am not conceited enough to think that my complexes are unique. What do we know about the source of their interest, anyhow?

As to Adler I agree with you that there may be much in his idea, but it needs much working out. It does not seem very practically applicable at present, owing to the vagueness of the Minderwertigkeitbegriff.[6]

I hope you will have a very pleasant and refreshing holiday. With kindest Regards

Yours most sincerely

Ernest Jones.

[1] Freud was vacationing at Noordwijk.

[2] Jones, "The Therapeutic Effect of Suggestion." Read before the first International Congress of Medical Psychology and Psychotherapy, Brussels, August 8, 1910. See *Journal de Psychologie und Neurologie* (Leipzig), 17 (1910), Ergänzungsheft [Supplement], 427–431; *Canadian Journal of Medicine and Surgery*, 29 (February 1911), 78–87.

[3] August Forel (1848–1931), Swiss psychiatrist and psychotherapist, predecessor of Eugen Bleuler as director of the Burghölzli, Zurich, and professor of psychiatry at the University of Zurich. He had spoken at Clark University in 1899 and had met Putnam then. See Putnam to Adolf Meyer, May 9, 1899, the Meyer Papers, The William H. Welch Library of Medicine, The Johns Hopkins University, and Ernest Jones to Forel, July 14, 1910, and July 18, 1910, in Hans H. Walser, ed., *August Forel, Briefe: Correspondance* (Bern and Stuttgart: Huber, 1968), pp. 407–408. Forel had founded the Society for Medical Psychology and Psychotherapy in Salzburg in 1909.

[4] See Jones to Putnam, July 1, 1910.

[5] Charles Loomis Dana (1852–1936), professor of neurology at Cornell University Medical College. Putnam's letter is missing.

[6] The concept of inferiority developed by Alfred Adler, who left the Vienna Psychoanalytic Society in 1911 and founded Individual Psychology.

112
Jones to Putnam
[August 14, 1910]

Aug/14/10.
The Portland Hotel.
London.
W.

Dear Dr. Putnam.

I thought you might care to have a few lines from me on my travels, which have been very enjoyable and interesting. I had a few days in London and Paris and then attended the Congress of French neurologists at Brussels.[1] It was unusually poor, but as a compensation we had a very agreeable three days tour (en auto) in the Ardennes. Then came the Internat. Congress of Med.

Psychol. at Brussels. Janet sent a paper, but didn't turn up. Bernheim, Forel, Vogt, Bérillon, Lévy, Hartenberg, Dupré, Mohr and thirty or forty others were there. The psycho-analysts were Seif of Munich (a most excellent man), Wittenberg (do.), Muthmann (Bad Nassau) and De Montet (Vevey).[2] Three quarters of the whole proceedings related to ΨA which again shows the paramount interest taken in it. The discussions were on the whole quite friendly and open, and often very entertaining. I think we more than held our own. There were many interesting signs of yielding resistance, e.g. Forel put sexuality back to the age of five instead of puberty, but not earlier, Vogt admitted that in the neuroses sexuality played the predominating "and colossal" role,[3] but doubted that it was quite essential, others said Freud's views were mostly discovered before so that he didn't deserve all the credit, etc. etc.

I then went to Noordwijk in Holland and passed three days with Freud. His health is greatly better, and he was in excellent form. He talked continuously and illuminating on every subject I put to him, so you may imagine it was a highly instructive treat to me. Ferenczi joins him there next week and they sail from Antwerp to Sicily to spend there three weeks. Freud was a little puzzled at not having got an answer from you.[4] He was very clear about our forming a local branch of the Verein, and produced the following argument which had struck me forcibly in America. We are so likely to have the work damaged by amateurs and charletans that it becomes necessary to protect our interests by enrolling those with some proper knowledge of the subject in a rather official Verein, which would therefore be *some kind* of guarantee in a general way that the members knew what they were talking or writing about. It further gives us the right to attend the Internat. meetings, to receive the Korrespond-Blatt,[5] etc. etc.

However, we must see in the fall. I hope you will enjoy your holiday and benefit greatly from it.
With kindest regards

Yours very sincerely
Ernest Jones.

P.S. I shall be in Toronto Aug. 28.

[1] For the proceedings, see *Archives de Neurologie*, 2, 8e série (September 1910), 182–200.

² The International Congress of Medical Psychology and Psychotherapy was held in Brussels, August 7–8, 1910. See August Forel, *Out of My Life and Work,* trans. Bernard Miall (New York: W. W. Norton Co., 1937), p. 282; *Journal de Psychologie und Neurologie,* 17 (1910), Ergänzungsheft [Supplement], 307–433; for the discussions of psychoanalysis, see esp. pp. 412–419. Of the participants Jones lists, the best known were Hippolyte Bernheim (1840–1914), French expert on hypnosis and suggestion, a founder of the Nancy School, with whom Freud had studied briefly; August Forel; Oskar Vogt (1870–1959), German neurologist, editor of the *Journal de Psychologie und Neurologie,* director of the Kaiser Wilhelm Institut für Hirnforschung; Ernest Dupré (1862–1921), professor of clinical psychiatry at the University of Paris; Leopold Löwenfeld (1847–1924), Munich neurologist and a friend of Freud.

³ In the left margin Jones wrote, "All were agreed about this." Jones's account, especially in regard to Vogt, is contradicted by the discussion cited in n. 2 above.

⁴ See, however, Putnam to Freud, [late July, 1910].

⁵ *Korrespondenzblatt,* the newsletter of the International Psychoanalytic Association. It was merged with the *Zentralblatt für Psychoanalyse* by the Weimar Congress in 1911.

113
Jones to Putnam

[September 9, 1910]

Sept. 9/10.
407 Brunswick Avenue,
Toronto.

Dear Dr. Putnam.

I was glad to hear from you, and to know you were enjoying your well-earned holiday. I shall be very interested in the outcome of your philosophic reflexions. It bespeaks well for ΨA. that it has a wide appeal, to men of very varied interests. Hart,[1] for instance, has primarily philosophic interests, though of a different camp from yourself. I was recently urging him to take up the study of the current theories of Space and Time, which will evidently have to be revised in the light of our knowledge of the unconscious.

I was very shocked to hear, from you of James' death,[2] as I had heard nothing about it. He was a noble fellow, and his influence will endure. Fortunately his day was past, so that his loss will only be a personal one — to his friends, not to Science.

Will you make a note to look up when you return two good articles by Hart and White respectively, the former in the July no. of the Journ. of Ment. Science, the latter in the Sept. no. of the Interstate Med. Journ.[3] Have you had the Jahrbuch forwarded to you? The most novel of its contents is a short note by Freud on Gegensinn in Words — a fascinating topic.[4] The reason why you do not figure more prominently in my Bericht über die englische Literatur is that it was written last December.[5]

At present I am hard at work on my Nightmare brochure, for the Schriften.[6] My out-pourings of articles will probably cease for a couple of years, for I have decided, on Freud's advice, to attempt a Text-book of Psychiatry.[7] Do not smile at the ambitiousness of the proposal, for it need not be very advanced for English readers. I think of dividing it into two volumes, psycho-neuroses and psychoses respectively. Do you think that might work?

The Leonardo turned up safely. Thanks. I gather that we have decided to constitute a formal Ortsverein of the Internat. ΨA. Verein.[8] I strongly feel the necessity of some such formal move to counteract the numerous amateurs who are already beginning to spring up, and who will do the cause much harm. Membership will constitute some kind of guarantee that the person has at least some actual knowledge of the subject. I suggest that we send a simple little circular to the following, inviting their adherence. Stanley Hall, Hoch, Macfie Campbell, Holt, Hart, White, Coriat.[9] We must take in Meyer *if he desires it*, but need hardly ask him. Karplus and Ricksher I am rather against.[10] You must of course be President, but we mustn't bother you with more of the detailed work than is necessary. I suppose that you, Brill [11] and myself can constitute a temporary Committee till we hold a meeting; or do you think Hoch should be asked as well (I have said nothing to him on the matter.). I don't know if it will be necessary to have a secretary; if so, it would have to be Brill or myself, as we are in touch with the people in Europe. Brill has many claims in front of me, no doubt, but I am not sure that he would be in better touch than I would with such men as Hoch, Hall, White, etc. Still I am sure that there need be no feeling of competition, as it is too unimportant. If you agree I will draw up a circular as suggested, to be sent to you and Brill for revision and to be signed by us three. Would you propose any other names? Let me know your views on these points at your leisure.

It must be delicious in the woods just now. Toronto is more hateful than ever, after Europe.

With kindest Regards

Yours very sincerely

Ernest Jones

[1] Bernard Hart (1879–1966), British psychiatrist and psychopathologist.

[2] William James died August 26, 1910. Putnam's letter is missing.

[3] Bernard Hart, "The Psychology of Freud and His School," *Journal of Mental Science*, 56 (July 1910), 431–452; William Alanson White, "The Theory, Methods and Psychotherapeutic Value of Psychoanalysis," *Interstate Medical Journal*, 17 (September 1910), 643–655.

[4] "Über den Gegensinn der Urworte. Referat über die gleichnamige Broschüre von Karl Abel" [The Antithetical Sense of Primal Words. Review of a Pamphlet of That Name by Karl Abel], *Jahrbuch*, 2 (1910), 179–184; SE, XI, 153–161.

[5] "Bericht über die neuere englische und amerikanische Literatur zur klinischen Psychologie und Psychopathologie."

[6] "On the Nightmare," *American Journal of Insanity*, 66 (January 1910), 383–417. Constitutes part I of Jones, *Nightmares, Witches, and Devils* (New York: Liveright, 1951), pp. 13–54.

[7] Jones never wrote this proposed textbook.

[8] Local branch of the International Psychoanalytic Association.

[9] Of this group, previously unidentified are: Granville Stanley Hall (1844–1924), president of Clark University; Edwin Bissell Holt (1873–1946), assistant professor of psychology, Harvard University; William Alanson White (1870–1937), director of St. Elizabeth's, the Government Hospital for the Insane, Washington, D.C., from 1903 to 1937; Isador Coriat (1875–1943), Boston psychopathologist and later a psychoanalyst.

[10] Morris Jacob Karpas (1879–1918), neurologist, who became a charter member of the New York Psychoanalytic Society; Charles Ricksher (b. 1879), psychiatrist, who became a charter member of the New York Psychoanalytic Society and was then on the staff at Manhattan State Hospital, Ward's Island.

[11] Abraham Arden Brill (1874–1948), New York psychoanalyst, Freud's first official translator into English, who became the leader of the American psychoanalytic movement.

114

Putnam to Jones

[September 14, 1910]

IX.14.

106 Marlborough Street

Dear Doctor Jones

Thank you for your letter. I have ordered the Jahrb.[1] forwarded and shall read it with grt. pleasure. I brought up Karl Pearson[2] and some books on the Hegel philosophy, and was deep in them when I was invited [in fact I was on the point of suggesting the same thing] to write a paper on James for the Atlantic Monthly.[3] This I have largely done, but I am starting to look over his books again, a delightful but often not especially profitable task. I do not accept his philosophy any more than you do, but I love the man and believe it true, as he says, that it always will be true that 'temperament' will give the bias to reasoning. I am puzzled to know whether I am blind and crazy in believing that my views about the nature of mind and the necessary presuppositions of all thinking go back even of the deductions from the discoveries of ΨA. I must get my slow mind working clearly and then talk with you about the matter. As I feel at present, I am inclined to write a critical review of Hart's excellent article on conceptual thinking.[4]

I agree with you in all you say about the branch society, though I suppose Prince will not like it.[5]

Indeed we have drifted a little apart for the moment (I fear), for which I am very sorry.[6]

Do be secretary yourself. It will be better on all grounds. I respect Brill and have written an *envoi* for his translation of the Drei Abhandlungen.[7] But he writes atrocious 'English' (if one must call it such) and would not give us as good standing as you could.

I am very glad to hear of your proposed book.

It is plain that a deeper knowledge of the Unconscious must underlie *every* thorough study of the mind, in illness or in health. The division into ps.^{ses} and ps.n^{ses} seems imperative.[8] There is surely a gulf, though not a wall, between — for example — the sadness of even a moderate 'true' melancholic phase of a manic-depressive, constitutional condition, and the sadness of neurasthenia. Of course, I believe that the ps.an. of the distant future, and still more the ps.therap., will have to consider not only the origin but the destiny, of our mental life as we see it. I do not think that, as intelligent men, we are justified in going on without framing a view of the nature of universe. Or, to put it in another way, I do not now see how we can think without studying the necessary conditions of thinking, nor how, if we do that, we can help arrival at universal laws, and at the conclusion that the universe is personal in *all* its parts.

Sincerely
James J. Putnam

¹ See preceding letter where Jones had advised Putnam to read Freud's "Über den Gegensinn der Urworte."

² Karl Pearson (1857–1936), British mathematician, a founder of modern statistics, and author of *The Grammar of Science* (1892).

³ "William James," *Atlantic Monthly,* 106 (December 1910), 835–848.

⁴ Bernard Hart, "The Conception of the Subconscious," *Journal of Abnormal Psychology,* 4 (February–March 1910), 351–371.

⁵ See preceding letter; Prince to Putnam, November 22, 1910.

⁶ On the left margin Putnam wrote, "I think we ought to get Hoch into the committee if we can." See preceding letter.

⁷ "Introduction to Brill's Translation of Freud's *Drei Abhandlungen zur Sexualtheorie*" [Three Contributions to the Theory of Sex], Nervous and Mental Disease Monograph Series No. 7 (New York: Nervous and Mental Disease Publishing Co., 1910), pp. ix–xii.

⁸ Jones considered dividing his proposed book into two volumes, one on the psychoses, the other on the psychoneuroses. See preceding letter.

115
Jones to Putnam
[September 23, 1910]

Sept. 23/10.
407 Brunswick Avenue,
Toronto

Dear Dr. Putnam.

Just a word about your postscript.¹ It was very kind of you to express the wish that I were in Boston. My attitude to the question is a very simple one. I should decidedly prefer to be in Boston than here, largely on account of the more active and congenial intellectual life there, but it would be folly for me to think of coming unless it were made worth while. I have got known here in the past two years, and am consolidating my practice; I have been promised an Assoc. Professorship and expect to get it at the Senate meeting in a week or two. To go to Boston means in addition losing six months over examinations (gynecology, materia medica etc.) as well as a huge cost in transportation and damage to my library and furniture.

Southard ² at one time seemed very keen on having me, and sounded me in detail, but from his hostile attitude in Washington and New York last May (altogether, I think, on account of my Freudian views). I surmised he had changed his mind, and dismissed the matter from my thoughts.

I might add that I am now negociating to build a house which will take all my capital, and expect to buy the "lot" for it next week. Therefore if there is any definite proposal in view I should naturally like to have some idea of it as soon as possible, for later on my being so firmly rooted here would exert an almost decisive influence with me.

With kind regards

Yours vy. sincerely
Ernest Jones

[1] Putnam's letter is missing.
[2] Elmer Ernest Southard (1876–1920), Bullard Professor of Neuropathology at Harvard Medical School, 1909–1920, and director of the Boston Psychopathic Hospital which opened in 1912.

116
Jones to Putnam
[September 27, 1910]

Sept. 27/10.
407 Brunswick Avenue,
Toronto

Dear Dr. Putnam.

I enclose for your correction the tentative circular, and list. When you have amended or added to it will you send it on to Brill (97. Central Park West: N.Y.) and ask him to return it to me, so that it may be sent out.[1] We will of course all sign it, and I have written to Hoch to ask him if he will join in this.

As to philosophy, well you know my disgracefully empiric position in the matter. It proves at least one thing, that it is possible for a relatively sane person to get along without a philosophy. I strongly suspect that at present all philosophies are but the refined and intellectualised projections of personal complexes, and that we shall only get light on the more ultimate problems from thinkers who have first performed a careful self-analysis — in fact just those who are at present most shy of such problems. I hope this does not shock you; it is the attitude of a very plain man.

I really don't know about the gulf between the psycho-neuroses and the psychoses.[2] It seems to me that the main distinction is a purely practical one based on the greater loss in the psychoses of

the corrective power of consciousness over internal complexes (?
weaker inhibiting censure or stronger complexes). At all events
the pure clinicians are rapidly breaking down the separation, e.g.
between M.D. insanity via cyclothymia and "constitutional Verstimmung" [3] and hysteria. Cf. an excellent article by Reiss in the
Zeitschr. Neur. Psychiatr. Originalien Bd. II. S. 347.[4]

Which article of Hart's did you refer to as suggesting a criticism.
Have you seen his in the Jour. of Ment. Sc. for July? [5]

Will you be kind enough to let me have a reprint of your paper
in the Boston J. of July, as I do not take the Journal? [6]

Very sincerely yours
Ernest Jones.

[1] An invitation to join in founding an American branch of the International
Psychoanalytic Association; see Jones to Putnam, September 9, 1910.

[2] See Putnam to Jones, September 14, 1910.

[3] Depression.

[4] E. Reiss, "Konstitutionelle Verstimmung and manisch-depressives Irresein;
klinische Untersuchungen über den Zusammenhang von Veranlagung und Psychose"
[Constitutional Depression and Manic-Depressive Insanity; Clinical Research on the
Relationship between Constitution and Psychosis], *Zeitschrift für die gesamte
Neurologie und Psychiatrie*, 2 (1910), 347–628.

[5] "The Psychology of Freud and His School."

[6] "On the Etiology and Treatment of the Psychoneuroses."

117
Jones to Putnam

[October 11, 1910]

Oct. 11/10.
407 Brunswick Avenue,
Toronto.

Dear Dr. Putnam.

Thank you for the reprint. I read it again with the greatest
enjoyment. As to my Epilepsy paper, I am sending a copy by
this post.[1]

Many thanks for the information re the Psychopathic Clinic,
etc. I gathered from Hoch that Southard would, from his position as Director, become Professor of Psychiatry. It sounds logical,
though it is a pity that his psychiatric training has been along
such narrow and non-clinical lines.

I haven't seen Ellis' paper, but will look it up. He recently sent
me a reprint from the Pop. Sc. Monthly on Symbolism in Dreams.
I presume you have read his new volume on Sex and Society?[2] It
is very fundamental, bold, calm and yet conservative. I think I
agree with about all of it, and should be most interested to hear
your opinion of it.

Brill tells me (a letter received today) that he has not yet got
the circular from you.[3]

I should be against either Taylor or Waterman[4] being asked
to sign it, for we want not so much a petition, as in the case of
the A. Pp. A.,[5] as a more authoritative document. I am even very
dubious about the wisdom of accepting them at all, at least for
the present. Taylor is a broadminded and highly capable man,
and has a sympathetic attitude, though he does not seem very interested in psychological questions. Is he taking up psychoanalysis any
more than before? Waterman, on the other hand, is rather disappointing. Last May he showed to me very great resistances
against psychoanalysis (I think personal, for he has strong complexes), and a complete ignorance of the subject. When one finds
a young neurologist so wrapped up in practice that he won't even
take the trouble of learning German — and how can one begin
neurology without that first indispensable step? — it is not very
hopeful. However it is our duty to be as charitable as possible,
and personally I should like nothing better than to hear of some
evidence that he was taking a real interest in psychopathology,
especially psychoanalysis. By the way, Coriat has written a good
article for the St. Paul's Med. J.,[6] which you have probably seen.
His last article in the Journ. of Abn. Psychol. was "recht
schwach." [7]

With kindest Regards

Yours very sincerely
Ernest Jones

P.S. Would you kindly let me have Holt's[8] initials and address.
Hitschman has asked me to find a translator for his recent book
"Freuds Neurosenlehre." [9] Could you suggest anyone?

---

[1] Ernest Jones, "The Mental Characteristics of Chronic Epilepsy." Read before
the National Association for the Study of Epilepsy, Baltimore, May 7, 1910. *Maryland
Medical Journal,* 53 (July 1910), 223–229; PPsa, 2nd ed.

[2] Henry Havelock Ellis, M.D. (1859–1939), editor of *Contemporary Science,* 1889–

1915; author of *The Psychology of Sex*, seven vols., 1897–1928. See *Sex in Relation to Society, Studies in the Psychology of Sex*, VI (Philadelphia: F. A. Davis Co., 1910), and "The Symbolism of Dreams," *Popular Science Monthly*, 77 (July 1910), 42–55, esp. p. 49.

[3] Announcing the foundation of an American branch of the International Psychoanalytic Association. See Jones to Putnam, September 9, 1910, and September 27, 1910.

[4] Edward Wyllys Taylor (1866–1932), Putnam's successor as professor of neurology at Harvard Medical School; George Waterman (1873–1960), Boston neurologist and Putnam's former assistant.

[5] The American Psychopathological Association.

[6] "Hysteria in the Light of the Analytic Method," *St. Paul Medical Journal*, 12 (September 1910), 413–425.

[7] Very feeble. "The Psycho-analysis of a Case of Sensory Automatism," *Journal of Abnormal Psychology*, 5 (August–September 1910), 93–99.

[8] Edwin Bissell Holt, author of *The Freudian Wish and Its Place in Ethics* (New York: Henry Holt and Co., 1915), one of the first popular books about psychoanalysis.

[9] Eduard Hitschmann (1871–1957), Viennese psychoanalyst; see *Freuds Neurosenlehre: Nach ihrem gegenwärtigen Stande zusammenfassend dargestellt* [Freud's Theories of the Neuroses: A Synthesis of His Present Conceptions], Leipzig and Vienna: F. Deuticke, 1911, published as *Freud's Theories of the Neuroses*, authorized trans. Charles R. Payne, Nervous and Mental Disease Monograph Series No. 11 (New York: Journal of Nervous and Mental Disease Publishing Co., 1913).

118

Jones to Putnam

[October 13, 1910]

Oct. 13.
407 Brunswick Avenue,
Toronto

Dear Dr. Putnam.

I have just read Prince's article on dreams,[1] which is quite interesting, but which through the weight of his authority may do much harm in giving a false impression of his having thoroughly investigated Freud's theory. (When I last saw him — after this paper was written he had not read the Traumdeutung).[2] I am writing to ask you if you would think it advisable for either you or me to send a few comments on it to the next number of the Journal.[3] The lines that occurred to me as being expedient to follow are: congratulation that such an eminent man as Prince sees the importance of dream study; importance of it in general; ready accessibility of material, value of self-analysis etc.: protest against Prince's use of the term psychoanalysis; question of technique; fact that all his analyses may be true and his interpretation correct without excluding possibilities of deeper ones (layers of mind etc.); correction of one or two misunderstandings, etc.

I should be glad to hear from you at your early convenience, as to catch the next number demands some haste.

Yours very sincerely

Ernest Jones

[1] "The Mechanism and Interpretation of Dreams."

[2] Freud, *Die Traumdeutung* [The Interpretation of Dreams], Leipzig and Vienna: F. Deuticke, 1900; 2nd ed., 1909; SE, IV, V.

[3] See Jones, "Remarks on Dr. Morton Prince's Article: 'The Mechanism and Interpretation of Dreams,'" *Journal of Abnormal Psychology*, 5 (February–March 1911), 328–336.

119

Putnam to Jones

[October 14, 1910]

Dr. Ernest Jones,
    407 Brunswick Ave.,
        Toronto, Canada.

Dear Dr. Jones, —

You are certainly the most energetic, precise and prompt and efficient individual I have ever met. I only wish you could have brought me up by military discipline some fifty years ago.

It is a mistake about Southard's becoming professor of psychiatry. He recognizes that it would not be suitable and will only give such instruction as is needed to carry things along.

The list[1] goes to Brill today. I wanted to know what you would say about Waterman before sending it and did not suppose that there was immense haste.

Holt's address is E. C. Holt,[2] 13 Chauncy St., Cambridge, Mass., and his title is assistant professor.

As regards the translator, I would suggest Dr. Linenthal,[3] unless a better candidate turns up. As you may know, I love good English and do not believe that anyone can make a really good translator except somebody who is born to the language in which he is to work and who realizes that to make a good translation means to render the author's meaning in the best terms.

I think better of Waterman than you do. He certainly has complexes but he is earnest and interested and does fair work.

I enclose as a matter of interest, Freud's last note to me. It took me quite by surprise and gave me, of course, much pleasure.[4] I do feel that I have the theory of the matter fairly well rubbed in and that I am slowly getting a better touch in practice. Still, there are some cases that stick hard, especially those of the neurasthenic type, and I am continually conscious that the job could be done better than I do it. With kind regards,

Yours sincerely,
James J. Putnam

Oct. 14, 1910.

[1] The list of those invited to join the American branch of the International Psychoanalytic Association; see Jones to Putnam, September 9, 1910.

[2] Holt's correct initials are E.B.

[3] Henry Linenthal (1876–1954), Boston internist, who was graduated from Harvard Medical School in 1904, and in 1930 became professor of clinical medicine at Tufts College Medical School.

[4] See Freud to Putnam, September 29, 1910.

120
Jones to Putnam
[October 17, 1910]

Oct. 17/10.
407 Brunswick Avenue,
Toronto

Dear Dr. Putnam.

I am in the fullest agreement with the whole tone of your letter,[1] and quite share your "harmony-complex," if it is one. There are very few things in life that would give me greater pleasure than to find Prince coming over in our direction. In fact so strong is my wish that my heart makes me very optimistic about it, though my head makes me gravely doubt it, for he is so "logical" and argumentative that his attitude towards ψA is far from being the most satisfactory. As you know I am very averse to futile controversies, and am so eager to avoid the risk of getting Prince's back up that I will trespass on your kindness to the extent of asking you to read through critically my comments.[2] I have written to him complimenting him on being the first to make a step towards a rapprochement between the different points of view—he is really to be congratulated on that—, and asking permission, which I do not doubt he will give, to comment on his article.

I have also written a complimentary letter to Waterman[3] (as compension[4] for my remarks to you about him). He has struck an unworked field in the matter of symptoms dating from dreams, and if he has the ability to follow it up, will do some valuable work. Perhaps my opinion of him partakes a little of personal disappointment, in that when I was first in Boston I singled him out in my mind as being the most likely of the younger men to take up ΨA. How do you manage with him personally? Can't you help him over his difficulties and resistances in learning? Personal assistance and explanation is invaluable, isn't it?

I enclose Freud's letter.[5] His genuine appreciativeness is very characteristic of the man, and although you more than deserve his compliments it must have been none the less gratifying to you. By the way, how ever do you read his handwriting? I had to get my wife to translate it for me. I always make him write in English to me, which he very patiently does.

The trouble about Linenthal is that he knows nothing of ΨA, which is a grave disadvantage in a translator. However, I will see. Thank you for suggesting him.

The President of the University here has just got me an Associateship in Psychiatry, and has promised me a professorship in a year's time. As Clarke[6] doesn't like lecturing, I am to give all the lectures (once a week for six months), which will be rather onerous. I am promoted to the magnificent salary of *$100* a year.

Yours very sincerely
Ernest Jones.

[1] Missing.

[2] "Remarks on Dr. Morton Prince's Article: 'The Mechanism and Interpretation of Dreams.' "

[3] See Waterman, "Dreams as a Cause of Symptoms." Read at the first annual meeting of the American Psychopathological Association, Washington, D.C., May 2, 1910. *Journal of Abnormal Psychology*, 5 (October–November 1910), 196–210. See Jones to Putnam, October 11, 1910.

[4] Jones meant "compensation."

[5] Probably Freud to Putnam, September 29, 1910.

[6] Charles Kirk Clarke, M.D. (1857–1924), dean and professor of psychiatry in the University of Toronto.

121
Jones to Putnam
[October 20, 1910]

407. Brunswick Avenue.
Toronto.
Oct. 20/10

Dear Dr. Putnam.

My "forgetting" to enclose Freud's letter the other day was of course unconsciously motivated; it is not worth while relating how, for it concerns only a trivial matter between my wife and myself and had nothing to do with either you or Freud. It is certainly a letter to be proud of.[1]

I have had to spin out my remarks on Prince's article more than I intended.[2] I should be very glad to have your opinion of them (you can write corrections on the paper if you wish, for I have another copy). It has cost me an effort to tone it down, for the original draft was much more vigorous. The more carefully I read Prince's article the more annoyed I get at his presumptuousness in being sure we are all hopelessly wrong, and I can't forget his telling me last May (after the analyses were made and the paper written) that he had not yet read the Traumdeutung. Fancy his saying that the latent content is not always the fulfilment of a wish, but sometimes of an "aspiration." I believe my remarks have definitely convicted him in a sachgemäs[3] manner, and I sincerely trust he will take them in a true scientific spirit, putting personality aside. You will see from his enclosed letter[4] that he does not wish any public interpretation of the dreams, and indeed this is a most reasonable condition, and one which I had naturally thought of myself. I am sure that you can divine a good deal from the dreams and the associations (the temptations, the exhibitionism, the birth phantasies, the jealousy and strong transference to Prince, etc.).

Collins' article is really a staggerer, isn't it?[5] I have a private theory of the whole events in his mind, but it is too uncharitable to make it right for me to mention on the meagre evidence we have. One thing is fairly sure. Collins is a man who generally jumps on the right side of the fence, so we may surmise that in his opinion psychoanalysis is going to "arrive." I anticipate that he will remain now an advocate of Freud, but I may be quite wrong.

Have you read my review in the Jahrbuch, by the way?[6] It will be excellent to see your article in the Zentralblatt.[7]

Yours very sincerely
Ernest Jones.

PS. Would you be kind enough to let me have the ms back as soon as you conveniently can, for I am eager to send it in in time for the next number if possible.

E.J.

[1] See Freud to Putnam, September 29, 1910.
[2] "Remarks on Dr. Morton Prince's Article: 'The Mechanism and Interpretation of Dreams.' "
[3] Relevant.
[4] Missing, but see Prince to Putnam, October 21, 1910.
[5] Joseph Collins, "The Psychoneuroses: An Interpretation," *Medical Record* (New York), 78 (July 16, 1910), 87–92.
[6] Jones, "Bericht über die neurere englische und amerikanische Literatur zur klinischen Psychologie und Psychopathologie."
[7] Probably Putnam, "On the Etiology and Treatment of the Psychoneuroses," trans. Freud, "Über Ätiologie und Behandlung der Psychoneurosen," *Zentralblatt*, 1 (1911), 137–154.

122
Jones to Putnam
[November 6, 1910]

407. Brunswick Avenue.
Toronto.

Nov. 6.

Dear Dr. Putnam.

Many thanks for your letter.[1] I am very glad you thought my paper would suit. So far as I can judge from his letter Prince seems to have taken it all right, but I am a little afraid he may publish a counter-reply.[2] I hope he will consult you or me first, for otherwise he would probably argue about definitions and perpetuate misunderstandings in a way that would lead to endless — and not very profitable — public discussions. I am eager to know the result of your talk with him, and hope you may be able to keep in continual touch with him on the subject. You struck an important point when you referred to his living on the past, and being no longer engaged in practice. Still that might be turned against his resistance if you appeal to the natural "retiring" complex ("Surely you are not giving up etc.").

You ask me about the omission and alteration of letters in writing. I have no analytic experience of it, but would think of a general "innere Unsicherheit"[3] rather than a localised complex.

I will get hold of your sketch of James.[4] Did you read the very admirable one Claparède wrote in the last number of his Arch. de Psychol.?[5] I suppose you saw Bruce's silly paper on "Masters of the Mind" in the Nov. no. of the American Monthly, — it has a sickly adulation of Sidis.[6]

I will send with pleasure those of my non-psychiatric papers that may perhaps be of interest to the Social Service Dept.[7] I am addressing them to you in two packets; perhaps you will be kind enough to see about their proper distribution.

I got some reprints from Freud this week, and suppose you got the same. You must have been especially interested in the social aspects of his psychotherapy paper,[8] for he so rarely enters into such questions; I found the whole paper particularly suggestive, it opens up many lines of thought.

Yours very sincerely
Ernest Jones.

[1] Missing.

[2] See Prince, "The Mechanism and Interpretation of Dreams — A Reply to Dr. Jones," *Journal of Abnormal Psychology*, 5 (February–March 1911), 337–353.

[3] Inner insecurity.

[4] "William James."

[5] Edouard Claparède, "William James," *Archives de Psychologie*, 10 (1910), 96–105.

[6] H. Addington Bruce, "Masters of the Mind: Remarkable Cures Effected without the Aid of Drugs or Surgeon's Tools," *American Magazine*, 71 (November 1910), 71–81, one of the first popular articles to discuss psychoanalysis.

[7] The Social Service department of the Massachusetts General Hospital was established in 1905, and Putnam added psychiatric social work in 1907.

[8] See Freud, "Die zukünftigen Chancen der psychoanalytischen Therapie" [The Future Prospects of Psycho-Analytic Therapy], *Zentralblatt*, 1 (1910), 1–9; SE, XI, 139–151.

123

Jones to Putnam

[November 8, 1910]

407. Brunswick Avenue.
Toronto

Nov. 8/10.

Dear Dr. Putnam.

I fully agree and sympathise with you in the difficulties you describe, and can only trust that you will make them act as an incentive to efforts that will diminish or overcome them. How little the general profession know of the difficulties of the psychotherapeutist when they talk lightly of "only hysteria." The intrinsic ones we are on a fair way to overcome, and the extrinsic ones will be dealt with only after an educative campaign in the profession and public. The paper of Freud's I referred to in my later[1] of yesterday will be doubly welcome to you at such a juncture, and no doubt his approaching book on Methodik will give us many[2] help, and light in dark places.[3]

Now to answer more concretely, as best I can, the questions you put.

First, I am not at all hopeful about cases that one cannot see regularly, at all events three times a week. Once a week puts it quite out of the question, and all that one can then do is to be helped by one's general knowledge gained from analysis of similar cases. With patients attending three times a week I have had several very good results. I have a difficulty in understanding how you come to have so many patients who can attend only so rarely. Often one can see business men, etc., between five and eight.

One has to be cautious of course with patients such as the lady you mention, with a severe, long-standing neurosis, and with whom one cannot carry the matter through, but for a reason I will presently give, I don't think you need reproach yourself. I had last year a rather similar case, a lady who had been confined to bed for years. I treated her for eight months in a nursing home, and then funds gave out and she had to return home. We went slowly to work, owing to her prostration, but she got considerable benefit, although the secondary motives of krankheitsgewinne[4] were too strong to lift her out of her old groove — at least in that time.

You put an important question about the method of recovery, and you quite see the difficulty of describing cases from that point of view in detail. One point I would lay much stress on, and that is the extraordinary way patients get benefit *after* the whole treatment is over. Instances. Last winter I treated a girl of 25 for four months, when she had to return to her home in the South. At that time although most of her (hysterical) symptoms were better she was in such a depressed state that I felt not very happy about her future. She has regularly written to me since, and fully. After she had been home for a fortnight she began to feel her new capacity for dealing with her very unfortunate domestic squabbles, and ever since then says that she had never been so well in her life and is quite happy. (No external sublimation) Another case, a severe Zwangneurose[5] in a man of 24 who had been in consequence unable to work for months. I treated him for seven months, and when I left for Europe left him very tremulous about going to work. I saw him on my return in September and he is thoroughly successful in his work, also never felt so well in his life, had never known before what it was to be free and what an enjoyable world this could be, etc. These both show a marked Nachwirkung.[6]

The Abreagieren[7] is quite an antiquated idea, at all events in its original sense. As you remember, the conception arose in dealing with the discharge in hypnosis of massive affects; nowadays one doesn't see that. The truth that remains is that when patients *actually realise* a given important point they naturally show signs of emotion, and I suppose in occasional cases an eingeklemmte Affekt[8] may work itself off more explosively. Freud puts the change in technique very well when he says that nowadays our main efforts should be directed not so much to a blind Eindrängen[9] towards unknown memories, nor even the discovery of complexes, but to the divining of the cause of each resistance as it presents itself. One is as a rule slightly ahead of the patient, being more objective, and therefore can help him in penetrating his unconscious. Again an example: In giving me an infantile theory of the origin of children a patient recalled the idea of two vague supernatural huge figures behind a gooseberry bush who worked away together moulding some material between them till it took a child's form. They used for each not an arm or leg but a lump of flesh of a certain shape (which soon brought a penis — erect — to his mind). (I had formerly learnt that he imagined women had a penis as well as men. At the age of six when seeing his sister bathe he exclaimed: Look, it's been cut off and piled all round!) The material was brown, of a putty consistence, and *fell from them into something* (a vessel). He had not the faintest idea of the meaning of it all, but soon took it in when I pointed it out to him.

I think it is important not to argue with a patient. If they don't accept a point, the analysis of it is not completed. If they accept it with their lips, but not with their hearts, either they need a little time, or the analysis of it is not complete. One certainly demands considerable conscious effort on the part of the patient — or I would rather say, *attention.*

Your last question is the hardest. One must write, I suppose, on the aspects that spontaneously appeal to each of us as being capable of exposition. Your suggestion of a paper to family physicians strikes me as eminently practical and important. I am daily expecting the appearance of my paper on education in the Journal of Educational Psychology,[10] but that is addressed to teachers. I fancy sublimation would be much harder, but I know it is a pet theme of yours.

Prince has postponed my "remarks" till the February number, and as Friedländer's paper comes in that I shall add a footnote of a general character to meet it — a pretty vigorous one.[11] I know Friedländers will be an unpleasant pill for us to swallow, and we must prepare ourselves not to take it too much to heart.

I wish I could answer your letter more usefully; talking is so much better, but I am only too delighted if I can be of any service at all.

Yours,

E.J.

---

[1] Letter.

[2] Much.

[3] Freud planned a book on the technique of psychoanalysis which he did not complete. However, he published a series of essays on method beginning with "Die Handhabung der Traumdeutung in der Psychoanalyse" [The Handling of Dream Interpretation in Psychoanalysis], *Zentralblatt,* 2 (1911), 109–113; SE, XII, 83–171.

[4] Secondary gains from illness.

[5] Compulsion neurosis.

[6] Aftereffect.

[7] Abreaction.

[8] Strangulated affect.

[9] Searching.

[10] Jones, "Psycho-Analysis and Education," *Journal of Educational Psychology*, 1 (1910), 497–520; PPsa, eds. 1–2.

[11] Jones did not add the footnote. See Jones, "Remarks on Dr. Morton Prince's Article: 'The Mechanism and Interpretation of Dreams'" and A. Friedländer, "Hysteria and Modern Psychoanalysis," *Journal of Abnormal Psychology*, 5 (February–March, 1911), 297–319. First published as "Hysterie und Moderne Psychoanalyse," *Psychiatrisch-neurologische Wochenschrift*, 11 (1910), 393–396, 406–408, 424–426, 435–436, 442–445.

124
Jones to Putnam
[November 20, 1910]

407. Brunswick Avenue.
Toronto.

Nov. 20/10.

Dear Dr. Putnam.

I have just read with great pleasure your Washington paper in the Nov. no. of the J. N. M. D.[1] It will surely do much good. I had sent Freud a copy of the discussion of it in the Oct. no.,[2] thinking he might be interested to see it, though I expect he will say in regard to many of the objections raised what he once said in a similar connection (at Worcester): "I seem to have heard something of the kind before."

I have just got an invitation to give an address in January before the joint meeting of the Chicago Neurol. Soc. and the Chicago Med. Soc., and to stay with the President of the former (Hecht).[3] It is just the occasion for your broad way of dealing with the subject, and I eagerly wish I could borrow the use of your easy pen and graceful style. The more so, as I have selected a subject especially adapted to that, namely "Reflections on Some Criticisms of the ΨA Method of Treatment."[4] I have felt inclined to ask whether you would not go instead, but I suppose one should not shirk these things and I must do what I can. It is a good sign of the times, I think.

I want to say just a word about the translation of some passages in my suggestion article.[5] When Prince wanted me to translate them I held out, for a number of reasons that are not worth repeating. As a compromise he offered to get them translated, suggesting your name. I said I wouldn't dream of being so presumptuous as to give you the trouble, repeated my objections and left the whole matter in his hands. I heard nothing more about it till I got the proof not long ago. Then finding a few of the translations not *literal* enough for my special purpose I altered them back again. I did not know they were yours and naturally intended no reflection on your work, which was in fact too good an English translation for my purpose; further I want to apologise to you that you should have bothered yourself in the matter, and to assure you that it was against my wish.

Have you read Pfister's latest contribution to the Schriften, and do you know his earlier work? [6] It will be most interesting to see how his clerical colleagues receive it.

By the way, in your paper you twice write Seelenlehre for Seelenkunde.[7] Can you discover the source of your unconscious preference for the former?

With kindest regards

Yours very sincerely
Ernest Jones.

[1] "Personal Experience with Freud's Psychoanalytic Method," *Journal of Nervous and Mental Disease*, 37 (November 1910), 657–674.

[2] See *Journal of Nervous and Mental Disease*, 37 (October 1910), 630–639.

[3] D'Orsay Hecht (1874–1915), Chicago neurologist, associate professor of nervous and mental disease and medical jurisprudence, Northwestern University Medical School. See Hugh T. Patrick, "D'Orsay Hecht," *Journal of Nervous and Mental Disease*, 42 (October 1915), 657–659.

[4] "Reflections on Some Criticisms of the Psychoanalytic Method of Treatment." Read before a joint meeting of the Chicago Neurological Society and the Chicago Medical Society, January 18, 1911. *American Journal of the Medical Sciences*, 142, n.s. (July 1911), 47–57; in PPsa, eds., 1–3.

[5] "The Action of Suggestion in Psychotherapy," *Journal of Abnormal Psychology*, 5 (December 1910–January 1911), 217–254; PPsa, eds., 1–4.

[6] Oscar Pfister, *Die Frömmigkeit des Grafen Ludwig von Zinzendorf: ein psychoanalytischer Beitrag zur Kenntnis der religiösen Sublimierungsprozesse und zur Erklärung des Pietismus* [The Piety of Count Ludwig von Zinzendorf: A Psycho-Analytic Contribution to the Study of Religious Sublimation Processes and Pietism], *Schriften zur angewandten Seelenkunde*, VIII (1910).

[7] Seelenkunde, psychology; seelenlehre has didactic connotations equivalent to "psychological doctrine."

125
Jones to Putnam
[December 11, 1910]

Dec. 11./10.
407 Brunswick Avenue,
Toronto.

Dear Dr. Putnam.

I will answer your letter in a detached way, point by point.[1]

Freud's little paper[2] was certainly very stimulating to thought; he has a remarkable faculty that way. Did you not think that the first number of the Zentralblatt was very promising? [3] I have sent a short review of it to Prince for the Journal.[4] Could you find time to do the same for the Da Vinci brochure and for Pfister's (Heft 8 of the same series)? [5]

I should like to hear how your papers go off, and of course you will be kind enough to let me have reprints of them. Re the Amer. Med. Assoc. at Los Angeles you will not let that clash with the May meeting of the Psychopathological and Psychoanalytic, where your presence will be indispensable. They are to follow the Amer. Neurol. meeting. Do you yet know the date and place of this? Is Prince really accepting the Philadelphia proposal? It is very curious. I shouldn't be surprised to hear that some opposition from Dercum would drive him more into our camp.[6] He quite refused to discuss things with me, saying that there were forty statements of fact or theory that he objected to in my criticising article! [7] I have lately given him a rest, and left the steady hammering to you. Has it had much effect? What do you find to be his main objections?

With regard to the new Assoc.[8] I think it must surely strengthen the older one by arousing a greater interest in psychopathology. All our members will join it, except perhaps the pure psychologists. It will be practically as you say a wheel within a wheel, but it is impracticable to make it formally so owing to the need for union with Europe. Also there are so many questions that should be discussed, as Meyer[9] puts it, en famille. Acceptances are coming in well, and it looks as if we shall have 25 members straight off.

White, Meyer and Stanley Hall are very cordial in their support, especially Hall. The only refusal so far comes from Jelliffe.[10]

You must read an essay by Chase, Prof. of Phil. in N. Carolina, in the Sept. no. of the Pedagogical Seminary on Ψa and the Unconscious.[11] He gives a sympathetic account of Freud's work, but explains the facts in a curious way, excluding repression and mental conflict.

Many thanks for sending me your paper on James, which I found exceedingly interesting and human. It was a model example of how such obituary reviews should be written.

I am glad you agreed about the translating of the passage from Janet in my article.[12] Apart from general objections there were in this case special ones as well. I wanted to prove from Janet's writings that his findings point to the sexual nature of transference and hypnotism, although he does not draw that inference. It was therefore practically impossible to make a translation that would be fair to him, in not strengthening his expressions re sex, and at the same time to my argument by not weakening them. Literal quotation is always fairer, and really one cannot be expected to bother much about psychologists who do not read even French.

Dr. Reed's[13] letter to you is very gratifying, and I have sent him one of our circulars. Such an earnest and sympathetic interest is surely worth more than mere knowledge alone, for this is bound to follow in its train. I had a very similar letter from Dr. Curran Pope[14] of Louisville, with him I had previously had a little correspondence. By the way would you mind letting either Brill or myself have the reference to the article he refers to, so that it may be abstracted for the Zentralblatt.

I am glad to say that my practice is again picking up, and I have several patients from influential circles, including Z.[15]

Yours most sincerely

REPRINTS   Ernest Jones.

P.S. Reed's failures are possibly due to his failure to deal with the Übertragung,[16] at which he hints.

[1] Putnam's letter is missing.
[2] Probably Freud, "Die zukünftigen Chancen der psychoanalitischen Therapie."
[3] The *Zentralblatt für Psychoanalyse* was first published in September 1910.

⁴ See the *Journal of Abnormal Psychology*, 5 (February–March 1911), 356–357.

⁵ Freud, *Leonardo da Vinci*; Pfister, *Die Frömmigkeit des Grafen Ludwig von Zinzendorf.*

⁶ Francis Xavier Dercum (1856–1931), Philadelphia neurologist. See The Philadelphia Neurological Society, "Symposium on Freud's Theory of the Neuroses and Allied Subjects," February 24, 1911, *Journal of Nervous and Mental Disease*, 38 (August 1911), 491–497. The major speaker on behalf of psychoanalysis was Sidney I. Schwab, a St. Louis neurologist, who had graduated from Harvard Medical School in 1896 and had studied briefly with Freud. See Schwab, "An Estimate of Freud's Theory of the Neuroses and Its Value to the Neurologist," *Interstate Medical Journal*, 18 (September 1911), 938–948. See also Dercum, "The Role of Dreams in the Etiology of the Psychoneuroses," *Journal of the American Medical Association*, 56 (May 13, 1911), 1373–1376.

⁷ "Remarks on Dr. Morton Prince's Article: 'The Mechanism and Interpretation of Dreams.' "

⁸ The proposed American Psychoanalytic Association. See Jones to Putnam, September 9, 1910.

⁹ Adolf Meyer.

¹⁰ Smith Ely Jelliffe (1866–1945), New York neurologist, joined the American Psychoanalytic Association in 1912 and with William Alanson White founded the *Psychoanalytic Review* in 1913.

¹¹ Harry Woodburn Chase, "Psychoanalysis and the Unconscious," *Pedagogical Seminary*, 17 (September 1910), 281–327.

¹² Jones, "The Action of Suggestion in Psychotherapy," pp. 241–243.

¹³ Ralph Reed (1879–?), Cincinnati physician, who joined the American Psychoanalytic Association in 1912; see his "From Mesmer to Freud, A Review of Psychotherapy," *Cincinnati Lancet-Clinic*, 103 (April 2, 1910), 355–367.

¹⁴ Curran Pope (1866–1934) Louisville, Ky., physician, who joined the American Psychoanalytic Association in 1912.

¹⁵ Information to identify this patient has been withheld.

¹⁶ Transference.

126

Jones to Putnam

[December 30, 1910]

Dec. 30/10.
407 Brunswick Avenue,
Toronto.

Dear Dr. Putnam.

Would you be so good as to give me your advice in the following matter? The enclosed letter will explain itself. The proposal ¹ looks to me a hopeless undertaking, and I do not feel at all inclined to undertake it. It is evidently animated by a desire to harm our work rather by any serious desire to learn anything about it. Prince's presence might also be embarrassing, as he would be tempted to revenge himself for my criticism that would be published a fortnight before the meeting, and the opponents might make merry over our differences.² I am also afraid I should not cut a good figure under such circumstances, for owing to my juniority in years and standing I have not the equanimity I would wish. However I might go if I thought it would really do some good. Would you care for me to suggest that you went? They are evidently afraid of you, for they cannot jump on a man like you in the way they could on me. In any case I would be very grateful to have your views.

With best Xmas and New Year greetings from myself and wife.

Yours vy. cordially

Ernest Jones.

¹ The letter is missing. The proposal probably was an invitation to speak at a "Symposium on Freud's Theory of the Neuroses and Allied Subjects," held by the Philadelphia Neurological Society, February 24, 1911. Sidney I. Schwab defended psychoanalysis. See *Journal of Nervous and Mental Disease*, 38 (August 1911), 491–497.

² See Jones to Putnam, October 20, 1910.

127
Putnam to Jones
[January 5, 1911]

Dear Dr. Jones, —

If I, being a pacific individual, may suggest a little further, I should say that your cue, or rather our cue, is to overcome prejudice by the obtaining, so far as possible, the admission of certain fundamental principles, of which the following seem to me particularly important:

1 — Those who accept in general terms the work of Freud are not compelled to give their adherence to every statement or interpretation that he has made. I mention this because Prince seemed to think that we were so obliged.¹

2 — Freud's doctrines are not a "theory" but a series of provisional conclusions based on observations.

3 — The main purpose of psychoanalysis is to do in a more thorough manner what every conscientious physician strives to do by less good methods.

4 — Everyone, doctors and patients alike, ask whether there is

little therapeusis beyond making the analysis. To this I should say that personally I stimulate and set him to work, etc., etc., just as I did before, with increased hopefulness, because I am able to show him his troubles in a different light. I have just had a very remarkable case of this sort where the outlook seemed distinctly that of an incurable paranoia.

5 — The most important application of psychoanalysis is in the *serious cases* which nothing else will touch, or touch with equal effectiveness.

6 — Some of the special facts that cause so much animadversion, so far from being suggested, come out spontaneously in statements and reports of dreams, even dreams of young children.

Finally — I think from my experience at our local meeting a few weeks ago,[2] we ought to guard ourselves as carefully as possible from criticising other methods or minimizing their value.

I suppose you have seen the report of the Congress of Neurologists where Freud was thoroughly pitched into?[3]

Yours very truly,
James J. Putnam

Jan. 5, 1911.

[1] See Prince to Putnam, November 26, 1910.

[2] Putnam read a paper, "Studies in Psychoanalysis" to the Boston Society of Psychiatry and Neurology, December 15, 1910. See the Society's Minutes in the Francis A. Countway Library of Medicine, Boston.

[3] See proceedings of the fourth annual meeting of the Society of German Neurologists, Berlin, October 6–8, *Neurologisches Centralblatt,* 29 (November 16, 1910), 1262–1263, 1266, and *ibid.* (December 16, 1910), p. 1364.

128
Jones to Putnam
[January 8, 1911]

Jan. 8/11.
407 Brunswick Avenue,
Toronto.

Dear Dr. Putnam.

Many thanks indeed for your prompt and useful advice. It has had the effect of making me practically decide to accept the invitation, and I am writing to Allen tentatively to that effect.[1]

I think Prince is wise in not accepting, for he must by now realize that his judgement on the matter is not ripe enough to pronounce on it definitely. It is good that he is approaching us more, but I should not be inclined to underestimate the gulf that still separates us.

With principles enunciated in your second letter[2] I should of course agree, though probably I would prefer to state some of them in a slightly different way. For instance it is only *in some respects* that the aim of ΨA is the same as that of the physicians; if one defined it — and quite accurately — as the translation of mental processes from the unconscious to the conscious level, most physicians would not find much common in it and their endeavours. Still I see your point.

The principle I would be inclined perhaps to cavil at is the stress laid on the value of ΨA for the *most serious* cases. These are just the cases where the results are least satisfactory, though they are certainly better than with other methods. I would lay more stress on the value of ΨA for prophylaxis, in preventing slight cases from ever becoming serious. It seems to me that this is its true place, for no other method can effect this with the same certainty and precision.

Southard wants me to read a paper at Los Angeles,[3] but I am afraid it is too far for me. Besides you are going there and will do all that is necessary.

Addington Bruce[4] called on me recently. He did not impress me favourably.

Thank you very much for sending me Dr. Reed's[5] reprints, which I am returning. They are very promising.

With best wishes for the coming year

Yours very sincerely
Ernest Jones

[1] Putnam's letter of advice is missing. See Jones to Putnam, December 30, 1910.

[2] See preceding letter.

[3] The sixty-second annual session of the American Medical Association was held in Los Angeles, June 27–30, 1911.

[4] H. Addington Bruce (b. 1874), journalist, an editor of the *World's Work,* and popularizer of psychotherapy and mental healing. See Jones to Putnam, November 6, 1910, n. 5.

[5] See Jones to Putnam, December 11, 1910.

129
Jones to Putnam
[January 13, 1911]

Jan. 13/11.
407 Brunswick Avenue,
Toronto.

Dear Dr. Putnam.

Your points I shall find most useful in the preparation of my Chicago paper, which I am beginning tonight.[1] By an odd chance I was quite prevented from writing to Allen[2] on the day I last wrote to you, and on the next day I got your other letter and one from Prince strongly urging me not to accept. (A curious Verschreiben)[3] I then wrote to Allen, not absolutely refusing, but suggesting it be postponed till next year, when further general knowledge of the subject should make it riper for discussion; I have not yet had his reply.

You will be grieved to learn that this week very serious personal trouble has arisen here: to put it quite shortly, a woman whom I saw four times last September (medically) has accused me of having had sexual intercourse with her then, has gone to the President of the University to denounce me, is threatening legal proceedings, and has attempted to shoot me. At present I am being guarded by an armed detective.

She is a hysterical woman, who has been divorced for adultery, and whose main complaints on coming to me were (1) being haunted by erotic thoughts concerning a certain woman with whom she used to sleep (she is pronouncedly homosexual) and (2) general mental confusion and tension arising from fear that she might satisfy her desires by appealing to some man on the street. I did not treat her by Ψa, but got her to talk, tried to calm her etc. Unfortunately she had an acute fit of Übertragung[4] (she was a stranger here, and I was the first man she had spoken to for months), and made unmistakeable overtures. She broke off coming, in high dudgeon at being rebuffed, and I heard nothing of her for over four months. In the meantime she got into the hands of some doctors of doubtful reputation, as well as of a woman doctor of very severely strict views; the latter fell in love with her and it was reciprocated. They were people who had cooked up rumours about my "lax" views and harmful treatment (stupid stories about my prescribing adultery, illicit intercourse, etc.), and a regular incubation of delusions took place all round. I foolishly paid the woman $500 blackmail to prevent a scandal, which would be almost equally harmful either way.

You may imagine I am very worried indeed, and dreadfully tired, so I cannot go further into details. I have gone to the best lawyer here, and he is hopeful of pulling the matter through all right. Still!

With kind regards

Yours very sincerely
Ernest Jones.

P.S. I am writing a short note to Prince to the same effect.

¹ Jones, "Reflections on Some Criticisms of the Psychoanalytic Method of Treatment."
² Alfred Reginald Allen (1876–1918). Former assistant of Silas Weir Mitchell, Allen was one of the few Philadelphia neurologists sympathetic to psychoanalysis and became a member of the American Psychoanalytic Association in 1913. He was killed in the Great War. See Jones to Putnam, December 30, 1910.
³ Slip of the pen.
⁴ Transference.

130
Jones to Putnam
[January 23, 1911]

Jan. 23/11.
407 Brunswick Avenue,
Toronto.

Dear Dr. Putnam.

Thank you very much indeed for your sympathy, though I felt some of it beforehand.¹ I would of course have felt happier about the support of the medical profession here had I not known of the rancorous hostility towards and misunderstanding of my views as regards the sexual aspects of the neuroses. Indeed I have just heard that a chief instigator of this very woman was one of the three Professors of Medicine in the University. Fortunately it looks at present as if the trouble will subside. I am to see tomorrow the President of the University,[2] whose attitude towards the matter has been very sensible. Nothing else has happened, and my legal advisor is considering the question of writing a warning letter to the woman doctor who is responsible for the bother. He is a very reliable and shrewd man, and I feel safe in his hands. I am obliged for my wife's sake to keep detectives here, and it is that uncertainty that is one of the most trying aspects of the matter.

I don't know if you recollect an analysis I published eighteen months ago of a case of hypomania, with some sexual details. It has aroused the fiercest opposition here. The Provincial Minister to whose ears it has come had a stormy scene with Dr. Clarke about it last week, and declares he would have prevented such "filthy stuff" going through the mails had he known of it. It is likely that questions will be put concerning it in the House of Commons that meets this week.[3] The attitude in Canada towards sexual topics has I should think hardly been equalled in the world's history; slime, loathing, and disgust are the only terms to express it.

The Chicago expedition[4] was a great success, and I had a most cordial reception. You will be glad to learn that Patrick,[5] who is certainly the leading neurologist there, is definitely sympathetic to ΨA, having been converted, so he says, by your paper in Washington and the talks he had with me there. He has a young assistant[6] working at the treatment, who is really getting a proper grasp of the subject. Curran Pope was the only other man I met who seemed thoroughly to understand the principles. He is enthusiastic over it, but unfortunately is not a strong man otherwise. At the meeting all the speakers supported me, except Sidney Kuh,[7] who made a very stupid and ill-mannered attack. "He couldn't agree with Freud's logic that because Frauenzimmer in German means woman, therefore to dream of rooms means something sexual," etc. etc. Unfortunately for himself he laid himself badly open, and as I had much pent-up Affekt that was crying for Abreagieren[8] I let myself go, and exposed his ignorance mercilessly. It was perhaps not the most politic thing to do, but one is not always dictated by wisdom. The other neurologists enjoyed it immensely, and I became very popular, for Kuh seems to be greatly disliked.

Prince also appears to have been travelling. He tells me that he got Allen to see the difficulty of discussing ΨA in Philadelphia at a single meeting.

With kindest regards

Yours very sincerely
Ernest Jones.

[1] See preceding letter. Putnam's letter is missing.

[2] Sir Robert Alexander Falconer (1867–1943), an ordained minister of the Presbyterian Church in Canada and president of the University of Toronto, 1907–1932.

[3] Jones, "Psychoanalytic Notes on a Case of Hypomania," *American Journal of Insanity*, 66 (October 1909), 203–218. Sir James Pliny Whitney (1843–1914), was prime minister of Ontario, 1905–1914. The issue was not raised in the House. See *Official Report of the Debates of the House of Commons of the Dominion of Canada*, Third Session, Eleventh Parliament, 1–2 George V, vol. XCVIII, November 17–January 18, 1910–1911; vol. XCIX, January 19–February 20, 1911; vol. C, February 21–March 22, 1911 (Ottawa: Printed by C. H. Parmelee, printer to the King's Most Excellent Majesty, 1910–1911).

[4] Jones addressed a joint meeting of the Chicago Neurological Society and the Chicago Medical Society on January 18, 1911, on "Reflections on Some Criticisms of the Psychoanalytic Method of Treatment."

[5] Hugh T. Patrick (1860–1939), Chicago neurologist, president of the American Neurological Association in 1907.

[6] Possibly Ralph Hamill (1877–1961), who studied in Vienna after graduating from Rush Medical College in 1902. He was assistant to Hugh T. Patrick and a founding member of the American Psychoanalytic Association.

[7] Sidney Kuh (1866–1934), Chicago neurologist.

[8] Abreaction.

131
Jones to Putnam
[February 5, 1911]

Feb. 5/11.
407 Brunswick Avenue,
Toronto.

Dear Dr. Putnam.

My troubles seem to be slowly settling, provided that no fresh explosion takes place. The woman doctor again called on the President and urged him to save the youth of Toronto by dismissing me, but he told her he was convinced the whole story was nonsense and flatly advised her to keep her mouth shut otherwise she would find herself involved in a serious legal action. I had a most satisfactory interview with him. We are collecting information about the patient's past, and hope to get her deported as an undesirable alien. She is certainly very psychopathic, is a morphinomaniac, has attempted suicide, quarreled with all her employers etc.

Your warm-hearted sympathy has been of the greatest help to me, and Prince was equally kind.

The racial question you raise is a very involved one. You know that in England we take the opposite view, and make a byword of American prudery. I do not subscribe to this, and think it is more a question of specific racial complexes, with each, Verdrängung[1] has taken a different line. I should resent any comparison being drawn between English and Canadians; the former are much nearer to Americans. The blood here is three fourths Scotch, and that is a main source of their "unco' guidness." which makes me think how difficult it is to make an objective racial psycho-analysis (I know I am full of prejudices in this direction), much needed as such a study is.

I am delighted to hear that you have decided to go to Europe in June. We must form a goodly American contingent for the Lugano Congress in September.[2] You will be greatly lionised over there, I may warn you. I am sending you copies of the Korrespondenzblatt, by the way.

Yours ever sincerely
Ernest Jones.

P.S. Certainly you may show Prince any of my letters you think fit. If there are times any reasons for not doing so you will appreciate them as well as I.

---

[1] Repression.
[2] The third International Psychoanalytic Congress, originally scheduled for Lugano, was held in Weimar, September 21–22.

132
Jones to Putnam
[February 19, 1911]

Feb. 19/11.
407 Brunswick Avenue,
Toronto.

Dear Dr. Putnam.

Well, what do you think of the Feb. no. of the Journal? I hope you will not be put out by Friedlanders article. It is quite stale, having already appeared in several German journals, a fact unacknowledged by the editor.[1] No doubt you read Bleuler's excellent paper in the Jahrbuch refuting it. Don't you think a translation of the latter should be published in the Journ. of Abn. Psych.?[2]

Badger[3] has kindly appended to my article a series of references taken from another as yet unpublished article I recently sent in. As both were on dreams, the fact is not obvious, which is unfortunate as detracting from the effect of the present article. Prince's reply[4] is very interesting. It is so weak that it cannot have much effect. It is strange that his much vaunted logical mind should have so completely burked the only point of my criticism — that he did not get Freud's results because he did not use Freud's method. Instead he pours out a stream of personalities which are quite irrelevant to the point at issue. He is very unfair in repeatedly imagining replies on my part that I would never make. If you glance at P. 342, line 14, note where he inserts his interrogation mark.[5] You must agree it is no evidence of fair-mindedness. I am hurt that he did not send me his reply first, or even tell me of it, for I could have pointed out to him such avoidable misunderstandings, as he did when I submitted my criticism to him. Also by all etiquette I should have been allowed the last word. Do you think it worth my replying to in the next number?

I am afraid the effect of his reply will be to accentuate the cleft between the two schools, especially by his uncalled for remarks about "cult," "faith," etc. If so, the blame is on his shoulders, for I feel I have striven for friendly reconciliation as conscientiously as my convictions will allow. It must now come to our founding a separate journal, and in any case I feel inclined to disassociate myself from his, on account of his discourtesy.

I should be very glad to hear your comments.

Yours very sincerely

Ernest Jones.

P.S. Brill has started a society in N.Y. with 16 members, including Hoch.[6] I hope it will be affiliated to the general American branch.

---

[1] See A. Friedländer, "Hysteria and Modern Psychoanalysis."

[2] Eugen Bleuler, "Die Psychoanalyse Freuds: Verteidigung und kritische Bemerkungen" [Freud's Psychoanalysis: Defense and Critical Remarks], *Jahrbuch,* 2 (1910), 623–730. For Jones's review, see *Journal of Abnormal Psychology,* 6 (February–March 1912), 465–470.

[3] Richard G. Badger, Boston publisher of the *Journal of Abnormal Psychology.*

[4] "The Mechanism and Interpretation of Dreams — A Reply to Dr. Jones."

[5] Prince had, in fact, inserted an exclamation mark: "Dr. Jones, in his paper, says, 'Dr. Prince's curious [sic] finding (pp. 143–144, 146), that many forgotten memories could be recovered by hypnotism, but not by Freud's method, is thus easily explained. It is well known to everyone [!] who has used both methods that far deeper memories can be recovered by psychoanalysis than by hypnotism, a fact which was one of the main reasons why Freud long ago abandoned the use of the latter.' " Prince continued, "Dr. Jones does not speak from the standpoint of wide experience, of that larger knowledge of hypnotism which researches of recent years and the newer conception of hypnotism have offered us."

[6] For the New York Society see, *Journal of Abnormal Psychology,* 6 (April–May 1911), 80; *Zentralblatt,* 2 (1912), 236; and Minutes of the New York Psychoanalytic Society, February 12, 1911. It voted to remain independent and was recognized as such by the Weimar Congress.

133

Putnam to Jones

[February 24, 1911]

Dr. Ernest Jones,[1]
407 Brunswick Avenue
Toronto, Canada.

Dear Dr. Jones, —

I have read Friedlander's article and also yours and Prince's with much sorrow and dismay.[2] Bleuler's rejoinder to Friedlander[3] I have not seen for the reason that it is obviously in the Jahrbuch which I have not yet received. All I can say is that at the present crisis I should regard that man as really public-spirited who would be willing to utterly sink all personal feelings and even to overlook what seemed to him unjust attacks on principles which he regarded as of paramount importance, for the sake of a future unity. I think it would be utterly unfortunate if those of us who really care about psychopathology in the large sense, should drift apart, no matter what the provocation.

I have just written at great length to Prince.[4]

Yours sincerely,
J. J. Putnam

Feb. 24, 1911.

[1] This letter was forwarded by Jones to A. A. Brill and transcribed for this edition by Edmund Brill.

[2] See preceding letter; Friedländer, "Hysteria and Modern Psychoanalysis"; Prince, "The Mechanism and Interpretation of Dreams — A Reply to Dr. Jones"; and Jones, "Remarks on Dr. Morton Prince's Article: 'The Mechanism and Interpretation of Dreams.'"

[3] Eugen Bleuler, "Die Psychoanalyse Freuds."

[4] Putnam's letter is missing. In this typed letter, Putnam changed the period after Prince to a comma in ink, and continued "and hope you will stay on. Of course, the rejoinder to your paper gives you plenty of opportunity for comment but I rather hope you will not feel obliged to make it: I think Bleuler's article ought to appear; certainly a copious extract." Jones added in pencil after the words "stay on": "(with the Journal)," and wrote in the left margin, "I suggested I be translator for the Journal." Jones in fact continued to serve as one of the editors.

134
Jones to Putnam

[February 27, 1911]

Feb. 27/11.
407 Brunswick Avenue,
Toronto.

Dear Dr. Putnam.

This is a great moment for studying our own complexes and motives. You have before now remarked on what you called your "unity-complex." [1] I have always been bothered by, amongst other less reputable complexes, one that might be called "truth for truth's sake." No doubt there is need in the world for all sorts of cultural complexes, but at the present moment I am admiring yours a good deal more than my own. Still one cannot help seeing that things tend to happen in spite of individual complexes, i.e.

they get taken out of one's own hand. I fully agree with you that it is mean-spirited to put personal feelings in front of principles, but I do not feel specially guilty of any desire to succumb to such a temptation. It is true that I feel sore at the ungrateful way Prince has treated me, and am surprised at it in a man of his generosity of heart. I console myself, however, with the knowledge that such behaviour indicates weakness; he knows he is being pushed into a corner. I do not feel at all inclined to answer his last article.[2] It would obviously mean much quibbling and back-biting, with no real gain, and I think that to people who count it is obvious that he has given himself away rather badly, with his flood of irrelevancy and abuse. Sidis' remark[3] is of course unpardonable, and Prince should not have allowed it to be printed; one will be bound to ignore him in the future. One thing above all else I hope, and that is that in America abusive language (Dercum, Collins,[4] Prince, Sidis, etc.) will remain the monopoly of our opponents. Then it is bound to react on them in time, while if any of us were to reply in the same strain it would lead to a never-ending muddle. So long as we maintain a dignified attitude we are safe, and the onlooker will soon see which side has the fanaticism and high feeling. The only man I am afraid of here is Brill. I had a heated letter from him this morning, but think I shall be able to hold his hand.

With regard to unity, that is on the lap of the gods. No one desires it more warmly than I do, except at the price of self-respect and honest convictions. I suppose no big movement can proceed harmoniously, without involving some alienation. Pour faire une omelette il faut casser les oeufs.[5] But it is very evident that here the disruption is coming entirely from the other side. Such language as the current number of the Journal contains makes it very difficult to keep the peace, and for such a situation Prince is altogether responsible. I trust you were very cross with him in your letter to him. I am exceedingly anxious to hear what he has to say to you. Probably he will show you the letter I wrote him. I should be very much obliged if you would keep me in touch.

Yours sincerely
Ernest Jones.

¹ See preceding letter.

² "The Mechanism and Interpretation of Dreams — A Reply to Dr. Jones."

³ In "Fundamental States in Psychoneurosis," *Journal of Abnormal Psychology*, 5 (February–March 1911), 320–327, Boris Sidis wrote: "In other words, slippery and mutable as Freud's statements are, he clearly declares in the last edition to his *magnum opus* the far and wide reaching generalization that all psychoneurosis is based on sexual wish-impulses (Wunschregungen) coming from infantile life. Suppression of sexual experiences can be easily observed (by competent observers, of course), in infants of a few months old. If you miss the process of suppression in the baby, you can easily trace it by means of psychoanalysis to the early recollections of tender infancy. It is certainly lack of comprehension that induces Ziehen to doubt Freud's speculation as Unsinn [nonsense].

"Some of Freud's admirers, with a metaphysical proclivity, are delighted over the theory of suppressed wishes. The wish is fundamental and prior to all mental states. This piece of metaphysical psychologism is supposed to be based on clinical experience. 'If wishes were horses, beggars would ride.' The Freudist manages to ride such horses" (p. 322).

⁴ Joseph Collins (1866–1950), New York neurologist. According to Jones, Collins had attacked Putnam's first paper on psychoanalysis as made up of "pornographic stories about pure virgins." See Jones, *Sigmund Freud*, II, 115; and Francis Xavier Dercum, "An Analysis of Psychotherapeutic Methods," *Therapeutic Gazette* (Detroit), 32 (May 15, 1908), 305–316.

⁵ You can't make an omelette without breaking eggs.

135

Putnam to Jones

[March 2, 1911]

III.2.1911
106 Marlborough Street

Dear Dr. Jones

It is rather amusing that the last of the patients spoken of by Sidis in his paper¹ has just come under my care, quite as badly off as ever, and that he himself told, without urging, of strong sexual tendencies (desire for exposure, with reference to older women — perhaps originally nurse or mother) dating back to *earliest* childhood.

Sidis and Prince should not, however, be spoken of as on the same plane, though in my optimism, I believe both of them are 'curable.'

It is rather funny that I find myself in the position of a buffer. First Prince writes, that he considers himself ——d by you, and then you write that you consider yourself ——d by him. I have written several long letters to him,² striving in³ induce broader attitudes, and I do think that patience is necessary on a large scale. We must all put ourselves into 50 years ahead.

I am insisting more and more, with my patients, that to get well from a psychoneurosis should mean not only losing symptoms but becoming broader and more reasonable and more moral persons.

I insist also that the *practice* of ps.an. tends in the same direction.

Prince is a fighter by nature and loves the rough and tumble of a battle for its own sake, and he cares less intensely for the issues than you and I do in this case. For, ignorant though I am I do care more intensely for these issues than for any others for a long time, except certain ones rangeable as philosophic, in a broad sense. But Prince has strong virtues and much real generosity and public spirit.

He is not an expert in ps.an[c] questions; is less of an expert even than he thinks; and so (*being* a fighter) he says things which he should not say and does not recognize the obligations which we see.

He might well have turned down Sidis, as you say, but I think he believes it best to let all combatants enter the arena.

Yours sincerely
James J. Putnam

[1] "Fundamental States in Psychoneurosis." See preceding letter.
[2] Missing.
[3] Putnam must have intended to write "to."

136
Jones to Putnam
[March 5, 1911]

Mar. 5/11.
407 Brunswick Avenue,
Toronto.

Dear Dr. Putnam.

All I was told about the Munich Congress was that it would be held "early in October." [1] I shall be writing again to the Secretary,[2] and will let you know the exact date if they have settled it.

I am glad to see that you are apparently less depressed and even optimistic in regard to the recent situation.[3] The trouble with Prince is that the very qualities that make him so loveable personally, his boyish love of fighting and his irrepressible irresponsibility, are harmful factors for a man placed in the responsible and influential position he is. One is always torn between the desire to forgive him everything, and the knowledge that in his wilful innocence he is bringing about an undesirable state of affairs.

It is the same thing over publishing questions: I simply cannot get him to take anything seriously. He laughs lightheartedly at careless blunders and inaccuracies that make my blood run cold, and yet I always imagined I had a fairly philosophic sense of humour. But my Weltanschauung (or what does duty for one) does not allow me to view *everything* as a joke; I could even, in private, subscribe to the platitude that "life is real, life is earnest." Or, put in a more acceptable way, I feel that there are things worth doing, and worth doing well.

Yours very sincerely
Ernest Jones.

[1] Probably a reference to the International Congress for Medical Psychology held in Munich, September 25–26, 1911.

[2] Probably Hans von Hattingberg (b. 1879), Munich neurologist and psychotherapist and, with August Forel, a founder of the International Society for Medical Psychology and Psychotherapy.

[3] The controversy over psychoanalysis involving Prince. See all the letters from Prince to Putnam; Putnam to Jones, January 5, February 24, and March 2, 1911; and Jones to Putnam, February 19, February 27, 1911.

137

Jones to Putnam

[April 7, 1911]

April 7/11.
407 Brunswick Avenue,
Toronto

Dear Dr. Putnam.

Dr. Madison Taylor[1] tells me that he finds much interest in psychoanalysis amongst the clergy, and suggests I should write a suitable article for some such journal as the Churchman. It is out of my capacity, and if you think it worth doing it is obvious that you are the man to do it.[2] You could give a review of Pfister's writings as well, which by now are pretty numerous.[3]

What a feeble production that is of Coriat's in this number of the Journal.[4] It maddens me to hear this people weighing the good and bad of Ψa, calmly assuming that they have nothing to learn as they know all about it. They harm more than downright opponents, but we shall have to get used to them, I suppose.

Have you read Stekel's great production "Die Sprache des Traumes?" It is a storehouse of symbolism, but I don't expect you will agree with him in regard to "telepathic dreams."[5]

Might I suggest that you write for the Journ. of Abn. Psych. a general review of the first ten Hefte of the Schriften zur-ang. Seelen Kunde?[6] You could do it beautifully, and so far only one of them has been noticed in the Journal.

The local situation here is, I am glad to say, clearly[7] considerably, but it is an unpleasant atmosphere for a free thinker. I have been quite seedy of late with two attacks of influenza, but am now better and am starting an address on Dreams and the Psychoneuroses I have promised to give in Detroit early next month, also on a short "organic" paper for the A N: A.[8] My contribution to the A Pp. A symposium on Angst was sent to Badger last week.[9]

Do you agree about May 9, 2 pm, as the date for our psychoanalysis meeting, and have you any other suggestions to make before I send out notices? What do you think about the N.Y. Society?[10]

I should be very glad to hear from you.

Yours very sincerely
Ernest Jones.

[1] John Madison Taylor (1855–1931), Philadelphia pediatrician, student of hypnosis and nervous diseases, and a member of the American Therapeutic Society which had sponsored the symposium on psychotherapeutics at New Haven in 1909. He had been an assistant of the neurologist S. Weir Mitchell for sixteen years.

[2] Putnam did not write the article for the clergy. See Jones to Putnam, April 15, 1911.

[3] Oscar Pfister (1873–1956), Swiss pastor and psychoanalyst, had written a dozen psychoanalytic papers in addition to reviews.

[4] Isador Henry Coriat, "A Contribution to the Psychopathology of Hysteria," *Journal of Abnormal Psychology*, 6 (April–May 1911), 33–65.

[5] Wilhelm Stekel, *Die Sprache des Traumes. Eine Darstellung der Symbolik und Deutung des Traumes in ihren Beziehungen zur kranken und gesunden Seele für*

Ärzte und Psychologen [The Language of Dreams. A Presentation for Physicians and Psychologists of the Interpretation and Symbolism of the Dream in Its Relationship to Both the Sick and Healthy Mind], Munich and Wiesbaden: J. F. Bergmann, 1911. Stekel believed in telepathic dreams, see *Die Sprache des Traumes,* pp. 506–512.

⁶ Several of the first ten of this series of twenty monographs became psychoanalytic classics: Freud's *Leonardo* and *Gradiva,* Karl Abraham's *Dream and Myth,* and Jones's *Hamlet.* See Ilse Bry et al., "Bibliography of Early Psychoanalytic Monographs," *Journal of the American Psychoanalytic Association,* 1 (1953), 519–525, 706–718. Putnam did not review the series.

⁷ "Clearer" was intended.

⁸ Jones, "The Relationship between Dreams and Psychoneurotic Symptoms." Read before the Wayne County Medical Society, Detroit, May 15, 1911. *American Journal of Insanity,* 68 (July 1911), 57–80; PPsa, eds. 1–5, and "The Deviation of the Tongue in Hemiplegia," *Proceedings of the American Neurological Association,* thirty-seventh annual meeting, Baltimore, Md., May 11–13, 1911 (New York), *Journal of Nervous and Mental Disease* (1912), 100–110.

⁹ "The Pathology of Morbid Anxiety." Read before the American Psychopathological Association, May 10, 1911. *Journal of Abnormal Psychology,* 6 (June–July 1911), 81–106; PPsa, eds. 1–4.

¹⁰ A. A. Brill founded the New York Psychoanalytic Society, February 12, 1911. See Jones to Putnam, February 19, 1911.

138
Jones to Putnam
[April 15, 1911]

April 15/11.
407 Brunswick Avenue,
Toronto.

Dear Dr. Putnam.

I quite agree that perhaps we had better steer clear of the clergy at least for a while, until the more scientific side of our work becomes better established. As to the Schriften,¹ my proposal was quite a modest one, merely a two page review indicating the contents and the lines along which the new knowledge was being applied. I hope that you will be able to do this some time in the summer.

I had this morning a letter from Hattingberg² saying that the date of the Int. Congress for Med. Psych.³ was not yet settled, but that they thought of holding it in Dresden at the time of the Hygiene Exhibition.

I am thinking of attending the German Neurol. Soc.,⁴ which meets at Frankfurt on Oct. 2. Will you come to that?

I shall be greatly interested in the two sets of papers you adumbrate. They will only do good. It is striking how free Ψa work leaves everyone to develope his own personal points of view. We have a system of thought, but no dogma. There is no reason why you shouldn't expound your conception at Lugano.[5] The President would translate it to those who don't follow English, but I am not sure that it would give rise to much discussion, being perhaps foreign to the trend of thought of most of the audience.

Coriat is evidently running with the hare and coursing with the hounds, and he is further hampered by a terrific Ich-complex.[6] I doubt that we shall make much out of him.

I am issuing notices for our meeting at the Belvedere Hotel, Baltimore at 2 p.m. May 9 (Tuesday). Will you kindly note the date. Next week we shall get the reports of the symposium of the A. Psychopathol. Assoc.[7] I am afraid you will find my contribution very elementary, but perhaps it is better so.

Of late I have been interested in working out three cases of "break-down from business overwork." It is remarkable to note the extent to which business can gratify tendencies which in other countries would find artistic or military outlets.

Brill's wife[8] has been dangerously ill with puerperal septicaemia. She is better now, but he has naturally been thrown off his work. My sister, whom you met here, has also just had a baby, and my other sister — the Boston one — is about to be married.[9] I hope to bring my wife to Baltimore, for I want to show her Washington.

With kindest regards

Yours ever sincerely,
Ernest Jones.

P.S. I have just been astonished to read a remarkably sympathetic review of my nightmare article in such a hostile quarter as the Zeitschr. f. Psychologie[10] (Bd. 58. S. 315).

---

[1] See preceding letter.

[2] See n. 2, Jones to Putnam, March 5, 1911.

[3] The Congress was held in Munich, September 25–26, 1911. See *Journal für Psychologie und Neurologie*, 19 (1912), Ergänzungsheft [Supplement], I; II, 273–388.

[4] For the proceedings on October 2–4, 1911, see *Neurologisches Centralblatt*, 30 (1911), 1185–1214.

[5] The third International Psychoanalytic Congress was held in Weimar instead of Lugano on September 21–22, 1911. Putnam read in German, "Ueber die Bedeutung philosophischer Anschauungen und Ausbildung für die weitere Entwicklung der psychoanalytischen Bewegung" [The Role of Philosophical Views and Training

in the Further Development of the Psychoanalytic Movement], *Imago*, I (May 1912), 101–118; Ad Psa, 79–96.

⁶ Ego complex.

⁷ The first meeting of the American Psychoanalytic Association. See Jones, *Sigmund Freud*, II, 87–88. The Psychopathological Association held a symposium on the pathogenesis of morbid anxiety May 10, 1911, see *Journal of Abnormal Psychology*, 6 (June–July 1911), 81–181.

⁸ Rose Owen Brill (1875–1963).

⁹ Jones's sister Elizabeth married the British surgeon Wilfred Trotter. Sybil Jones was a student in Boston. See Jones, *Free Associations*, p. 181.

¹⁰ Jones's article "On the Nightmare" was reviewed by R. Hennig in *Zeitschrift für Psychologie und Physiologie der Sinnesorgane*, 58 (1910–1911), 315–316.

139
Jones to Putnam
[June 1, 1911]

June 1/11.
407 Brunswick Avenue,
Toronto.

Dear Dr. Putnam.

I have only just seen the number of the J.A.M.A. Dercum's paper is merely a repetition of his former one. As for Lloyd, he is a vulgar and ill-bred fellow who doesn't even know how to express himself.¹ I have been asked to reply to his paper, but I cannot really descend to take notice of such stuff, and I am sure you will agree it is better not.

The Detroit meetings were very successful, and I also spent a day at Ann Arbor with Barrett, where I saw Pillsbury and others.²

It has been decided to hold the meeting at Weimar on Sept. 16 or 21, probably the latter.³

When do you sail? Perhaps you will be able to spend some time with Freud before the date of the Congress. I am sure it would give him great pleasure.

Did you see Mendel's review of Stekel's book in the Neurol. Centralbl. No. 9. S. 491?⁴ I notice that Pfister is having a controversy in the Zeitschr. f. Religionspsychologie.⁵

My wife greatly enjoyed her trip, and wishes to be kindly remembered to you.

With kind Regards

Yours sincerely
Ernest Jones.

¹ Francis Xavier Dercum, "The Role of Dreams in the Etiology of the Psycho-neuroses" and "An Analysis of Psychotherapeutic Methods" (1908); James Hendrie Lloyd (1853–1932), "The So-Called Oedipus Complex in Hamlet," *Journal of the American Medical Association,* 56 (May 13, 1911), 1377–1379. Dercum and Lloyd were neurologists in Philadelphia.

² Jones had addressed the Detroit Academy of Medicine May 16, 1911, on "The Psychopathology of Everyday Life." See *American Journal of Psychology,* 12 (October 1911), 477–527; PPsa, eds. 1–5. Albert Barrett (1871–1936), professor of psychiatry and nervous diseases and director of State Psychopathic Hospital, later the Neuro-Psychiatric Institute, University of Michigan. Walter B. Pillsbury (1872–1960), professor of psychology, University of Michigan.

³ The third International Psychoanalytic Congress.

⁴ Kurt Mendel, "Die Sprache des Traumes von Wilhelm Stekel" [Wilhelm Stekel's *The Language of Dreams*], *Neurologisches Centralblatt,* 30 no. 9 (May 1, 1911), 491–492.

⁵ See Oskar Pfister, "Hat Zinzendorf die Frömmigkeit sexualisiert?" [Has Zinzendorf Sexualized Piety?] *Zeitschrift für Religionspsychologie,* 5 (1911), 56–60, and *Zentralblatt,* 1 (1911), 432.

140

Putnam to Jones

[June 14, 1911]

VI.14.1911
106 Marlborough Street

Dear Dr. Jones

I have just been reading Mendel's notice of Stekel.¹ Of course, it is what it is, and of no use to the seekers for truth. Still, I confess Stekel makes me uncomfortable.

He too is frivolous, though in a different way from Scripture.²

He seems to me to start in with a very low view of man in general and if I dared and thought it wise I would take him as an example of the (as I think) pernicious tendency of the psycho-genetic method used to the exclusion of the personal-universe-and-free-will method, which alone I regard as scientific.

We should be observant, we should be honest, we should be courageous, but we should not be so sensitized that we see only the beast in a man, or his dreams even, and if we must, *as we must,* publish the facts as they are, we are also under obligation to do this reverently and not to roll the unpleasant morsels (unpleasant at least to others) under the tongue, as Stekel does. Would that I had the power to bring this to the clear consciousness of Freud and of Stekel himself, without offending them.

I can see and select the good and valuable (very valuable) in the *Sprache des Traumes,*[3] but I can well believe that many a person might be driven out of our camp by it.

You will be interested to know that the 'Harvey Society for the promotion of useful knowledge' (Dr. S. J. Meltzer, Pres., Dr. Simon Flexner, and others) have chosen Freud's work as the subject for next winter's lecture, and have asked me to give it.[4]

Sincerely

James J. Putnam

VI.14.

[1] Kurt Mendel, "Die Sprache des Traumes von Wilhelm Stekel." Stekel (1868–1940), Viennese psychoanalyst, editor of the *Zentralblatt,* resigned from the Vienna Psychoanalytic Society in 1912.

[2] Edward Wheeler Scripture (b. 1864), associate in psychiatry at Columbia University, 1909–1914, and a charter member of the New York Psychoanalytic Society.

[3] Wilhelm Stekel, *Die Sprache des Traumes.* See a translation by James S. Van Teslaar of part I, *Sex and Dreams: The Language of Dreams* (Boston: Richard G. Badger, 1922).

[4] Samuel James Meltzer (b. 1851), bacteriologist and pathologist on the staff of the Rockefeller Institute; Simon Flexner (1863–1946), biologist, director of the Rockefeller Institute for Medical Research, 1903–1935. See Putnam, "On Freud's Psycho-Analytic Method and Its Evolution" delivered before the Harvey Society, November 1911. *Boston Medical and Surgical Journal,* 166 (January 25, 1912), 115–122; Ad Psa, 97–122.

141
Putnam to Jones

[June 20, 1911]

106 Marlborough Street

Dear Dr. Jones

I send a line just to say that of course I entirely agree with the essence of your excellent statement on sublimation, etc. vs. "beast." [1] The only possible differences between us c⁴ be — not that I halt on the "beast" idea, but that, as I think, I give, i.e. my principles give, motives for progress which are nowadays strangely overlooked. You have, so far as I can see, no scientific justification for 'will.' Everything *is* because it *becomes* so. When you get your 'superman,' what next? Does he, tired of ennui and Rotation, commit suicide? However, everyone really does believe in will, and appeals to it, and I have no doubt but that as a practical idealist and courageous worker for reforms, you are far ahead of me.

Thank you sincerely for your sister's address.[2] If it is in any way possible I shall call on her.

I mean to carry some Bernard Shaw. Could you tell me, even by telegraph, or by note to care of *Brown, Shipley & Co.* London what you would suggest.

I read Man and S.man[3] last year and I had planned to take along the latest volume or to buy it in England.

Sincerely and with best thanks
James J. Putnam

[1] In the left margin, Putnam wrote, "Stekel seems rather to revel in showing up the beast without seeing the 'statue in the marble.' However I can take him at his best, with little feeling even of repulsion." See preceding letter.

[2] Sybil Jones.

[3] Bernard Shaw, *Man and Superman: A Comedy and a Philosophy* (London: A. Constable and Co., 1903). Another edition was published in 1911 in Constable's Sixpenny series.

142
Jones to Putnam
[October 29, 1911]

October 29, 1911.
407 Brunswick Avenue,
Toronto.

Dear Dr. Putnam:

I am glad to hear that you experienced the same stimulating effect as I did from the Weimar congress.[1] It certainly gave one to think, and I trust we shall both be able to transmute what you describe as excitement into a stream of useful activity.

I greatly doubt my capacity to help you much as regards dream interpretation, for the simple reason that in a man of such rich mentality and numerous experiences of life and reading as yours the dreams are bound to be extremely involved. With the comments you pass on the dreams related in your letter I throughout agree. The first one, about the mud bath, is doubtless an excretion phantasy in the main.[2] I would draw your attention to a detail confirming this by hinting at the well-known relation between money and faeces; namely, the scene is in a luxurious house ("much more so than my own") in *Beacon St.*[3] One cannot help connecting this with Prince's well-to-do-ness, and a very natural envy of all that this connotes in the way of leisure, etc.

You ask about bicycle dreams. I have found them to indicate both heterosexual and auto-erotic wishes, but perhaps more often the latter. The one you depict, riding through a defile of earth with a man rolling two stones (testicles) towards you, is, I should say, certainly a homosexual dream with analerotic aspects; it portrays a conflict between male and female tendencies as regards the form of functioning.

The case you refer to sounds very interesting. I would suspect that the wooden doll's legs in the dream about the sister might refer to a death wish against the latter (children are equally struck about dolls by the fact that they are alive and also dead — double phantasies). The dream of the old lady suggests the same thing, and I daresay she has transferred the wish to a number of lady friends, though no doubt your interpretation of her fear and distress also applies. The phobia of being buried alive is, as you of course know, always the expression of a Mutter-leib[4] phantasy, and I have generally found this to be also connected with death-wishes as well as with the birth-phantasy that it strictly means. In general I do not think one can overestimate the extraordinary connection between birth and death in the imagination. They are simply the same thing. I have recently come to the conclusion, interesting also philosophically, that *without exception* no one at heart believes in permanent annihilation of his own personality. I say "permanent" advisedly, for, as indeed you point out in this very case, the idea of loss of consciousness or rather of self-consciousness usually means rapturous ecstasy and is of course frequent enough. Otherwise the idea of death is always transformed into a peaceful creeping back to the mother, usually to the womb, i.e. being born again. Rank has beautifully illustrated this in his book I got last week on the Lohengrin saga,[5] which by the way you must certainly read for it contains a stream of new suggestions. He remarks amongst other things on a matter that might have a bearing on a detail of your patient's dream, namely the falling of the house into pieces; this may be connected with the infantile idea that the child is built inside the mother bit by bit, to which there are of course many variations.

I sent Prince last week for publication a dream of my own in which I was much interested; perhaps if he has not yet sent it to the printers you might look at it.[6] It was a beautiful combination of the typical Oedipus motive with the saving phantasy to which attention has so much been called of late. Of especial interest was the fact that analysis of the dream brought to memory a forgotten dream of the same night in which the childhood conflict was solved in a different way; the one, namely, was heterosexual the other homosexual. In one I solve the riddle of the sphinx by repudiating my father, marrying my mother, and actually beget myself like the gods of old; in the other a replacement figure of the father, beautifully determined, appears and gratifies my desire for knowledge about the mysteries of birth and life in a way that unfortunately was not true in reality. The connection between the two dreams was remarkable; in the analysis of the first I lighted on the thought of someone of whom I really had not had in my mind so far as I know since I was a child, and lo and behold in the other dream this person appears in the flesh!

I am sending you a few reprints most of which you will have already seen. The one on everyday life, however, will I hope bring many little things of interest, and I should be much indebted for a criticism of my neurological attempts at the "tongue in hemiplegia" problem if you have the time or inclination to read about such things.[7]

At present I am thinking much about the question of homosexuality in relation to alcohol and drug habits on which I have had some good experiences with private patients. I am sure we are on the way to the solution of what everyone considers a grave social problem, and it is not unreasonable to expect that in that case a great deal will be done for the happiness of humanity, for really the married lives of such people that I have observed constitute something as near to a nightmare as can be offered by waking life. By the way I spoke again to Abraham in Berlin about his article.[8] He said that all his reprints were exhausted but that he thought it probable that Hirschfeld [9] the editor might still have some copies of that number of the Zeitschrift left; if you get a copy sent you would you be good enough to let me know. And one other business point.

As the subscription to the Internat. Soc. will now be 15 marks to enable the Zentralblatt to be distributed gratis I calculate that we shall have to charge five dollars to our members to cover expenses.[10] If it proves to be too much we can lower it next time. May I therefore ask you kindly to forward me the sum, so that I may remit a cheque to Riklin.[11]

Yours very sincerely
Ernest Jones.

[1] The third International Psychoanalytic Congress held in Weimar September 21–22, 1911.

[2] Putnam's letter to Jones is missing, but see Putnam to Freud, October 20, 1911.

[3] Morton Prince, who was independently wealthy, lived at 458 Beacon Street, a new and fashionable quarter of Boston.

[4] Womb.

[5] Otto Rank, *Die Lohengrinsage: ein Beitrag zu ihrer Motivgestaltung und Deutung* [The Lohengrin Legend: A Contribution to Its Motivation and Interpretation], *Schriften zur angewandten Seelenkunde*, XIII (Leipzig: F. Deuticke, 1911).

[6] See Jones, "A Forgotten Dream: Note on the Oedipus Saving Phantasy," *Journal of Abnormal Psychology*, 7 (April–May 1912), 5–16. "The subject of the analysis," Jones wrote, "is a university teacher of a branch of biology, is quite normal, and presents no neuropathic traits."

[7] Jones, "Beitrag zur Symbolik im Alltagsleben" [Contribution to Symbolism in Everyday Life], *Zentralblatt*, 1 (1911), 96–98; and "The Deviation of the Tongue in Hemiplegia."

[8] Karl Abraham (1877–1925), founder of the Berlin Psychoanalytic Society. See "Die psychologischen Beziehungen zwischen Sexualität und Alkoholismus"; in Karl Abraham, *Selected Papers*.

[9] Magnus Hirschfeld (1868–1935), pioneer German investigator of human sexual behavior, author of *Men and Women: The World Journey of a Sexologist*, introduction by A. A. Brill (New York: G. P. Putnam & Sons, 1935).

[10] The International Psychoanalytic Association. Fifteen marks was the equivalent of $3.75.

[11] Franz Riklin (1871–1938), Swiss psychiatrist, secretary of the International Psychoanalytic Association, and later a follower of Jung.

143
Jones to Putnam
[October 31, 1911]

407 Brunswick Avenue,
Toronto

Oct. 31.

Dear Dr. Putnam.

No doubt you got my letter of Sunday, although I believe I addressed it to 106 Marlborough St. I fancy I forgot to thank you for sending on the Tr. D,[1] which arrived quite safely.

Re your last note[2] two or three points occur to me. The being prevented from seeing (by the cross-piece) is evidently to be read reversed as being enabled to see, i.e. being shown. The shape of the curious structure on the handle bar seems to be female. You are being initiated into the mysteries by someone. Was your brother older or younger, and was[3] of his wife? Was he married before you or not? [4] I would think of a transference to her. The whole act of riding down hill is plainly a coitus, the bicycle being both the person underneath, and the instrument with which the riding is performed.

I have met several dreams (of my own and patients) of a masculine nature, but in which a man (father) shows the person how to achieve the aim. The latter is I think a pretty common wish of children. (help).

Yours sincerely,
Ernest Jones.

---

[1] Freud, *Die Traumdeutung*, 3rd ed., enl. and rev., 1911.
[2] Putnam's note is missing.
[3] Jones intended "what."
[4] Charles Pickering Putnam (1844–1914) was two years older than James Jackson Putnam and married Lucy Washburn, who was also a friend of the younger brother, in 1889. Putnam married Marian Cabot in 1886.

144
Jones to Putnam
[November 6, 1911]

November 6, 1911.

407 Brunswick Avenue,
Toronto

Dear Dr. Putnam:

I am very happy indeed that you found my few remarks of some value.[1] It shows how little experience is necessary to convince one of how useful it would be to have a small circle where one could interchange views and experiences and talk out difficulties, both personal and general.

With regard to your question about the matter of help from dream analysis I agree with your remark that often one cannot see why it should help when it does. Or rather I should prefer to put it that one doesn't see the *immediate* connection between the help and the analysis. In general I think one should concentrate a little more on the analysis itself for its own sake and not ask at every step "what is the direct use of this particular piece of information?" In this respect it is a little like much scientific research in that one cannot always see the immediate practical application of given work, but on the other hand we all know what happens to the investigator who has his eye constantly fixed on "results" to the exclusion of all other considerations.

But I think we can after all be a little more specific in this matter. To take a particular instance, that of homosexual tendencies: the great advantage a detailed analysis possesses over the mere fact of knowing about such tendencies is not only that it convinces one in one's heart much more completely of their existence — replacing a lip-assent by a thorough knowledge — but that laying bare the precise experiences and reactions whereby it became established in the first place automatically gives one more control over any unfortunate reactions in daily life that may have resulted from their operation. Here dream analysis is of peculiar value in its near relation to the childhood basis.

Did the reprints I despatched arrive safely?

> yours very sincerely
> Ernest Jones

P.S. Thank you for the enclosure. I am writing today to Riklin, so we should get the Zentralblatt before Xmas.²

---

¹ Putnam's letter is missing.

² *The Zentralblatt für Psychoanalyse. Medizinische Monatsschrift für Seelenkunde* [The Journal for Psychoanalysis. Medical Monthly for Psychology], was the official organ of the Association and began publication in September 1910.

145
Putnam to Jones
[October 24, 1912]

October 24, 1912

Dr. Ernest Jones,
London, England.

Dear Dr. Jones:

Thank you for your letter,¹ which as always was very interesting.

I made two attempts to meet Dr. Jung in New York, and the last one was in so far successful that I heard his address, though unfortunately missing the first part of it; and I had a few words with him afterwards.² I am sorry I did not see the work referred to in the letter which I enclose for your edification. What Dr. Jung said, in effect, was that while he still held to the importance of the psychoanalytic technique, he had come to rate the infantile fixations as of far less importance than formerly as an etiological factor, and, indeed, as I understood him, as an almost negligible factor in most cases — though I hardly think he could really maintain this if he were pushed for a positive opinion. At any rate, the point on which he seems now inclined to lay emphasis is the difficulty of meeting new problems and environmental conditions which arise at the time of the actual onset of the neurosis. It seems to me that we all recognize the importance of these influences, and I cannot as yet feel that anything is won through minimizing the significance of the other factor. However, I want very much a chance to read his position in extenso.

He seems to me a strong but egotistic man (if I may say this in complete confidence), and to be under the necessity of accentuating any peculiarity of his own position for his own personal satisfaction. I cannot think that any serious breach would be occasioned by this present movement on his part. I have talked with Dr. Brill about it, and will send you a letter[3] received a short time ago from him, asking you, at the same time, to send it back to me. The point which seemed to me to indicate most strongly the idea of a breaking off on his part was that he said, if I understood him rightly, that he thought the significance of the whole conception of infantile sexual tendencies in Freud's sense had been overrated; that all persons, sick or well, have about the same fantasies, and that, for example, he did not any longer believe that the sensations which a nursing child has could be classified as sexual in any sense, but only as related to nutritional necessities.

This does not coincide with my present beliefs, but of course it will go far (although possibly in an unfortunate way, in some respects) toward gaining adherents for the psychoanalytic method. Perhaps, after all, that is the important thing, because whatever ideas are really the most sound will *in the end*, far away, come most strongly to the front.

I am glad you liked my paper, and I can say the same for your "Zwangsneuroses," which I have been reading with great interest.[4] You have a wonderful insight into the complex relationships of these fantasies. I only wonder sometimes whether the number of possible associations and relationships is not really infinite, and whether, on the other hand, we could get along, therapeutically — sometimes, at any rate — with less than it is fairly possible to bring out. In other words, what seems to be aimed at is by no means a complete result. If it was complete, this would show itself in the production[5]

[1] Missing.

[2] At the invitation of Smith Ely Jelliffe, Jung lectured in September 1912 in an extension course in neurology and psychiatry at Fordham University. The lectures described in detail his major disagreements with Freud and were published as "The Theory of Psychoanalysis," in the first two volumes of the *Psychoanalytic Review*, 1 (1913–1914), 1–40, 153–177, 260–284, 415–430; 2 (1915), 29–51.

[3] The letter is missing.

[4] See Putnam, "A Clinical Study of a Case of Phobia," *Journal of Abnormal Psychology,* 7 (October–November 1912), 277–292; Ad Psa, 156–174; and Jones, "Analytic Study of a Case of Obsessional Neurosis." Read before the American

Psychoanalytic Association, Boston, May 30, 1912. In PPsa, eds. 1–4. In German as "Einige Fälle von Zwangsneurose," part I, *Jahrbuch,* 4 (1912), 563–606; and part II, *Jahrbuch,* 5 (1913), 55–116.

⁵ The remainder of the letter is missing.

146
Putnam to Jones
[September 2, 1913]

September 2, 1913.

Dr. Ernest Jones,
    London, England.

Dear Dr. Jones:

Thank you for your interesting letter.¹ I am almost sorry that I did not carry out my intention of writing to Janet,² urging him not to adopt so hostile an attitude as you say he did. I rather thought, from my conversation with him, in the summer of 1911, that he had changed his views considerably; but prejudice for his own views, and against those of others which he realizes himself unable fully to understand, has evidently been too much for him.

I was much interested also in what you said about Jung, — the more so that I have been reading, with entire sympathy, Ferenczi's review of his book.³ The only criticism I would make of this latter is that I think he draws too hard and fast a line between what the psychoanalyst may and may not suitably undertake for the purpose of promoting sublimation. After all it is impossible to avoid the kind of influence which goes with the treatment of such a man as Ferenczi, and I see no reason why any one who chooses to prepare himself to do so may not study out what the essence of this influence is.

I was struck with one passage in Ferenczi's review, in which he seems, unless I strangely misread it, to endorse the *possibility* of a real prophetic power. This goes even beyond me, prepared as I am to admit the possibility of telepathy.

I have exchanged letters with Pfister about his book,⁴ and have been struck with his strong feeling, as well as Maeder's, in favor of Jung; or rather, I do not particularly wonder at the feeling, but do not quite understand the special grounds on which they base it. They would seem to say that Jung is devoting much more attention to "reality"; but I should like to know whether *practically* this is true. Jung's feeling about the prophetic dream seems to be positive with him. He has been treating a former patient of mine for the past year, and utilized her dreams as a means of deciding whether she ought to return to America for a visit. This seems queer, and the more so that during his absence just a little later, she analysed her own dreams, and came to the conclusion that a different meaning was to be asserted for them in this respect!! [5]

I am to review Pfister's book for one, and possibly a second journal here. The "one" is the Harvard Theological Review; the other, Prince's journal.[6]

I have also been reading, of course with much interest, the philosophical number of the "Imago," and hope to have it finished in a day or two. I agree entirely with Hitschmann's paper,[7] except that I do not see why he goes out of his way, as especially in the last paragraph, to express sentiments about philosophizing in general, which do not seem to me at all warranted. Whatever one may conclude about the temperament of the philosopher — and I am sure the diagnosis of neuropathic does not by any means suit all of them — it is certain that the philosophizing habit is very apt to have excellent practical results; also, that philosophy in the best sense furnishes a definite and scientific mode of approach to very important matters.

The next paper, on the history of philosophy,[8] I object to very much, because it seems to me clear that the writer does not really grasp the meaning of some of the principles of which he speaks — especially Plato's doctrine of ideas, and the subject-object nature of[9]

[1] Missing.

[2] Pierre Janet (1859–1947), French neurologist and psychopathologist. See Janet, "Psychoanalysis," *Journal of Abnormal Psychology*, 9 (1914–1915), 1–35, 153–187.

[3] Ferenczi, review of Carl Gustav Jung, *Wandlungen und Symbole der Libido: Beiträge zur Entwicklungsgeschichte des Denkens* [Changes and Symbols of the Libido: Contributions to the Developmental History of Thought], Leipzig and Vienna: F. Deuticke, 1912; *Zeitschrift*, 1 (1913), 390–403.

[4] Oskar Pfister, *Die psychoanalytische Methode: eine erfahrungswissenschaftlich-systematische Darstellung* [The Psychoanalytic Method: An Empirical, Scientific and Systematic Exposition], Leipzig and Berlin: J. Klinkhardt, 1913.

[5] In the left margin, Putnam wrote, "I do not understand that. Neither Maeder or Adler [whose reply to Maeder you have doubtless seen] consider dreams prophetic in any other sense than that our feelings may be acuter than our knowledge." For their views of the dream see Alphonse Maeder, "Über die Funktion des Traumes (mit Berücksichtigung der Tagesträume Spieles, usw)" [Concerning the Function of the

Dream (with consideration of daydreams, play, etc.)], *Jahrbuch*, 4 (1912), 697–707; Alfred Adler, "Traum und Traumdeutung" [Dream and Dream Interpretation], *Zentralblatt*, 3 (1912–1913), 574–583. For the controversy see Maeder, "Zur Frage der teleologischen Traumfunction. Eine Bemerkung Zur Abwehr" [On the Question of the Teleological Function of the Dream. A Note in Opposition], *Jahrbuch*, 5 (1913), 453–454, and Adler, "Erwiderung" [A Reply to A. M.], *Zentralblatt*, 3 (1913), 564–567.

⁶ Putnam, review of "Pädagogicum, Band I: Die Psychoanalytische Methode, von Dr. Oscar Pfister, Pfarrer und Seminarlehrer in Zurich: mit einem Geleitwort von Prof. Dr. S. Freud. Verlag von Julius Klinkhardt, Leipzig u. Berlin, pp 490," *Harvard Theological Review*, 7, no. 2 (April 1914), 261–268.

⁷ Eduard Hitschmann, "Schopenhauer: Versuch einer Psychoanalyse des Philosophen," *Imago*, 2 (April 1913), 101–174.

⁸ Dr. Alfred Frh. v. Winterstein, "Psychoanalytische Anmerkungen zur Geschichte der Philosophie" [Psychoanalytic Observations on the History of Philosophy], *Imago*, 2 (April 1913), 175–237.

⁹ The remainder of the letter is missing.

147

Putnam to Jones

[December 16, 1913]

December 16, 1913.

Dr. Ernest Jones,
   London, England.

Dear Dr. Jones:

You will remember, I am sure, that I have spoken several times of the illness of my children. I now write a line to say that one of them, a very promising, vigorous-minded girl, of rather rare balance, and exceedingly healthy up to within a couple of years, has just died, after a short illness.¹ We discovered, two years ago, that she had diabetes, and although she had not had much suffering in consequence of it, still that was beginning, and would have come in greater force had not an intercurrent illness broken the nutritional balance and brought matters to a crisis.

If you will pass this note on to our friend, Dr. Freud, I shall be very much obliged. I think he would remember her, because she was at the Adirondacks when he was there, and I well recall a pleasant picture of her sitting next to him at the table and chatting happily, as it seemed to me, with him. She was singularly free from self-consciousness, and met every one, including strangers, with a natural simplicity and appreciation of their good qualities. Of course at the time of Freud's visit she was only twelve years old, and he may not recall her.

Strangely enough she seemed, up to the time when this trouble was discovered, to be the strongest member of our family.

Yours sincerely,

James J. Putnam[2]

[1] Frances Cabot Putnam (1897–1913).

[2] Below the closing of this typed letter, Putnam added in ink: "This is not the daughter of whom I have several times written to Dr. Freud, with reference to attacks that must be called epileptic [Louisa Higginson Putnam (1895–1958), see Putnam to Freud, September 30, October 6, October 20, November 14, 1911]. We think this latter is improving, although but slowly. Our three older children are perfectly well." [Elizabeth Cabot Putnam (1888–   ), James Jackson Putnam (1890–   ), Marian Cabot Putnam (1893–   ).]

148
Putnam to Jones
[July 17, 1914]

Boston

July 17 [1]

I had no right to bother you with my doubts, and have indeed decided to go ahead and do my best, trusting my instinct that I have something to say. I have also begun to read the very interesting accounts of Bunyan and propose to carry on the two jobs together.[2] At the same time, I wish to make no serious blunders or to follow any path that I shall have to retrace. So that if at any time you have a suggestion or two to make, from your point of vantage, it will be very welcome.

I shall look carefully for outcries from the friends of those whom Freud struck at, with his crushing sincerity.[3] I know however that it had to be.

Yours sincerely

James J. Putnam

VII.17

[1] On the address side of this postcard there is this note: "*Please tear up*. E. J."

[2] Probably a reference to *Human Motives* (Boston: Little, Brown and Co., 1915), which Putnam had begun to write. The Bunyan project was not carried out.

[3] See Freud, "Zur Geschichte der psychoanalytischen Bewegung" [On the History of the Psychoanalytic Movement], *Jahrbuch,* 6 (1914), 207–260; SE, XIV, 2–66.

149
Putnam to Jones
[August 19, 1914

Aug. 19, 1914
106 Marlborough Street

Dear Dr. Jones

I have your war letter[1] and thank you for it very much. We here can hardly think or talk of anything but war and everyone feels at liberty to become a war-critic if not a Napoleon or a Moltke, or a Cassandra. It is horribly interesting to glance at the whole situation from the standpoint of a psychologist, but heart-rending to think of it from most other standpoints.

Think of men who might have rendered incalculable service in the cause of sublimation, going down before a stray bullet or a bayonet, fired or used presumably by no unfriendly hand! Suppose it had all happened twentyfive years ago, and Freud had been the victim. Well, the only consolation is that sublimation does *on the whole* gain (doesn't it?) as the centuries roll on; and perchance some future Germany if really in fear of some Slav power will conciliate a future France instead of furiously dashing itself against her!

It seems as if this might have been so easily accomplished! And then, why should not the Slav consciousness have a chance? Are Russians and Servians, with all their fine qualities to be *forever* pushed aside from the world's table?

Thank you for telling me about our various friends; may no harm come to them!

I have, by the way, two young nephews in England or Wales, and a sister and brother in law in Switzerland, but unless the conflagration spreads inconceivably they are safe enough.[2]

I trust that Lord Kitchener is really the genius that he used to seem, and that he may be as good in organizing as in detailed performance.[3]

I am not surprised at Jung's success in England and although of course I wish he had been a sounder and more unselfish man, yet on the whole I think we may be glad.[4] He is engaging and dominating and the best of those who follow him may go still further, though not without some effort.

Very sincerely

James J. Putnam

[1] Missing.

[2] The nephews cannot be identified; the others were the sister of Marian Cabot Putnam, Mrs. Arthur Lyman, her daughter, Margaret Lyman, and her brother, Stephen Perkins Cabot.

[3] Horatio Herbert Kitchener (1850–1916), Field Marshal and Secretary for War, who organized the British Armies in 1914. He had been commander in chief in Egypt in 1892 and reconquered Khartoum in 1898.

[4] Jung read "The Importance of the Unconscious in Psychopathology" to the section on Neurology and Psychological Medicine at the eighty-second annual meeting of the British Medical Association, July 29–31, 1914. See *British Medical Journal*, 2 (December 5, 1914), 964–966.

150

Putnam to Jones

[November 1, 1914]

Finished, Nov. 1. 1914

106 Marlborough Street

Dear Dr. Jones

It is delightful to get yr. letter[1] and to feel in touch with you again.

I shd have written to you before but I felt that you might be Heaven knew where and doing Heaven knew what — perhaps medical service in the army — and that in face of so many bigger interests a letter would seem almost an intrusion. Yr. acct. of the people who are carrying on their work unmoved — and the enterprises of all sorts that are being carried out without change, especially the ps.an^c publications,[2] is highly interesting and instructive and presumably stimulating.

I was, at any rate, just about to read Cramb's book, and although that one of Russell's of which you speak is yet to be read, I did hear his whole course of Lowell lectures, last winter, and have read several articles in Hibbert's Jr. by him, so that I feel acquainted with his drift.[3]

I had not heard of Federn's[4] troubles and if you know how I can communicate with him I will write to him. He sent me a note just before he sailed, as I believe I told you.

I have found the events of the war, with all their collaterals, not only immensely engrossing, and painfully interesting, but exceedingly depressing, so much so as to interfere somewhat seriously with work and sleep at times. Finally, I concluded that this attitude was unmanly and neurotic and have called a halt on it, but thus far, or until recently, newspapers and kindred literature had the floor, not wholly, indeed, but in large measure.

A couple of days ago I went to hear Prof. Francke[5] — a good fellow — make an address on Germany's ideals, which on the whole was eloquent and well done.

But, impressive though it was to hear the apotheosis of the German strivings for the success of their national ideals, and easy though it was to feel, as by radiation, the glow and warmth of F.'s enthusiasm, the ultimate effect was to make me feel all the more [as I used to feel with reference to Nietzsche's superman idea] the intolerability and the tragedy of the situation.

Francke indeed admitted, himself, in conversation with my brother in law, that — while he could not agree that Germany wished the war or had planned a pan-Germany — yet it was true and tragic that the ideals of the military party did involve, almost necessarily, the crowding out of 'uncomfortable neighbors' (whose ideals and civilization they do not understand). In other words, the world cannot stop at nationalism but must pass on to cosmopolitanism, in the best sense.

This gives a distinct interest to a little book just published by Josiah Royce, called, The War and Insurance,[6] which is a working out, on the philosophical side, of his theory of loyalty.

I am thankful to hear you say that Germany cannot absolutely win out, in your judgment, and should be glad if some cause — unlikely enough I fear — brought about our interference on your side, so that Germany might be 'crushed.' What calamities will follow if this does not happen, or if — through big guns and Zeppelins — the reverse happens; or, on the other hand, what new and almost unforeseeable form of civilization may arise, it is idle now to think of.

If you all can be cheerful and courageous, surely we should be. May Kitchener[7] prove himself the host that we have thought him.

Later.

Since writing the above I have read Cramb — of course with the greatest interest — and also several thoughtful papers in the last issue of Hibbert's Jr. which form I think [I have Jacks's article especially in mind] a good supplement to the book.[8] I have also been indulging myself in attending a number of the lectures on Nietzsche, by the French exchange professor — Lichtenberger — and have enjoyed them very much.[9]

Both from them as well as from Salter's[10] paper in the Hibbert Jr., I conclude that he was by no means the monster he is usually made out to be, although I can easily imagine that his countrymen have drawn inferences from his writings to feed their Jehovahism, which has certainly grown large.

But enough of the war, with all its horrors and its splendors. May your people be strong, brave, inventive and persistent and SUCCESSFUL! Faulty as the course of England has often been, we love her and what she has stood and still stands for, with all our hearts, and realize that she is apt to do best when her back is fairly against the wall. A Russian here [Prof. Wiener],[11] speaking on Russian ideals, has brought out the view, with which, I think, all of us must agree; namely, that no nation lives for itself alone but is at its best itself when giving out its best to other nations and getting, too, their best from them. That is, of course, the real sense in which we want to possess Germany, and to be possessed by her.

———

Our small ps.a.ᶜ group has resumed its meetings, and if we do not illumine the world, we sharpen at least each others' wits.[12]

I have been reading Prince's book[13] and am impressed with the voluminousness of his data and the luminousness of his style. At the same time I find it dry reading, because — I suppose — of the very quality which recommends his work to himself; namely, that it lacks — not wholly indeed but relatively to psychoanalysis — the connecting thread of human interest. However, I could not have written it, and he has, and each one must utilize his contributions as he can. I have also read, though not word for word or as fully as I should wish, Silberer's Symbolik der Mystik,[14] and found much in it to admire and, I hope, to use.

What an excellent and interesting piece of work Rank and

Sachs's study of the extra medical contributions of ps.a. is!¹⁵ I have been over it once hastily but intend reading it again shortly.

I am extremely sorry to hear of your physical troubles and trust that the operation of which you speak will set you right.

Taking the whole year together, you have had, I judge, an unusual amount of handicap in the illness line. But your life is still ahead of you, whereas I have just passed my sixty eighth birthday. I do not complain, but it is also, and naturally, the case that fatigue comes far more quickly than it once did. I hope to finish one small, and I fear you will say inadequate book this winter¹⁶ and, if it is possible, which I doubt, to go over the same ground more thoroughly, later on. I do not feel quite sure that Freud is right in limiting the amount of contribution that ps.a may make even to the teaching of ethics, because I cannot yet, separate sharply men's 'symptoms' from their faults and their shortcomings.

Very sincerely

James J. Putnam

¹ Missing.

² See Jones, *Sigmund Freud*, II, 181, 187.

³ John Adams Cramb, *Germany and England* (New York: E. P. Dutton and Co., 1914). Possibly Bertrand Russell, *War, The Offspring of Fear* (London: Union of Democratic Control, 1914). Russell's Lowell Lectures, delivered in March and April, 1914, were published as *Our Knowledge of the External World* (Chicago: Open Court Publishing Co., 1915). See also Russell, "The Essence of Religion," *Hibbert Journal*, 11 (October 1912), 46–62, and "Mysticism and Logic," *ibid.*, 12 (July 1914), 780–803.

⁴ Paul Federn (1872–1950), Viennese psychoanalyst, had been lecturing in America and had difficulties returning home. His ship was turned back to New York, and he finally arrived in Trieste on a neutral vessel. See Jones, *Sigmund Freud*, II, 173.

⁵ Kuno Francke (1855–1930), professor of the history of German culture, Harvard University.

⁶ *War and Insurance* (New York: The Macmillan Co., 1914).

⁷ See n. 3, Putnam to Jones, August 19, 1914.

⁸ L. P. Jacks, "Mechanism, Diabolism and the War," *Hibbert Journal*, 13 (October 1914), 29–49.

⁹ Henri Lichtenberger (1864–1941), professor of German literature at the Sorbonne, author of *La Philosophie de Nietzsche* (1898).

¹⁰ William Mackintire Salter, "The Philosopher of 'The Will to Power,'" *Hibbert Journal*, 13 (October 1914), 102–123.

¹¹ Leo Wiener (1867–1939), professor of Slavic languages and literatures, Harvard University.

¹² Probably a reference to the Boston Psychoanalytic Society founded in 1914 with Putnam as president and Isador Coriat as secretary. See *Journal of Abnormal Psychology*, 9 (April–May 1914), 71.

[13] Prince, *The Unconscious: The Fundamentals of Human Personality, Normal and Abnormal* (New York: The Macmillan Co., 1914).

[14] Herbert Silberer (1882–1922), *Probleme der Mystik und ihrer Symbolik* (Leipzig and Vienna: H. Heller, 1914), trans. by Smith Ely Jelliffe as *Problems of Mysticism and its Symbolism* (New York: Moffat, Yard and Co., 1917).

[15] Otto Rank and Hanns Sachs, *Die Bedeutung der Psychoanalyse für die Geisteswissenschaften* (Wiesbaden: Bergmann, 1913); *The Significance of Psychoanalysis for the Mental Sciences*, trans. Charles Rockwell Payne, *Psychoanalytic Review*, 2 (1915), 297–326, 428–457; 3 (1916), 69–89, 189–214, 318–335, Nervous and Mental Disease Monograph No. 23 (New York: Nervous and Mental Disease Publishing Co., 1916).

[16] *Human Motives.*

151

Putnam to Jones

[May 12, 1915]

106 Marlborough Street

Dear Dr. Jones

Your letter[1] was forwarded to me in New York, just at the close of the meetings — about which I will tell you. Before I do so let me say that the Psychopath. Soc.[2] unanimously and gladly placed your name on the list of honorary — I believe literally "associate" — members. I was not in the room when the motion was made though I came in time to vote. I understand however that it was offered by Stanley Hall[3] who spoke of you as the chief pillar of the enterprise, or in similar terms, — a sentiment which I am sure every person felt as sound and true.

It is very certain that I should not be taking the position I do take, and that my last four years would have been very different affairs, had it not been for two or three eventful talks with you in the spring of 1910, followed as they were by the momentous visit of Freud, Jung and Ferenczi to Worcester and later to the Adirondacks.[4]

Perhaps I should be earning a larger income if I had gone along on the old paths, but that is another matter. (My practice just now is nothing to boast of.)

Let me say also, before I begin on New York, that we had the terrible news of the Lusitania disaster.[5] I will not try to swell the list of adjectives or to apportion blame. The whole situation makes one too dizzy to contemplate it with justice. But the pressing question is What can we *do* to help? and this is far more easily asked than answered.

I believe I told you that I have a nephew in the automobile ambulance service, and that my son[6] is going over with a friend, to work as orderly in the American Hosp. in Paris until something else turns up for them to do. They do not claim that they go as doctors but certainly sympathy with you all is one motive.

By the way, you speak of your membership in the A. Ps.A.,[7] but I assure you that no one would dream of considering you out of it, as long as you are willing to let your name remain. There is in fact no one who can take your place with any adequacy, though Brill is honest, courageous and sound. White and Jelliffe have their good points, and McCurdy is at times really brilliant and full of energy.[8]

Hoch's paper[9] was a critical study of Freud's pronouncements on the subject of "repression and Object-libido." I am fond of Hoch and think him genuine and sympathetic. Also, *perhaps,* his primary contention is sound, that we ought to look closely at what Fr. has *said,* and not be too ready to read between the lines what we may think he meant, which is sometimes what we *think.* However, I am more in the mood of going as far as possible on this very — latter — path, so that in fact I did not care so very, very much about the paper, except in so far as it made me think where the real truth lies.

The discussion was a good informal talk, but led to no conclusions, as of course.

In the evening Hall made a good impression with his paper on the fear of death, which I have heard before.[10] He bases this sentiment largely on the horror of putrefaction and had little or nothing to say about deeper ideas and repressions. The discussion was however interesting. Burrow's paper,[11] — in which he carried the notion of identification with the mother, through ante-natal impressions, to a far point, — aroused quite a talk. His idea, which is slated to explain one root of homosexualism, may be of great value; I dare say it is, but he trod on my philosophic corns by a few expressions such as that "Nature abhors self-consciousness."

This opinion is the equivalent of one which Stanley Hall has voiced and which I regard as not a sound one.

The idea is that *theoretically* evolution should go on in smooth-
ness and silence and that the inruption of consciousness and reason is a sign of theoretical failure of the plan. I wd take up the
gauntlet on this issue, for I think that evil belongs, not only
practically but theoretically, to the order of events. However, the
paper was noteworthy and I would not prejudice you against it.

The most important event of the Ps.path. meeting was the adop-
tion of a constitution etc. looking towards a drawing in of psychiatrists. It was proposed that the name of the society shd be
changed but in the end this was voted down.

Stanley Hall read an interesting paper[12] showing that not alone
sexuality but anger, and other instincts cd profitably be studied
à la Freud.

He always marshalls a vast array of facts but also always leaves
me with the feeling that he has emphasized points of secondary
importance.

Before you hear from me again you will receive my little
volume.[13] I wish I might see your face as you glance over it.

Alas, I wish also that I could hear some very solid critic say
that German submarines w^d never win the day.

Sincerely
James J. Putnam

[1] Missing.

[2] American Psychopathological Association, sixth annual meeting, New York, May
5, 1915. *Journal of Abnormal Psychology*, 10 (1915–1916), 263–292. Jones's letter is
missing.

[3] Granville Stanley Hall (1844–1924), President of Clark University and a member
of the American Psychoanalytic Association.

[4] The conversations took place in the spring of 1909, and Freud visited America
the following September.

[5] The Cunard liner Lusitania was sunk by a German submarine May 7, 1915, in
the Irish Sea, with 1,198 dead, of whom 124 were American citizens. A total of
761 passengers and crew were rescued.

[6] James Jackson Putnam.

[7] The American Psychoanalytic Association was founded at Freud's request by
Jones and Putnam on May 9, 1911, in Baltimore. See Freud to Putnam, June 16,
1910, Putnam to Freud, [late July, 1910].

[8] A. A. Brill; William Alanson White; Smith Ely Jelliffe; John T. MacCurdy
(1886–1947), lecturer in medical psychology, Cornell University Medical College.

[9] Hoch's paper does not appear in the *Proceedings* and was not published.

[10] G. Stanley Hall, "Thanatophobia and Immortality," *American Journal of Psychology*, 26 (October 1915), 550–613.

[11] Trigant Burrow (1875–1950), "Material Illustrative of the Principle of Primary
Identification," unpublished.

[12] "The Freudian Methods Applied to Anger," *American Journal of Psychology*, 26 (July 1915), 438–443.
[13] *Human Motives.*

152
Putnam to Jones[1]
[May 14, 1915]

Just a line more to say that I have been reading for the second time your Janet criticism and that I think very temperate, fair and good.[2]

I am very sorry about J., whom I know and am fond of, but he certainly has shown himself an unscientific and ungenerous opponent.[3] Do send me a few words of opinion on submar. prospects.

James J. Putnam

May 14.

[1] Possibly an addition to Putnam's letter to Jones of May 12, 1915. The evidence on this point is not clear.
[2] Jones, "Professor Janet on Psycho-Analysis: A Rejoinder," *Journal of Abnormal Psychology*, 9 (1914–1915), 400–410; PPsa, 2nd ed.
[3] See Pierre Janet, "Psychoanalysis."

153
Putnam to Jones
[July 21, 1915]

July 21, 1915.

Dear Dr. Jones.[1]

Thank you for your letter,[2] as always, so satisfactory and interesting. You will have seen that my last brief note was written just before your last arrived. I was rather dreading your comments on my little book and was greatly relieved that you were able to see it as I meant it.[3]

In fact, I am for psychoanalysis, root and branch, but wish and intend to find its place and meaning in terms of the marvellous Auseinandersetzungen[4] of Hegel.

Of course your criticisms are sound and could have been multiplied many times with justice. My "history" is responsible for much that is mischievous, there as elsewhere, and made me shrink timidly from saying what I believe — especially in a popular book — upon the sex in childhood question.

Sometimes I am tempted to try writing about it so clearly and carefully and reasonably and yet fully, that no one not an idiot could go wrong, but still I shrink.

I write now mainly to thank you, in the first place, and in the next place to try to answer your questions, to give a little — very little — gossip, and, most of all, to tell you, once again, a brief dream of my own, in the hope of a comment like the last, — when leisure serves you, — if it ever does!

You ask ab^t y^r civic duties with reference to the war, and refer to the strong reasons for not positively going into active service. I recognize the significance of what you say and feel as if the decision must depend upon the actual urgency of the need and on whether you c^d make effective use of the knowledge and skill in which you are especially equipped. A man might well feel, under some circumstances, that he c^d not stay at home even though he c^d not accomplish very much by going, but you are filling an extremely useful place, and one which practically no one else can fill and this fact ought to count for much in favor of staying where you are. Would it not be practicable for you to go to a certain place — perhaps even in France if need be — at regular intervals, for neurological consultations? I can conceive that this might be of real service, but perhaps your experience with the half-time plan would lead you to think differently.

Have you talked with anyone in authority, so that you know to what an extent the armies are suffering for lack of *medical* aid? Osler[5] of course wd know. It is tragic to consider what multitudes of lives that might have been so fruitful in some other field have been sacrificed or turned into less good channels.

Yet at moments one cannot count cost in ordinary terms and would use bankbills to light a fire. May we live long enough to see the evidences, that are sure to come, in the way of better harvests than are now visible.

I hope that Sachs and Rank go as physicians, not as soldiers.[6]

It is wonderful how vigorously Freud's mind still works. I thought his recent paper on Trieb u. Triebschicksale, and still more the Ratschläge,[7] as keen as anything he has written on such lines. I had a good though brief letter from him about ten days ago, in which he reiterates his lack of interest in philosophic questions and attitudes and — in the most friendly way — his disagreement with me about connection between psychoanalysis and ethics.[8] He does not see for instance why ps.^{ansts} sh^d be expected to be any more sublimated than ordinary people, whereas from my standpoint, and for reasons that you can readily understand, there is good reason why this result sh^d be expected — namely, bec^e infantile tendencies partially control every aspect of our lives.

I am just in receipt of a joint note from Pfister and Payne, asking permission to dedicate to me the translation of Pf.'s Ps.an.se.[9] It is a pleasant honor but I think that Brill — not to speak of y'rself — must think it strange that so late a comer and so feeble an advocate is chosen in place of a more aggressive and scientific worker. I note what you say about America in the eyes of European criticism and wish with all my heart that we could do, and had done, more. Still, one should imagine some other government in our place and then think — in the light of history — whether the result would have been very different.

This letter has run on so far that my dream must wait.

Sincerely

James J. Putnam

[1] On the top left margin Putnam wrote, "Have you, by the way, received quite a large sized cabinet photograph of myself?"

[2] Missing.

[3] *Human Motives*.

[4] Explanations.

[5] Sir William Osler (1849–1919), Regius Professor of Medicine at Oxford, and a friend of Putnam. Born in Canada, he had taught at The Johns Hopkins University, and had written on chorea and cerebral palsies in children, as well as on diseases of the spleen, blood, and heart.

[6] Freud's closest assistants during the war years, Otto Rank and Hanns Sachs, were inducted into the Austrian Army in 1915, but Sachs was released after twelve days' training.

[7] Freud, "Triebe und Triebschicksale" [Instincts and Their Vicissitudes], *Zeitschrift*, 3 (1913), 84–100; SE, XIV, 109–140; and "Weitere Ratschläge zur Technik der Psychoanalyse" [Further Recommendations on the Technique of Psychoanalysis] published in three parts: I, "Zur Einleitung der Behandlung" [On Beginning the Treatment], *Zeitchrift*, 1 (1913), 1–10, 139–146; II, "Erinnern, Wiederholen und Durcharbeiten" [Remembering, Repeating, and Working-Through], *Zeitschrift*, 2 (1914), 485–491; and III "Bemerkungen über die Übertragungsliebe" [Observations on Transference-Love], *Zeitschrift*, 3 (1915), 1–11; SE, XII, 121–171.

[8] See Freud to Putnam, July 8, 1915, and June 7, 1915.

⁹ Oscar Pfister, *Die psychoanalytische Methode*. Published as *The Psychoanalytic Method*, trans. Charles Rockwell Payne (New York: Moffat, Yard and Co., 1917). The American edition was dedicated to "Prof. James Jackson Putnam in appreciation of his service in introducing Psychoanalysis in America." Payne (1880–1926) was a psychiatrist, a translator, and member of the American Psychoanalytic Association.

154
Putnam to Jones
[October 1, 1915]

1/10/15
106 Marlborough Street

Dear Dr. Jones

Best thanks for yr. letter,[1] which, as usual, sets me thinking deeply.

I shall read with deepest interest yʳ paper on the war,[2] and congratulate you heartily that you can write so freely and so well and have so clear a mind.

Would that London were nearer Boston!

The chance of harm coming to Rank or Sachs is indeed dreadful to contemplate. But I imagine that the siege of Vienna is still far away.

You were right about the submarines, and I can imagine your rejoicings over the present news.

As regards the question of "religion" [wh. — you will understand — is no dogma with me] I feel bound to say my say about it just because the scientific attitude is so recalcitrant or hostile.

Of course it has a heavy load of sins to bear — so to speak — but one shᵈ not for that, I think, while glad to recognize the claims of "justice" and "honor" etc. etc., fail to admit those of the moving spirit that underlies justice and honor and makes them possible.

My God by the way is not "in the skies," as of course you know.

Furthermore, since the stream cannot rise higher than its source, and since we are "personal" yet have obvious possibilities of further progress, I can see no other possibility than that the universe is personal and may fairly demand a personal recognition.

However, no one, right or left, cares for generalizations such as these and I doubt much if I write more, on any subject.

Sincerely, as ever

James J. Putnam

¹ Jones's letter is missing.
² Jones wrote two papers on the war, "War and Individual Psychology," *Sociological Review*, 8 (1915), 167–180, and "War and Sublimation," which was read before the British Association for the Advancement of Science, Section of Psychology, Manchester, September 10, 1915, and was published in the *International Review*, 1 (1915), 453–461. Both were included in Jones, *Essays on Applied Psycho-Analysis* (London and Vienna: The International Psycho-Analytical Press, 1923, and London: The Hogarth Press and the Institute for Psycho-Analysis, 1951).

155

Putnam to Jones

[November 12, 1916]

Nov. 12 (finished Nov. 19), 1916
106 Marlborough Street

Dear Dr. Jones

It seems to me high time that we exchanged letters again. I am anxious for news of you and from you and sh^d like to know whether you received my paper on Adler¹ and if it seemed a fair presentation of the case. I have just come in from Cambridge where I had a long talk with an able young man (an applicant for Ph.D.) who was a close and favorite student of Josiah Royce — recently deceased — and is acting as his literary biographer.²

I have always been a friend and admirer of Royce and in substantial agreement with his philosophy, and I was pleased to find myself strengthened in my beliefs through this conversation.

I feel also confirmed in my intention of writing two or more suitable papers and then publishing the cream of all that I have thus far put out, in the form of a book entitled Introduction to Psychoanalysis. One portion of it w^d be the study — with the able collaboration of the patient, a lady — of a case which presents, I think, some points of interest.³

May my zeal not flag!

I have just received a card from Freud,⁴ and am glad to have it for I feared I should not hear from him again until the war was over. He gives no news of his sons, nor does he say whether, — or that — he received a book and paper that I sent him. I shall write to him today.

His Leonardo (translated by Brill) is out, as of course you know. I am sorry to say the translation seems to me extremely poor, mainly to be sure from the literary standpoint.

It seems to me a serious misfortune that Freud, whose writings and style, which though fine are sometimes hard to master, should have been presented so inadequately to his English-speaking public. I am somewhat surprised that Brill himself, who is conscientious, should not have seen this. However, so it is.

A patient of mine is now translating Das Seelenleben des Kindes[5] and I shall make it my business to see that it is well done.

I have been reading Kaplan's Gründz. d. Psa.[6] and find it interesting. What do you think of it?

Prince is at home again and I have met him once and talked with him several times by telephone.[7]

I believe he intends going abroad again but of this I am not sure.

Meantime he is making addresses here and there and is to give one soon for the benefit of the Social Service Dept. of the M. G. H., in which I am interested.[8]

I doubt if I have other news in which you would be interested. Your friend Dr. Payne, who is a neighbor of mine (25 miles away to be sure) in the country, brought over Jelliffe and White[9] for a good visit, in September, and I enjoyed them and learned afresh to admire their industry.

Their journal (the Psychoanalytic Rev.) seems to me to fill a good place and to gain in interest. I have just received an announcement from Stanley Hall that he is to edit a new periodical, dealing with applied psychology,[10] and this reminds me to say — what you probably know more about than I — that a certain amount of familiarity with psychoanalysis is rather rapidly on the increase in America, as witness frequent references in journals, books (Wallas's great society, for instance, The New Republic).[11] It is taken up also in certain courses and seminaries at Harvard, especially by Holt and Hocking.[12]

In a few weeks I am to give a talk to a group of Radcliffe students.

Some of the comments are misleading even though friendly and I have started a paper of explanation, one part of which will deal with Trotter's Herd Inst.[13]

By the way, I met Mrs. Toulmin yesterday, looking very well. She is just starting for Manchuria to shoot tigers!!!

Sincerely yours,

James J. Putnam

[1] "The Work of Alfred Adler, Considered with Especial Reference to That of Freud," *Psychoanalytic Review*, 3 (April 1916), 121–140; Ad Psa, 312–365.

[2] Possibly William Fergus Kernan (1892–   ), Royce's last graduate assistant. Royce died September 14, 1916.

[3] The project was not carried out. But see Putnam, "Sketch for a Study of New England Character," which utilized in part his patient's written account of her case, *Journal of Abnormal Psychology*, 12 (June 1917), 73–99; Ad Psa, 366–396.

[4] Probably Freud to Putnam, October 1, 1916.

[5] Hermine von Hugo-Hellmuth, *Aus dem Seelenleben des Kindes: eine psycho-analytische Studie* (Leipzig and Vienna: F. Deuticke, 1913).

[6] Leo Kaplan, *Grundzüge der Psychoanalyse* [Basic Principles of Psychoanalysis], Leipzig and Vienna: F. Deuticke, 1914.

[7] Prince was active in war work for the Allies and lectured on the war abroad.

[8] The department was founded by Richard Cabot at the Massachusetts General Hospital in 1905. Putnam added psychiatric social service in 1907.

[9] Charles Rockwell Payne, Smith Ely Jelliffe, and William Alanson White; White often spent part of the summer at Jelliffe's home at Hulett's Landing, Lake George.

[10] *Journal of Applied Psychology* (Worcester, Mass.), 1917–

[11] A vogue for psychoanalysis began among intellectuals around 1915. Graham Wallas's *The Great Society: A Psychological Analysis* (New York: Macmillan, 1914) was one of the first important appreciations of Freud by a philosopher. Wallas's student at Harvard Walter Lippmann and a classmate, Alfred Booth Kuttner, both wrote extensively on psychoanalysis for the *New Republic*.

[12] See William Ernest Hocking, "The Holt-Freudian Ethics and the Ethics of Royce," in *Philosophical Review*, 25 (May 1916), 479–506, and Holt, *The Freudian Wish and its Place in Ethics*.

[13] Wilfred Batten Lewis Trotter, *The Instincts of the Herd in Peace and War* (London: T. Fisher Unwin, 1916).

156
Putnam to Jones
[March 11, 1917]

March 11th 1917

106 Marlborough Street

Dear Dr. Jones

Fine! Fine! I congratulate you with all my heart. Life must indeed take on fresh color for you and we shall all reap a portion of the benefits. I shall write to Freud and tell him, but whether my letters will get through I cannot say. I have written three times already but have received no answer. What a honeymoon week you must have had! [1]

And to think of your enlisting for the army — for the medical service I assume! I trust they will reject you, but England is having several sorts of hard times just now, and I can understand that you would wish to go if needed over in France.

May it not be very long before your wife and you can come across to Boston for your greatly needed change.

Please accept and extend my most cordial wishes and greetings, and may good fortune smile on you.

Sincerely,
James J. Putnam

[1] Jones married Morfydd Owen, a young Welsh musician, in 1916. She died from delayed chloroform poisoning after an appendectomy in 1918. Hanns Sachs introduced Jones to Katherina Jokl; they were engaged in three days and married within three weeks, in October 1919. They had four children. See Jones, *Free Associations*, pp. 253–255, 259.

157
Putnam to Jones
[December 8, 1917]

Dec. 8. 17/
106 Marlborough Street

Dear Dr. Jones

I am delighted that this ridiculous period of silence is over and that our pleasant correspondence can begin again. As a matter of fact, I wrote to you, at considerable length, quite a time ago, but never sent the letter because I was not satisfied with it.

Since then I have thought of you innumerable times, and, about two weeks ago, I wrote a half a page, complaining of the blockage and taking the blame upon myself. Of course there has been some sort of inhibitory influence at work, of which 'laziness' would be an imperfect designation.

But I will not take the time to analyze it now, otherwise than to say that it goes with other inhibitions that are too numerous.

Last Sunday came McCurdy, and made me an exceedingly pleasant call, and on top of that came, a few days ago, your letter.[1]

McC. and I talked, of course, of you, and he made me feel in a measure, as if I had been eye-witness of your new menage.[2] I like him and his views and am reading with great interest his paper in the last number of the psychiatric bulletin.[3]

I am glad that you are getting out a new edition of your papers,[4] for everything that you write has real thought behind it and careful observation. I ought to write more, for I have but little practice and yet have material enough to use intensively, if the power was there. The leisure may not last however for the need of doing indirect war-work looms up, and indeed I greatly wish to be of service.

One job will be a limited amount of hospital service, to supplement that of our somewhat dwindling department, the other, helping to organize preparations for the care of men coming home mentally disabled. When I do write — and that goes on a little all the time — I drift strongly toward the old theme — that a man is a bigger thing, and impelled by more motives, that[5] most psychoanalysts conceive, and that the habit should grow, among the latter, of cultivating, primarily for their own edification, secondarily for that of their patients, idealistic views of life. I do believe that the scientific method, when it comes to a dealing with human notives, is somewhat inadequate and even stifling, marvellous though it is as an instrument in its place.

The way out, I think, and one which does not necessarily bring in metaphysics, is to keep alive the feeling that, *theoretically* a psa trt should not be regarded as complete until it had seen the patient landed (I will not say 'how,' for there trouble begins) on the shores of a somewhat advanced sublimation. I will write again soon.

Very sincerely,

James J. Putnam

[1] John Thomson MacCurdy, a member of the American Psychoanalytic Association; he made important studies of the war neuroses in England and from 1923 was lecturer in psychopathology at the University of Cambridge. Jones's letter is missing.

[2] See preceding letter.

[3] See MacCurdy, "War Neuroses," *Psychiatric Bulletin of the New York State*

Hospitals, 2 (July 1917) (State Hospital Bulletin Series II, vol. X), pp. 243–354, and his review of M. D. Eder, *War Shock, ibid.*, pp. 386–388.

⁴ See Jones, *Papers on Psycho-Analysis*, rev. and enl. ed. (London: Baillière, Tindall, and Cox, 1918).

⁵ Than.

IV

Ferenczi–Putnam Correspondence

Letters 158–168

Sandor Ferenczi, 1909–1914

Ferenczi was born in 1874 and practiced as a neurologist in Buda-pest for ten years before taking up psychoanalysis. His interest was aroused by a rereading of the *Traumdeutung* and the *Studies in Hysteria* and by a meeting with Freud in 1907. Ferenczi accom-panied Freud and Carl Jung to America in September 1909. It was Ferenczi who, in daily walks an hour before Freud was sched-uled to speak, suggested the topics he should take up in his Five Lectures on Psychoanalysis delivered ex tempore in German at the Clark Conference. Putnam's personal impressions of Ferenczi and Jung, as well as of Freud, dispelled lingering doubts about the integrity of the psychoanalysts.

Ferenczi's formal, almost courtly letters, described for Putnam exactly how psychoanalysis differed from previous therapies. Put-nam had been accustomed to encourage his patients to exercise their will and effort in overcoming their symptoms. Psychoanalysis avoided this on grounds that it would strengthen repressions. Ferenczi also clarified a point Freud had made at Clark: that as a result of psychoanalysis, a rational, conscious rejection should replace the unconscious repression of impulses.

One of the most original of the psychoanalysts, Ferenczi con-tributed interpretations of hypnosis and suggestion which Ernest Jones drew on for his own discussions of the subject in 1910. Ferenczi also made important studies of alcoholism, paranoia, and homosexuality.

Ferenczi criticized Putnam's paper, delivered at the Weimar Conference in 1911, on the significance of philosophy for psycho-analysis. Ferenczi argued that to attempt to make psychoanalysts accept any specific philosophy, such as Putnam's idealism, was premature and would hamper empirical investigation. Putnam re-plied that the youth of psychoanalysis did not preclude analysts from becoming aware of their own philosophical presuppositions. Yet, in some respects, Ferenczi sympathized with Putnam's outlook. Ferenczi often spoke of medicine as a soulless discipline, and his own major work was the highly speculative *Genitaltheorie,* published in 1924.

Ferenczi also was concerned, as Putnam had been, by therapeutic failures. He drastically modified psychoanalytic techniques in the 1920's. The therapist, Ferenczi believed, should play an active role; he attempted to give patients the sense of love they had longed for as children. Ferenczi died from pernicious anemia in 1933, just before his sixtieth birthday.

158
Ferenczi to Putnam
[October 22, 1909]

Budapest, VII, Erzsébet-Körut 54
22/X. 1909.

Dear Professor

Forgive my presumption, if I say that I must "abreact" the feeling of gratitude aroused by your friendly hospitality at "Putnam's Camp." [1] I am now trying to do this by very simple words of thanks for everything you did for us which so greatly enhanced our stay in America. Please express my thanks to all the ladies of your household as well as to Mr. Charles Putnam,[2] and give my best greetings to the young people. It will interest Mrs. Putnam to learn that my friend Dr. Thuolt (the judge in Budapest) is actually a relative of that Hungarian friend of the Putnam family.

With repeated sincere greetings,

Yours ever,

Ferenczi

[1] Ferenczi with Freud and Jung had visited Putnam Camp in the Adirondacks in September 1909, after the Clark Conference.

[2] Charles Pickering Putnam, M.D. (1844–1914), brother of James Jackson Putnam, and one of America's first specialists in pediatrics.

159
Ferenczi to Putnam

[November 27, 1909]

Budapest, VII, Erzsébet-Körut 54
d. 27 November, 1909

Dear Professor

Thank you heartily for your detailed letter:[1] I am happy to learn how great your interest is in the new directions in psychology and psychotherapy. The countless problems which obtrude especially when one first takes up psychoanalysis unfortunately can't be dealt with adequately within the narrow limits of correspondence. However, I assure you from my own cases, that with increasing experience much becomes simpler than it seemed to be at the outset. Inevitably other equally difficult problems arise; definitive and all-embracing knowledge never can be attained.

As for cases of impotence, you will find some information in the article I enclose and in the one I have sent already.[2] In my opinion, it is much better not to influence the patient in any way during the analysis. In this way one helps him to obtain a complete insight into his unconscious and to look at the darker aspects without any pangs of conscience. Of course that does not imply that the impulses he has previously repressed can be allowed unlimited expression. The patient should be told that he ought to *acknowledge* what he has denied up to now, and then, *for appropriate, practical reasons consciously reject it.* Freud puts it this way: conscious condemnation should take the place of repression.

Part of the libido then will find its own way to natural erotic satisfaction. The part which cannot be satisfied will be checked by consciousness (this kind of resolution by means of conscious thought is in fact also a form of sublimation), on the other hand, the patient then instinctively will look for and find objects from which he can derive sublimated pleasure. It is difficult to make general rules; methods of sublimation differ in each case.

In principle I believe that it is important to make a strict distinction between sublimation and repression. If a patient who has not had an analysis or has not completed an analysis is persuaded to overcome the compulsiveness of a symptom by an "effort of will", one does to him what he would have done instinctively himself, i.e., the symptom is repressed a bit more. But that is not a cure, because whatever has been repressed will become manifest in another form. Cures by "re-education" and suggestion (without analysis) suppress the symptoms which then are replaced by new ones.

The analysis itself, I believe, is the first and most important thing. If it has reached a certain depth, ways and means of sublimation always will come up for discussion. But these must not be *forced* on a patient.

All this is only my personal opinion, and I cannot know definitely whether Professor Freud agrees with me on *every* point; however, I believe these views accord with the spirit of his writings. (The conversations I have had with him on these subjects reinforce this opinion).

With sincere greetings to you and those of your family whom I have met.

Yours most sincerely,
Dr. Ferenczi

P. S. The second volume of Jung's Assoz. Stud. has not yet appeared.[3]

¹ Missing.

² See Ferenczi, "Analytische Deutung und Behandlung der psychosexuellen Impotenz des Mannes" [Analytic Interpretation and Treatment of Psychosexual Impotence], *Psychiatrisch-neurologische Wochenschrift*, 10 (1908), 289–301, 305–309.

³ See C. G. Jung, *Diagnostische Assoziationsstudien: Beiträge zur experimentellen Psychopathologie*, [Studies in Word Association: Experiments in the Diagnosis of Psychopathological Conditions], 2 Bd. (Leipzig: J. A. Barth, 1910).

160
Ferenczi to Putnam

[February 1, 1910]

Budapest, VII, Erzsébet-Körut 54
Den Feb. 1, 1910

Dear Professor,

The photographs which you so kindly sent me are a pleasant reminder of our stay in America and more particularly of our visit to the hospitable Putnam Camp. Thank you sincerely for your kindness.

I am equally grateful to you for graciously mentioning my name in your article in the *Journal of Abnormal Psychology*,[1] which I saw the day before yesterday at Prof. Freud's. I would be greatly obliged to you if you could send me a reprint. At Prof. Freud's there was much talk of America, and we frequently mentioned the friendly reception which you accorded not only to us personally but also to psychoanalysis. It seems that the fight will be no less hot in America than here. However, the participation of important men such as you and Stanley Hall [2] will restrain the injudicious and uncritical attacks of our enemies.

You probably already have heard that this year's Psychoanalytic Congress probably will take place in Nuremburg on March 30–31. [3] We hope for a sizeable contingent from America.

With many greetings to you and to the members of your family, I am, as ever, faithfully yours,

Ferenczi

[1] Putnam, "Personal Impressions of Sigmund Freud and His Work, With Special Reference to His Recent Lectures at Clark University," *Journal of Abnormal Psychology*, 4 (December 1909–January 1910), 294; Ad Psa, 2.

[2] Granville Stanley Hall (1844–1924), president of Clark University.

[3] See Ferenczi to Putnam, April 1, 1910.

161
Ferenczi to Putnam
[March 8, 1910]

Budapest, VII, Erzsébet-Körut 54
den 8 Marz 1910

Dear Professor,

You were kind enough to write me a second letter even before I had answered the first.[1] I thank you warmly for both of them as well as for graciously mentioning me in your article.[2] I have already learned of this from Prof. Freud and look forward with much interest to the reprint you promised to send. I find your doubts about the success of therapy in reality unwarranted. We have learned by means of analysis both to understand and to help incomparably more than before. In addition, if one takes the time, (and to complete a cure often requires one to two years, although lighter cases can be considerably improved in three to four months), one can justifiably dismiss patients as "cured." Slight setbacks are possible, but are easy to remove. But it cannot be denied that there are cases in which at a certain stage, for example, in the transference, the cure faces insuperable difficulties. Sometimes external circumstances cause an undesirable interruption; in certain cases psychotic traits emerge from behind the neurosis, for example, paranoid tendencies, which hardly can be influenced therapeutically. But these are the exasperating exceptions. For the most part *very much indeed,* and in a practical way, everything can be accomplished if one is only patient and persistent. The most difficult phase is always the resolution of the transference. One makes many mistakes before learning the proper tactics. Knowledge must be paid for. — I now have had two patients in treatment for more than a year, one of them, an impotent man, has brought me nothing but resistances since October. There was no trace of any improvement. In the last two or three weeks he is at last giving up his resistances and he has erections. In the practice of psychoanalysis one must get accustomed to such time intervals.

With hearty thanks and many greetings to your honored family,

Yours ever,
Dr. Ferenczi

¹ Both letters are missing.
² See n. 1, preceding letter.

162
Ferenczi to Putnam
[April 1, 1910]

Budapest, Erzébet-Körut, 54
den 1 April 1910

Dear Professor

I have just returned from the second Psychoanalytic Congress which met yesterday and the day before in Nuremburg, to find your letter.[1] I hasten to thank you for it, as well as for the two issues of the *Journal of Abnormal Psychology*.[2] It is for us analysts a pleasure after all the attacks (which we suffer patiently and consider inevitable but by no means enjoy) finally to meet with recognition from a man whose love of the truth is more powerful than any preconceived resistances. I am convinced that your example will cause others to examine all these matters for themselves, and whoever does this *must* join us. Facts cannot be denied.

I owe you special thanks for the way you referred to me and for the favorable course you predicted for my scientific future.[3] Be that as it may, the joy of having stood at the cradle of this young science cannot be taken from us. I am still full of my impressions of the Congress. There were about 60 (55?) participants. Freud opened the Congress with most instructive observations on the future of psychoanalysis.[4] Abraham (Berlin), Maeder (Zurich), Honegger (Zurich), reported on analyses of fetishists and paranoiacs. Marczinowsky (Kiel) spoke on the role of dissociations of consciousness in neurosis; Löwenfeld on hypnosis (according to him this should be retained in conjunction with analysis). Stegmann (Dresden) discussed the way in which general practitioners could utilize psychoanalysis. Adler (Vienna) talked on psychosexual Hermaphroditism; Jung (who came directly from America where he had to make a hurried call on a patient) described his impressions.[5] I gave the reasons for my proposal to found an International organization.[6] This was accepted after lively discussion together with my proposals to make Zurich its headquarters and Jung, its president. We shall from now on be called the International Psychoanalytic Association, which at the moment consists of Associations in Vienna, Zurich, Berlin and Budapest. Probably there will also be a branch in Munich shortly. Would not one or more such groups be possible in America? It would be splendid if you could take this up with Jung. Again my hearty thanks for all your kindness.

Yours sincerely,

Ferenczi

₁ Putnam's letter is missing. At Freud's request, Ferenczi had presented plans for organizing the International Psychoanalytic Association. See Jones, *The Life and Work of Sigmund Freud*, 2 vols. (New York: Basic Books, 1955), II, 66–72, and Ferenczi, "Referat über die Notwendigkeit eines engeren Zusammenschlusses der Anhänger der Freudschen Lehre und Vorschläge zur Gründung einer ständigen

internationalen Organisation" [Report on the Need for a Closer Alliance of the Members of the Freudian School and Proposals for Founding a Permanent International Organization], *Zentralblatt*, 1 (1910), 131; in Ferenczi, *Final Contributions to the Problems and Methods of Psychoanalysis* (New York: Basic Books, 1955), 299–307.

² Putnam, "Personal Impressions of Sigmund Freud and His Work," in two parts, *Journal of Abnormal Psychology*, 4 (December 1909–January 1910), 293–310, and (February–March 1910), 372–379; Ad Psa, 1–30.

³ See respectively p. 294 in the *Journal of Abnormal Psychology* and p. 2 in Ad Psa in n. 2 above.

⁴ Freud, "Die zukünftigen Chancen der psychoanalytischen Therapie" [The Future Prospects of Psycho-Analytic Therapy], *Zentralblatt*, 1 (1910), 1–9; SE, XI, 139–151.

⁵ Of those listed, the following were the best known: Karl Abraham (1877–1925), founder of the Berlin Psychoanalytic Society; Alphonse Maeder (1882–   ), Swiss psychiatrist and psychotherapist; Leopold Löwenfeld (1847–1924), Munich neurologist; Alfred Adler (1870–1937), Viennese psychoanalyst, who left the movement in 1911 and founded Individual Psychology.

⁶ See n. 1 above.

163
Ferenczi to Putnam
[December 16, 1910]

Budapest, VII, Erzsébet-Körut 54
16. XII. 1910.

Dear Professor,

Please accept my sincerest thanks for sending me your articles. I have read them all with great pleasure and have learned much from them. The beautiful and warmly sincere obituary which you published about Professor James[1] was most interesting to me, not only because of its special content but also because, while reading it, I remembered the beautiful days spent with you in the primeval forests of the Adirondacks at your summer home.

With my sincere regards and many greetings to all those members of your family whom I met, Merry Christmas and Happy New Year;

Yours,
Ferenczi

[1] "William James," *Atlantic Monthly*, 106 (December 1910), 835–848.

164
Putnam to Ferenczi
[April 9, 1912]

April 9, 1912.

Dr. Ferenczi,
  Budapest, Hungary.

Dear Dr. Ferenczi:

Can you tell me, without too much trouble, about the standing and intelligence of Dr. Jenö Kollarits,[1] who has written recently on "Charakter und Nervosität"? I notice that he says:

"Ich muss ganz entschieden behaupten, dass heute die Freudsche Psychoanalyse zu den Hilfsbedingungen der Nervosität gerechnet werden muss, und es wird, wie es scheint, mit der Zeit noch ärger werden, wenn erst die Methode noch mehr verbreitet sein wird. Ein Gemüt, das gründlich psychoanalysiert wird, erträgt diesen brutalen Angriff nicht ohne Erschütterungen. Wir kennen alle schon Fälle, die diesem Verfahren zum Opfer gefallen sind. Solche Patienten verabschieden sich ohne Heilung und mit gesteigerter Nervosität von ihrem Psychoanalytiker. Ich kenne ein junges Mädchen, bei der die Psychoanalyse eine starke geschlechtliche Erregung hervorbrachte. Solche Fälle sind eine neue Abart der Unfallsneurose." [2]

Of course we all recognize that there are dangers in every treatment which is important enough to be placed in the front rank. It has also been my experience — and, I suppose, yours — that an imperfect treatment by psychoanalysis may have bad effects. I have thought sometimes of publishing my own failures from this standpoint. In spite of this, I imagine that these unfortunate results are decidedly exceptional, and one would like to know whether Dr. Kollarits, for example, can claim better ones.

Yours sincerely,

---

[1] Jenö Kollaritz (1870–1940), neurologist in Budapest. See *Charakter und Nervosität* (Berlin: Springer, 1912), p. 192.

[2] "I must assert categorically that today Freudian psychoanalysis has to be included among the treatments used for nervousness, and it seems to me that in time this unfortunately will increase, as the method spreads. A personality that undergoes a thorough psychoanalysis cannot stand such a brutal attack without shock. We all

know cases which have become victims of this method. These patients leave their analyst without being healed and with increased nervousness. I know a young girl in whose case psychoanalysis produced severe sexual excitement. Such cases are a new species of traumatic neurosis."

165
Ferenczi to Putnam

[April 29, 1912]

Budapest, VII, Erzsébet-Körut 54
29. IV. 1912.

Dear Professor:

Thank you very much for sending me your articles. They are all fitted to make a deep impression on your opponents, not only because of the logic of the arguments and the dignity of the style, but also because your name and previous record constitute a significant argument ad hominem. They will give pause even to Allen Starr.[1] [By the way, I learned from Professor Freud that he does not even know Allen Starr.]

As far as Kollarits'[2] comments are concerned, I can enlighten you in a few words. I know for certain that Kollarits has no knowledge of psychoanalytic literature, except for my Hungarian essays and perhaps Freud's *Five Lectures*.[3] He himself has *never* done *analysis*. The source of his attitude toward the etiology of the neuroses can easily be guessed on the basis of his naïve pronouncements on the subject; he believes everything his patients say and takes their utterances to be statements of fact. His chief, Professor Jendrassik,[4] a not unintelligent, but extremely vain person, whose own complexes render him hypocritical, had the book written; he likes paradoxes and therefore considers psychoanalysis to be paradoxical. He is struggling with a sexual complex and therefore is always trying to ferret out immorality in analysis. [A short time ago he married the mistress of a rich aristocrat, in spite of the fact that thereby he lost all social respectability. I do not blame him for this, but it is necessary to know these details in order to understand his kind.] Kollarits himself, a limited intellect, is tubercular, and, if possible, still vainer than Jendrassik, and is without a grain of independence in his make-up. I think I know one case to which he seems to refer. A twenty-four year old girl who was treated by me for two months had to interrupt treatment on the advice of Jendrassik during the phase of transference [the brother, who did not want to support the sister any longer in spite of his prosperity, arranged for this interruption through Jendrassik.] Such evil-minded delving into half-analyzed patients is the material on which Kollarits bases his authoritarian and partially lying statements. Professor Freud is quite right; lying and deceit have long ago found a path across the ocean to Europe.[5]

I have made it a matter of principle not to reply to such attacks and believe that this is the best tactic. One cannot count on any kind of fruitful discussion with people like that.

That is all I can reply to your question. I consider all these failures to be brought about by outward circumstances or my own ineptitude but they are not to be blamed on the method.

With best regards,

yours

Dr. S. Ferenczi

[1] Moses Allen Starr (1854–1932), New York neurologist, had denounced Freud before the section on neurology of the New York Academy of Medicine, April 4; see Putnam to Freud, June 4, 1912, and Freud to Putnam, June 25, 1912.

[2] See preceding letter.

[3] Freud, "Five Lectures on Psychoanalysis," delievered at Clark University in September 1909. See Über Psychoanalyse (Leipzig and Vienna: F. Deuticke, 1910), and "The Origin and Development of Psychoanalysis," trans. Harry Woodburn Chase, American Journal of Psychology, 21 (April 1910), 181–218; SE, XI, 2–55.

[4] Erno Jendrassik (1858–1921), neuropathologist in Budapest.

[5] Lüge und Schwindel haben längst den Weg über den Ozean nach Europa gefunden.

166
Ferenczi to Putnam

[September 6, 1912]

Hotel Regina, Vienna

Vienna, 6. 9. 1912

Dear Professor

When I allowed myself to criticize your fine philosophical article,[1] I did so, convinced that you, dear professor, would not misunderstand my presumption. I assumed you would consider it merely an expression of what I felt when I saw my own position attacked by a man of such reputation as yourself.

Therefore I asked the editor of *Imago* to let me know when my critique would appear in order that I might send you a copy of it before it was published. I now learn that the galleys already have been sent to you, and I can only assure you in this tardy letter that it was this very uncomfortable feeling of being unable to agree with your opinions, always so important to me, which was the motive for my comments.

I am writing to you to Boston, even though I imagine that you are still in your beautiful and comfortable camp in the Adirondacks, the memory of which is so dear to me. Please, dear professor, give my respectful greetings to all the members of your household whom I met.

Yours most sincerely,

S. Ferenczi

P. S. I am about to travel to Italy with Professor Freud. Originally we wanted to go to England, but circumstances prevented this, and we had to be content with a less extended itinerary.[2]

---

[1] Ferenczi, "Philosophie und Psychoanalyse. (Bemerkungen zu einem Aufsatze des H. Professors Dr. James J. Putnam von der Harvard Universität, Boston, USA)" [Philosophy and Psychoanalysis (Comments on a Paper of James J. Putnam of Harvard)], *Imago*, 1 (December 1912), 519–526; in Ferenczi, *Final Contributions*, pp. 326–334, and Putnam, "Antwort auf die Erwiderung des Herrn Dr. Ferenczi" [A Rejoinder to Dr. Ferenczi's Reply], *Imago*, 1 (December 1912), 527–530.

[2] See Jones, *Sigmund Freud*, II, 93–96.

167
Ferenczi to Putnam

[October 17, 1912]

Budapest, VII, Erzsébet-Körut 54

17.X.1912

Dear Professor

Please accept my hearty thanks for your exceedingly kind letter. It put a final end to my worry that my reply might have impaired our pleasant personal relationship.[1] At the same time let me thank you for the fine article in which you mentioned me so honorably.[2]

I too hope that the disagreement which separates us on this one point will disappear in time. Even if it does not, we still have so many other points of scientific contact where our goals are the same. Again, my sincerest thanks and greetings,

Yours ever,
Ferenczi

[1] See preceding letter. Putnam's letter is missing.

[2] Putnam called Ferenczi "one of the best and most experienced workers in the field." See "Comments on Sex Issues from the Freudian Standpoint." Read before the section in Neurology of the New York Academy of Medicine, April 4, 1912. *New York Medical Journal,* 95 (June 15, 1912), 1251; Ad Psa, 136.

168
Ferenczi to Putnam
[June 19, 1914]

Internationale Zeitschrift
für ärztliche Psychoanalyse
Budapest, June 19, 1914.

Dear Professor

I thank you for your kind letter[1] and for agreeing with me about the concrete problems confronting the psychoanalytic movement. It not only pleases me personally that you are with us in this very unnecessary and unpleasant inner crisis of the International Association, but it is no less important for the cause of psychoanalysis in the United States.[2] — This split should not be artificially kept from coming to a head: in science, compromises ought to be avoided. The sooner this crisis is over, the earlier we can resume our work undisturbed.

I greatly regret that you cannot come to this year's Congress;[3] I should have been delighted to invite you to Budapest and to have an opportunity to reciprocate your hospitality even though in a more modest form.

I have read your last article in the *Journal of Abnormal Psychology*[4] with great interest and have admired the patience with which you deal with ignorant antagonists.

With greetings and my repeated thanks,

Yours ever,
S. Ferenczi

¹ Missing.

² Jung resigned as president of the International Psychoanalytic Association in April 1914. See Jones, *Sigmund Freud*, II, 150, and *Zeitschrift*, 2 (1914), 405–406.

³ The fourth International Psychoanalytic Congress, scheduled for September 4 and then September 20, at Dresden, was not held because of the Great War which began in August. See *Zeitschrift*, 2 (1914), 483, and Jones, *Sigmund Freud*, II, 104–105, 170.

⁴ See Putnam, "Dream Interpretation and the Theory of Psychoanalysis," *Journal of Abnormal Psychology*, 9 (April–May 1914), 36–60; Ad Psa, 223–253.

V

Prince–Putnam Correspondence

Letters 169–172

Morton Prince, 1910–1911

The most original of the American psychotherapists, Morton Prince, witnessed the sudden growth of interest in Freud's psychoanalysis with misgivings. Ernest Jones suggested that Prince was piqued because he had missed so much that Freud had discovered in investigations of the psychoneuroses. To Prince the issue was one of a well-rounded scientific approach that took into account all the relevant data, including the findings of French psychopathology and his own studies of nervous disorders.

Prince's sympathetic interest in psychotherapy preceded Putnam's. In a series of brilliant papers in the 1880's and 1890's he had advanced what could be described as a behavioristic theory of the neuroses. Symptoms developed through accidental associations and became fixed through habit into rigid, repetitive patterns. By 1904 he welcomed Ivan Pavlov's first conditioning experiments as a corroboration of his own hypothesis. Putnam ranked Prince with Pierre Janet, Breuer and Freud, and Boris Sidis, among those who were making psychotherapy a scientific and rational discipline.

In 1905 Prince published his famous study of Sally Beauchamp, *The Dissociation of a Personality*, and the next year he founded the *Journal of Abnormal Psychology*. Although he had an international reputation as a psychopathologist, it was not until 1914 that he published his major work, *The Unconscious: The Fundamentals of Human Personality, Normal and Abnormal*.

Prince was especially annoyed in 1910 by what he considered the fanatical cultism of Ernest Jones and the other Freudians. Some of this annoyance was provoked by Jones's insistence that Freud's results could be obtained only by the use of Freud's method. Prince, on the other hand, argued that any valid method of investigation, especially hypnosis, could be used to test Freud's theories. If hypnosis could not corroborate them, they must be invalid. The controversy over method continued beyond the period of these letters and resulted in contrasting studies of the same patient by Prince and Putnam presented at a meeting of the American Psychopathological Association, May 29, 1912.

Prince's first letter concerned Ernest Jones's proposal to criticize Prince's evaluation of Freud's theory of dreams that had appeared in the October–November, 1910 issue of the *Journal of Abnormal Psychology*.[1] The remaining letters convey Prince's scientific and personal objections to Freud's theories which he judged to be a fanciful extension of Freud's actual evidence. In a letter of November 22, 1910, Prince assumed the pen name "Fiona McLeod" of the Scottish poet William Sharp to express freely his highly emotional reaction to the psychoanalytic issue. Despite these difficulties, Prince and Putnam remained friends until the latter's death in 1918. After the Great War Prince viewed psychoanalysis more sympathetically, although still rejecting Freud's sexual theories. Prince informed a symposium on psychoanalysis in 1921 that all psychotherapists were indebted to Freud for two cardinal principles — repression and conflict. Above all, the Freudians had belligerently championed a functional psychotherapy at the time when many neurologists still were hostile to it:

"This, to my mind, is the great gain for which we must be thankful to Freud — the acceptance of the dynamic approach and the dynamic conception of aberrations of the normal personality however manifested. It is the search for the 'Why', which is the final step in dynamic pathology." [2]

Prince, who, like Putnam, had attended Boston Latin School and Harvard College, in 1926 was appointed associate professor of the new Department of Abnormal and Dynamic Psychology at Harvard. With Dr. Henry A. Murray, Prince established the Harvard psychological clinic in the two years preceding his death in 1929.

---

[1] Three letters from Putnam to Prince from 1906 have been omitted.

[2] Morton Prince, "A Critique of Psychoanalysis." Read at the forty-seventh annual meeting of the American Neurological Association, June 1921. *Archives of Neurology and Psychiatry*, 6 (July–December 1921), 620–621.

169
Prince to Putnam
[October 21, 1910]

458 Beacon street
Oct. 21, 1910

Dear James,

I was glad to get and much interested in your letter.[1] I expected to get a withering criticism or to be treated with the contumely of silence.

I am pleased that you find something of value in the contribution and that you estimate it as such and appreciate the heroic self control and "repressed ideas" which I read between the lines. Seriously I think you are quite fair and am glad you find me impartial as I tried to be. I agree with you we ought to study these problems open mindedly and support the work of each other.

I am far from imagining that the dream problems have been solved by my humble communication — I would emphatically disclaim that.[2] In fact I think my conclusions can not be applied further than to those particular dreams and that particular case. I do not believe that they are likely to be true of all dreams. The dreams I have analyzed I am inclined to think are of a peculiar kind and pertain to a particular class of subjects perhaps few in number. Their value I think is in showing one kind of mechanism.

Further the why of that mechanism remains a good deal of a mystery. I do not think however Freud's "why" is applicable to them.

I should welcome a criticism by you and would like to publish it. The only condition I would make is this and not on my account —

I should not want to have possible *sexual* interpretations pointed out. As you might do in re *clubs* and wild men. Mrs. B is now known by quite a number of people and has yielded a good deal in allowing her dreams to be published at all, and if they are made the subject of public discussion over her sexuality she would feel it horribly as I think any one would. She would not only suffer but I should be deprived of future material (and she is a gold mine) for experimentation. It is a matter of expediency (on my part —) and playing square with her. She is not however squeemish in discussing the sexual aspect with me, but quite frank. Some of her sexual dreams are beauties but I could not publish them. They showed the same mechanism.

I hope this limitation will not prevent such criticism as you wish to make.

I can not close without congratulating you on your article (which I read in ms) on the work of English psychopathologists.³ It is extraordinarily impartial and generous in its exposition of another's views. Its only fault is the undeserved flattery of myself which I wish I could truly honestly feel I deserve. This is not the expression of an uberdrängt⁴ conceit but perhaps of a "wish".

Sincerely as ever,
M. P.

¹ Missing.

² See Morton Prince, "The Mechanism and Interpretation of Dreams," *Journal of Abnormal Psychology*, 5 (October–November 1910), 139–195.

³ Putnam did not write such an article. Probably Prince was referring to the praise in Jones, "Bericht über die neuere englische und amerikanische Literatur zur klinischen Psychologie und Psychopathologie" [Review of the Recent English and American Literature on Clinical Psychology and Psychopathology], *Jahrbuch*, 2 (1910), 316–337, *Archives of Neurology and Psychiatry* [London], 5 (1911), 120–147.

⁴ Prince may have meant to coin a word "überverdrängt," "overrepressed."

170
Prince to Putnam
[November 22–November 26, 1910]

Tuesday Nov 22/10
On board rr train.

Dear and beloved Jim

For I know Morton Prince or think I know him as much as any man can know the real self of any man and that is not much: for no man knows wholly even himself.

I know that he likes your bouquets, for he does not receive many, at least from those he cares about whose opinion he values, whom he loves and who are qualified as critics. Popular applause he scarcely listens to and values as much as the chirpings of crickets.

In this respect I think he keeps his head level and does not fool himself. I know too, because he has often told me this, that he has a warm spot in his heart — a little hearth stone reserved for you, where no one else shall sit. He would not say it himself as men don't; but I am his "Fiona Macleod"[1] and I can write over my name the thoughts of his inner self. For I am his second self.

It is because of this little hearth stone that he likes to hear you speak out — whether in blame or praise.

Later, Nov. 26

The train came to a stop and so did my letter and the moment never seems to have been propitious, the mood not to have returned till now — the serene mood of "Fiona" — when I could take up my theme.

I am glad of this opportunity — the one which your note has brought — to write what has been in his inner mind a long time and it is time that some one said it for him.

But first — let me say for him like Cassius "Thou wrongst me Brutus" in thinking that he feels that other people's ideas could not be *as* good (as his own) especially if it seems to tread on the corns of his. Of course this refers in particular to Freud. Now I happen to know that when he comes across something in Freud which to him seems to be true, to be supported by facts of observation and logic, a thrill of real delight goes through his somebody. And when he in his own observations finds something that supports Freud he also has great delight — And I am glad it is so. Otherwise it would be obstinacy and arrogance and jealousy which prevented him acknowledging that which is good in another.

I am sure these are not the reasons which prevent his accepting Freud's views. The real reasons I will tell you later. And here is something amusing and suggestive.

Sidis[2] complains to him that he is too much of a Freudian and Jones and Putnam complain that he is too much of an opponent of Freudians!

Indeed with Sidis he argues for certain fundamentals for which he gives Freud credit: when in the dream interpretation study he found Freud's symbolism it was a great joy to him why then this great difference of opinion? It is because of two things. First as a result of objective study he had accumulated a large mass of facts which the Freudians show themselves not to be possessed of and totally disregard. Hence he thinks from the standpoint of these facts which are stored in his mind and which rise into consciousness whenever psychopathological problems are discussed.

Do you remember that years ago when you and others were antagonistic to Janet's work you called J. and M. P. "a couple of cranks"; and when Courtney read a childish paper on hysteria and all applauded?[3] He, M. P., was astounded by the latter experience not realizing that none of you had the facts in mind. And so it is now. By the way do you remember he showed no obstinacy but enthusiasm in accepting Gurney's[4] and Janet's work, but could not accept Meyers'[5] theories which by the way are fundamental to Freud. The former was based on carefully observed data arrived at by scientific methods. Meyers' views were a philosophy not science.

The second reason for his not accepting F's theories is because of their absolutely different types of mind. He can only accept conclusions based on a consideration of *all* related data and drawn by logical processes of thought which do not admit any other possible conclusion. Or if the data are insufficient for such conclusions then only tentative hypotheses. In other words the inductive method. Freud's type of mind on the other hand formulates concepts satisfied with the attitude that if the concepts are true the facts could be explained. This is the method of philosophy. The result of this "method" is that wider and wider concepts are drawn. Concept is piled upon concept — until finally we have a structure which falls to the ground with the first crumbling of the foundation.

When he reads Freud he begins with keen interest and enthusiasm. Then presently he comes across a statement of fact which is contradicted by experience; then an interpretation which defies every law of logic, disregards other further interpretations, sets every logical process at defiance. At this point and not till this point he puts the book down in despair.

Now here comes in another difference in the two types of mind; it is a difference in attitude. He believes the Freud attitude a dangerous attitude. It is an attitude which has wrecked many splendid minds in their search for truth. It wrecked Dick Hodgson[6] who had one of the most beautiful minds I ever knew. When once Dick — one of the dearest fellows — had accepted the concept of spiritualism all his critical faculty was lost; his sense of perspective and proportion went with it. (of course only in connection with his problem) he found it easy to explain all phenomena through spiritualism, and to the spiritualistic concept everything was adjusted. He was right too if the concept was true everything was easily explained. (By the way Dick made the same criticism of M. P. that you do, but time seems to be showing M. P.'s head was level). Likewise many scientists have been caught by spiritualism. We see the same attitude of mind in Christian Science — and it was observable in the Emmanuel Movement.

M. P. was nearly caught once in the same way, years ago, when psychical research first came into being. He remembers it well. It was à propos of thought transference and the concept of forces transcending those of the phenomenal universe.[7] He remembers well the feeling the elation, that went with the acceptance of the concept — ; How easy by it to explain so much that was mysterious.

But a remark brought him to himself and he realized how near he had come to losing his mental grasp of the situation his mental equilibrium. Never again! Never again. M. P. thinks you Freudians do not realize how near most of you are to that attitude of mind — indeed that most have it. Jones is hopelessly lost, his judgment is gone. Jung ditto. You are raising a cult not a science. In principle the attitude of the school does not differ from that of the Christian Scientists and their dogmas and Mrs. Eddy.

We read continually, with oppressing repetition of the great strides that Freudian Psychology is making and the large number of converts. What of it? It is not surprising. Medical men are human like laymen. There is no limit to the numbers which any cult founded on concepts can attract. I myself, Fiona, could start a cult tomorrow with a metaphysical concept for a dogma and attract followers enough to rival Christian Science.

You only have to appeal to the imagination and offer a few practical consequences which benefit human happiness. Have you noticed that none of the followers of the cult are trained abnormal psychologists I mean men who have begun at the bottom and observed and accumulated the recognized data. What would a bacteriologist say to a clinician who offered theories of immunity without showing a first-hand knowledge of bacteriology. Look at the men. Jung — Jones — Brill — Maeder — Abraham, etc. None trained.[8] So much for M. P.'s point of view and attitude.

Now for his beliefs. It is difficult to say how far he is in accord with Freud, because the latter has piled so many concepts upon concepts has postulated so many theses that one might hold one and not the other.

M. P. holds that so far as we have gone the facts show that every mental event depends on antecedent events. That our life's experiences are to a large extent conserved as a "subconsciousness" or "unconsciousness", if you like those terms — better as neurograms or brain residua. At any rate the records of our mental lives are largely conserved somehow and somewhere.

That these conserved experiences largely determine the form which later experiences shall take.

They provide the formative material of the torch to which later experiences apply the match. (See the Unconscious Jr Ab. Psy) However our obsessions, fears etc. are largely determined by the experiences of our early life, and if it was not for these early experiences there would be no obsessions phobias, etc.
Hence it is desirable to discover these antecedent experiences and in M. P.'s crude way he has been doing it for years.
Upon this his "Educational Treatment" (1898) was based.[9] But his method was not as refined as is that of Freud's, nor as has been his own of recent years. (Jim Putnam showed years ago that traumatic neuroses depended upon the previous social education of the victim).[10]

In addition to all this however the principle of automatic memory plays a part in the mechanism of the psychoses. Now so far as these views are those of Freud, M. P. is in agreement with him. But when Freud conceives of the torch made up only of sexual experiences, of a *specific* Freudian mechanism of hysteria etc. that a cure can only take place through psychoanalysis, that the cure by p. a. is through bringing to the "light of day" the suppressed complexes etc., M. P. parts company with him.
Some of their statements are falsities. We are not nincompoops and we know a cure when we see one and have made them often. Cures can, have been and will be made without Psy. An., and Psy An does make use of the Educational Method and not only of the

principle of light-of-day. I challenge any one to use psychoanalysis without any educat. as we use it.

Theoretically and practically the personality can be altered at will without touching the submerged memories. If it were not so, the social organization would be impossible.

And now dear Jim I bring this long epistle to a close. You called it forth, but it seems to me (Fiona) that you have not taken the same pains to discover M. P's psychology that you have Freud's that possibly your attitude to him has been near that which you think is his to Freud.

In one respect M. P. is to blame. In all these years he has felt it unwise to raise discussions amongst the students of Abnormal Psychology; but that all, regardless of differences of opinion, should march against the indifference and antagonism of the profession. Hence he has not criticized in detail Freud's or others views — has not criticized Jones, Brill, Putnam, Sidis or insisted on his own theories by preference.

The time perhaps has now come to do so. He is sorry to see that a Freud Society is being formed, for it means the breaking up of those who should be united by a common bond.[11] If the Freud people can't bear discussion in a common society, what can they stand for but a cult?

I wish Jim you were with him now for he would like to have you by him so that he could talk it out heart to heart; for he is depressed under the hopelessness of the problem.

As ever

Fiona Macprince.

[1] "Fiona Macleod" was the pen-name of the Scottish poet William Sharp (1855–1905).

[2] Boris Sidis (1867–1923), American psychopathologist.

[3] Pierre Janet (1859–1947), French psychologist and psychopathologist who profoundly influenced the Boston School. Joseph William Courtney (1868–1929), Boston neurologist, an opponent of psychoanalysis. See Courtney, "The Genesis and Nature of Hysteria." Read before the Boston Society of Psychiatry and Neurology, December 19, 1907. *Boston Medical and Surgical Journal*, 158 (March 12, 1908), 340–346.

[4] Edmund Gurney (1847–1888), a founder of the British Society for Psychical Research and a friend of William James. Probably Prince was referring to Gurney's experiment with hypnotism. See "Recent Experiments in Hypnotism," *Proceedings of the Society for Psychical Research* (London), 5 (1888), 3–17, and "Hypnotism and Telepathy," *ibid.*, pp. 216–259.

[5] Although Frederick William Henry Myers (1843–1901) was one of the first English writers to publicize Freud's work, their views of the unconscious differed completely. A founder of the Society for Psychical Research, Myers believed that

the unconscious or subliminal self included phenomena ranging from routine memories to glimpses of the World Soul. See Myers, *Human Personality and Its Survival of Bodily Death*, 2 vols. (New York: Longmans and Co., 1904), esp. I, 50–56, for a discussion of Freud.

[6] Richard Hodgson (1855–1905) was born in Australia and studied with Henry Sidgwick, professor of Moral Philosophy, University of Cambridge, and a founder of the British Society for Psychical Research. Hodgson was secretary of the American Society from 1887 to 1905. In his second report on the medium Mrs. Piper, he concluded that she was in fact in communication with the dead. Hodgson, who loved puzzles and children, was a frequent visitor at Putnam Camp. See the obituaries by J. G. Piddington and Mrs. Henry Sidgwick, *Proceedings of the Society for Psychical Research* (London), 19 (1907), 356–367, and Hodgson, "A Further Record of Observations of Certain Phenomena of Trance," *ibid.*, 13 (1897–1898), 284–582.

[7] See Morton Prince, "Thought Transference," *Boston Medical and Surgical Journal*, 116 (February 3, 1887), 107–112.

[8] All had been trained chiefly as neurologists or psychiatrists. Alphonse Maeder (b. 1882) was a Swiss neurologist and psychiatrist, Karl Abraham (1877–1925), a Berlin psychiatrist.

[9] Prince, "The Educational Treatment of Hysteria and Certain Hysterical States," *Boston Medical and Surgical Journal*, 139 (October 6, 1898), 332–337.

[10] Putnam, "Typical Hysterical Symptoms in Man Due to Injury and Their Medico Legal Significance," *Journal of Nervous and Mental Disease*, 11 (July 1884), 496–501; "On the Etiology and Pathogenesis of the Post-Traumatic Psychoses and Neuroses," *ibid.*, 25 (November 1898), 769–799.

[11] See Jones to Putnam, September 9, 1910.

171
Prince to Putnam

[February 25, 1911]

458 Beacon Street
Boston, Mass.
February 25, 1911.

My dear Jim,

I thank you most warmly and from the bottom of my heart for your letter.[1] I always like to get such letters from you, and to have you tell me exactly what you think. I wish you would do it more often. I really sympathize entirely with your point of view and I should really like to coöperate with you in carrying it into practice, but, of course, sympathy in the abstract is one thing and in the concrete another.

Of course Jones has written to you as he has written to me, complaining of my treatment of him. His letter to me however is not only bitter but offensive, not to say insolent. However, I don't care. He is a nervous, highstrung, self-centered young fellow and takes everything one says as personal to himself. I do not know what he has written to you, but to me he makes a number of absolutely untrue statements of facts and charges regarding the publication of my reply.[2]

Now are you not a little bit unjust in assuming that I made the attack on Jones? The facts as I see them are these — and I have talked the matter over with Waterman,[3] laid your letter and Jones' before him, and he takes exactly the same ground. Jones wrote an entirely gratuitous criticism, not to say attack, upon my article, attempting to discredit my observations and work.[4] He went out of his way to do this, not in a contribution to the subject in hand of original observations with a comparison of results arrived at, and pointing out the discrepancies and the reasons therefor, but a pure criticism with an attempt, as I said, to discredit my work. This article, as he told me, was written as a consequence of interchange of notes between you, Brill, and myself.

Now what was I to do? What would any one do? Was I to remain silent and allow my work to be tacitly discredited? I did not begin the controversy; I made no attack upon Freud, him, or any one else in my original article on dreams but merely compared my results with those of others. I do not see therefore how I can be charged with stirring up animosities. The attack came from the other side. Jones seems to think that he is at perfect liberty to criticise somebody and then to feel hurt if he is criticised in return. I call it crying baby and if he were five years of age he might be taken on one's knee and petted — or the other thing.

Now as to my reply. Let me say first, however, that your memory has played you a trick in thinking that I claimed that my explanation of certain dreams was applicable to all dreams. O, Jim! Jim! I never thought that you, of all persons, would impute such claims to me. I said, distinctly, in my article on dreams, three times in three different places, that my conclusions were only applicable to those particular dreams, and I disclaimed any intention of applying them further, and said we were not justified in doing so. I do not know what more I could have said. I have been complimented on this reserve and have been told that a reviewer of the article for one of the *Journals* had laid particular emphasis upon and complimented this caution. As a matter of fact I do not believe the conclusions were applicable to all dreams.

As to a "satisfactory" cause of a phenomenon referred to in my reply, that is an entirely different question. If the cause is found it is satisfactory, if it is not satisfactory it is not the cause. However I will not go into that now.

As to the tone of the reply, as I was saying, I am astonished that Jones should take it as he did. I had no idea that he would be hurt and really supposed he would have a good laugh over it. I submitted the paper to two critics before publishing it asking them whether there was anything in it that was personal or that would offend, and I was assured that there was nothing of the kind in it and that it was particularly "courteous" "reserved" and "self-contained." I have since asked Waterman to give me his frank and unbiased opinion and he says the same thing. Therefore I am more than astonished that anyone's feelings should be hurt. The latter part of the article, which I suppose is what offends Jones and which you think is "banging and whanging," was written for the following reasons: I, and others, have been accused by all of you of not accepting Freud's doctrines because of ignorance, obstinacy, and arrogance. Now I wanted to show that those were not the reasons but that we were unable to accept the reasoning from the data, and that the data offered were insufficient for the conclusions. If these reasons were sound an explanation was needed as to why men of such eminent ability as yourself and Jones accepted the theories while we lesser lights did not. Here was a paradox and that paradox had to be explained, and I tried to explain it, and that's all there is to it. I had no wish and did not suppose that I had "banged" or "whanged" anybody.

I wish I could feel that your analogy of a "leading representative of chemistry" was applicable to me. I never dreamed in my wildest moments that I was any such representative, and that I had any corresponding responsibility. I am not really and truly conscious of having any special principles of my own which I wish to advocate beyond trying to find the truth, and I believe I would to-morrow turn around and advocate Freud's theories if I could see them in the same light that you do.

However, I do not want to have any controversies and would

not have hurt anybody's feelings if I had thought I was doing so. I really don't know what I am to do under similar circumstances.

I am sorry to hear you say that you were ashamed of losing your temper and talking back in the meeting.[5] You were never so splendid and you never talk so well as when you are mad, and I, for one, like to hear you, even when you hit me.

By the way, I think you are wrong in thinking that this controversy will hurt psychopathology and Freud's theories; on the contrary it will be a good advertisement, if read, and will awaken interest. It will turn the attention of people to Freud who otherwise would have been indifferent and passed by. Nothing like advertising, my boy.

Since writing the above a New York physician dropped into my office. He had read the articles and has a leaning towards psychoanalysis and I asked him to state his unbiased opinion. He saw nothing in my article that was not courteous but added that Jones attack was "trivial, petty and unprintable," meaning I suppose insolent — . I really did not mind Jones attack at all though I thought it uncalled for. I simply laughed, but I think that if any one goes into a controversy he ought to have enough sand to take blows as well as give them.

I am going to send you Jones letter as soon as I have answered it. You will see the *real* Jones come out. Of course I will publish Bleuler's article.[6] That is what the Journal is for.

Now to conclude. I will promise you I will try and take the position in the future that you want me to and will do all I can to help matters along.

Please don't think so poorly of me as to think that I don't accept Freud because I can't bear to see new views or leaders come along. On the contrary I *want* to believe.

But write Jones and tell him not to be a baby — and that he began it.

As ever
Affectionately
Morton.

[1] Missing.

[2] See Jones to Putnam, February 19 and February 27, 1911; Prince, "The Mechanism and Interpretation of Dreams — A Reply to Dr. Jones," *Journal of Abnormal Psychology*, V (February–March, 1911), 337–353.

³ George Waterman (1873–1960), Boston neurologist and psychotherapist and Putnam's former assistant.

⁴ Jones, "Remarks on Dr. Morton Prince's Article: 'The Mechanism and Interpretation of Dreams,'" *Journal of Abnormal Psychology*, 5 (February–March 1911), 328–336.

⁵ Possibly a reference to the meeting of December 15, 1910, or January 19, 1911, of the Boston Society of Psychiatry and Neurology.

⁶ Eugen Bleuler, "Die Psychoanalyse Freuds: Verteidigung und kritische Bemerkungen [Freud's Psychoanalysis: Defense and Critical Remarks], *Jahrbuch*, 2 (1910), 623–670; for Jones's review, see *Journal of Abnormal Psychology*, 6 (February–March 1912), 465–470.

172
Prince to Putnam
[March 3, 1911]
N. Y. & Nrth RR.

March 3
458 Beacon Street,

Dear Jim

Thanks for your letter, even more thanks than for the first.[1] I am going to have it framed and hung up. Of course I recognize that point of view — *attitude* I call it of Jones and the Freudians.

That is what I have been saying — all critics have been saying. It is what I said in my 'Reply'[2] in the last part and called 'attitude of mind.' I did not dare say it as boldly and frankly as you have said it. I would have been mobbed — or else the contrary effect, the infants would have sat down and boo-hooed. As you said Jones is a fanatic. It is the fanatic attitude — the attitude of Christian Science, Spiritualism, Suffragettism. It was the attitude of the Abolitionists, Martin Luther and reformers in general. You are quite right — Poor dear Dick Hodgson[3] latterly acquired the attitude.

But mind you, any one with that attitude may not be invited into the 'society of scholars' including scientists. It destroys the judgment. The capacity to weigh criticize, to see in perspective and true proportion. It is all right for a reformer in Religion or politics. But in science there is no common ground on which such a person can meet with a scientifically minded person again:

I admire the fanatic who goes forth to fight for the faith, to battle nobly, but then he must be prepared to lay down his life without whimpering. Can you imagine John Brown Luther Calvin, Edwards Garrison — Sumner, whimpering 'like a girl' because their opponents hit them back or because they would not believe? If you are going to battle for the faith do it manfully and don't cry when hit I am afraid Jones will never be a hero — poor dear. Now beloved Jim. I care a good deal about you. Please, please hold back before you get involved in that paralysing attitude. It is the grave of reputations. Hold what theory you want. Freudian — Buddhistic Confucian or any other. Nobody cares a rap what theories a man holds. What scientists do care about — all men care about — is the mental method by which theories are arrived at. Freudians think that objectors object to the conclusions. The real fundamental objections are to the methods.

You can hold to the most extreme sexual theories if you like and if your methods justify the theories, no criticism will hold. But if your methods are dictated by the attitude of mind you describe — then you are bound to suffer and I think — from the point of view of science — ought to suffer. As I have said before do let me implore you not to get so far involved with Jones and his crowd as to unconsciously slide into 'the attitude' — largely I am afraid from a mistaken sense of duty and loyalty.

You may hold any theory under heaven, for all I care but shun the attitude.

Voltaire called the attitude of Church and State in his time 'L'infâme'; Lawson called the attitude of financial interests 'The System'.⁴ What shall I call the attitude you so well describe — well just The Attitude.

I don't think you saw that the criticism of your paper at the Soc N and P. was of the attitude not the theory. Hence you did not meet the objections in the second paper.

Last call for the dining car

Done — Finished I have said my last word — Ring down the curtain.

Affecly
M. P.

Tell Jones to read the Life of John Brown.

¹ Both are missing.
² Prince, "The Mechanism and Interpretation of Dreams — A Reply to Dr. Jones," *Journal of Abnormal Psychology*, 5 (February–March 1911), 337–353.

[3] See n. 6, Prince to Putnam, November 22, 1910.

[4] See Thomas William Lawson (1857–1925), *Frenzied Finance* (New York: The Ridgway-Thayer Co., 1905), p. vii: "The 'System' is a process or a device for the incubation of wealth from the people's savings in the banks, trust, and insurance companies, and the public funds."

Chronology of Events

Chronology of the Letters

Selected Bibliography

Biographical Notes

German Texts of the Freud Letters

Index

Chronology of Events

1842 William James, b. January 11.
1846 James Jackson Putnam, b. October 3.
1854 Morton Prince, b. December 21.
1856 Sigmund Freud, b. May 6.
1874 A. A. Brill, b. October 12.
1876 Putnam dismisses George Beard's mental therapeutics before the American Neurological Association, June 8.
1879 Ernest Jones, b. January 1.
1885 Morton Prince, *The Nature of Mind and Human Automatism.*
1889 Janet, *L'Automatisme Psychologique.*
1890 William James, *Principles of Psychology.*
1891 Morton Prince, "Association Neuroses," May.
1893 Breuer and Freud, "The Psychic Mechanism of Hysterical Phenomena (Preliminary Communication)," January 1, 15. On April 21, F. W. H. Myers discusses the above before the Society for Psychical Research, London.
1894 William James reviews Breuer and Freud in March in the *Psychological Review.*
1895 Putnam's first paper on psychotherapy, May 23, mentions Janet, Breuer, Freud, and Christian Science.
1898 Havelock Ellis discusses Breuer and Freud in the St. Louis *Alienist and Neurologist.*
1900 Freud, *The Interpretation of Dreams.*
1902 The Freud circle organized in Vienna in the fall.
1903 Freud, *Three Essays on the Theory of Sexuality.*
1904 G. Stanley Hall, *Adolescence.*
        Pierre Janet lectures in Boston.
        Freud learns from Eugen Bleuler and Carl Jung that psychoanalysis is being tried at the Burghölzli, Zurich.
1906 Janet lectures in Boston again.

Putnam appraises psychoanalysis in the first issue of the *Journal of Abnormal Psychology,* April.

1908   The first Psychoanalytic Congress, Salzburg, April 26.

In September Ernest Jones sails for Toronto.

A. A. Brill returns from Zurich to New York in the fall.

1909   *Jahrbuch* begins in January.

The American Therapeutic Society symposium on psychotherapy, New Haven, Conn., May 6.

September 7–11, Freud lectures at Clark University.

A. A. Brill, first translation of Freud, *Selected Papers on Hysteria and Other Psychoneuroses.*

1910   International Psychoanalytic Association organized March 30–31 at Second Psychoanalytic Congress.

American Psychopathological Association founded May 2.

Putnam delivers first paper on psychoanalysis, May 3.

Freud proposes Putnam found American branch of the International Psychoanalytic Association, June 16.

William James dies, August 26.

Zentralblatt published, September.

Brill, translation of Freud, *Three Contributions to the Sexual Theory.*

1911   A. A. Brill founds New York Psychoanalytic Society, February 12.

American Psychoanalytic Association founded, May 9.

Third Psychoanalytic Congress, Weimar, September 20–21.

Freud announces Adler's resignation from the Vienna Psychoanalytic Society, October 11.

Freud, first paper on technique, "The Handling of Dream Interpretation in Psychoanalysis," December.

1912   *Imago* published, March.

Jung lectures in New York, September.

Freud announces Stekel's resignation from the Vienna Psychoanalytic Society, November 6.

1913   *Internationale Zeitschrift* published, January.

Ernest Jones returns to England in the fall.

The Fourth International Psychoanalytic Congress, Munich, September 7.

The *Psychoanalytic Review* published, December.

Brill, translation of Freud, *The Interpretation of Dreams.*

1914   Freud, "On Narcissism: An Introduction."

Jung resigns as president of the International Psychoanalytic Association, April 20.

Boston Psychoanalytic Society founded.

Freud publishes "On the History of the Psychoanalytic Movement," June.

Morton Prince, *The Unconscious.*

1915   Putnam, *Human Motives.*

Freud begins *Introductory Lectures on Psychoanalysis.*

Freud, first metaphysical paper, "Instincts and Their Vicissitudes," published.

1918   Putnam dies, November 4.

Chronology of the Letters

May 26 [1877]: James to Putnam
January 17, 1879: James to Putnam
March 2, 1898: James to Putnam
March 3, 1898: James to Putnam
March 4, 1898: James to Putnam
March 9, 1898: Putnam to James
August 19, 1908: James to Putnam
June 1, 1909: Jones to Putnam
October 22, 1909: Ferenczi to Putnam
November 17, 1909: Putnam to Freud
November 19, 1909: Jones to Putnam
November 22, 1909: Putnam to Jones
November 25, 1909: Jones to Putnam
November 27, 1909: Ferenczi to Putnam
December 3, 1909: Putnam to Freud
December 5, 1909: Freud to Putnam
January 13, 1910: Jones to Putnam
January 16, 1910: Jones to Putnam
January 28, 1910: Freud to Putnam
February 1, 1910: Ferenczi to Putnam
February 12, 1910: Jones to Putnam
February 15, 1910: Putnam to Freud
March 8, 1910: Ferenczi to Putnam
March 10, 1910: Freud to Putnam
April 1, 1910: Ferenczi to Putnam
April 9, 1910: Jones to Putnam
April 14, 1910: Putnam to Freud
May 19, 1910: Putnam to Freud
June 4, 1910: James to Putnam
June 16, 1910: Freud to Putnam
June 19, 1910: Jones to Putnam
June 25, 1910: Putnam to James
June 27, 1910: Jones to Putnam
June 29, 1910: Putnam to Freud
July 1, 1910: Jones to Putnam
July 12, 1910: Jones to Putnam
July 18, 1910: Jones to Putnam
[Late July, 1910]: Putnam to Freud
August 4, 1910: Putnam to Freud
August 14, 1910: Jones to Putnam

August 18, 1910: Freud to Putnam
September 1, 1910: Putnam to Freud
September 9, 1910: Jones to Putnam
September 14, 1910: Putnam to Jones
September 23, 1910: Jones to Putnam
September 27, 1910: Jones to Putnam
September 29, 1910: Freud to Putnam
October 10, 1910: Putnam to Freud
October 11, 1910: Jones to Putnam
October 13, 1910: Jones to Putnam
October 14, 1910: Putnam to Jones
October 17, 1910: Jones to Putnam
October 20, 1910: Jones to Putnam
October 21, 1910: Prince to Putnam
November 6, 1910: Jones to Putnam
November 8, 1910: Jones to Putnam
November 20, 1910: Jones to Putnam
November 22, 1910: Prince to Putnam
December 11, 1910: Jones to Putnam
December 16, 1910: Ferenczi to Putnam
December 26, 1910: Putnam to Freud
December 29, 1910: Freud to Putnam
December 30, 1910: Jones to Putnam
January 5, 1911: Putnam to Jones
January 8, 1911: Jones to Putnam
January 13, 1911: Jones to Putnam
January 20, 1911: Putnam to Freud
January 22, 1911: Freud to Putnam
January 23, 1911: Jones to Putnam
January 26, 1911: Putnam to Freud
February 5, 1911: Jones to Putnam
February 6, 1911: Putnam to Freud
February 19, 1911: Freud to Putnam
February 19, 1911: Jones to Putnam
February 24, 1911: Putnam to Jones
February 25, 1911: Prince to Putnam
February 27, 1911: Jones to Putnam
February 27, 1911: Freud to Putnam
March 2, 1911: Putnam to Jones
March 3, 1911: Prince to Putnam

March 5, 1911: Jones to Putnam
[Late March, 1911]: Putnam to Freud
March 27, 1911: Putnam to Freud
April 7, 1911: Jones to Putnam
April 15, 1911: Jones to Putnam
May 14, 1911: Freud to Putnam
May 30, 1911: Putnam to Freud
June 1, 1911: Jones to Putnam
June 14, 1911: Putnam to Jones
June 20, 1911: Putnam to Jones
July 15, 1911: Putnam to Freud
August 24, 1911: Putnam to Freud
September 30, 1911: Putnam to Freud
October 5, 1911: Freud to Putnam
October 6, 1911: Putnam to Freud
October 20, 1911: Putnam to Freud
October 29, 1911: Jones to Putnam
October 31, 1911: Jones to Putnam
November 5, 1911: Freud to Putnam
November 6, 1911: Jones to Putnam
November 14, 1911: Putnam to Freud
November 20, 1911: Putnam to Freud
Christmas (December 25, 1911):
    Freud to Putnam
March 2, 1912: Putnam to Freud
March 28, 1912: Freud to Putnam
April 1, 1912: Putnam to Freud
April 6, 1912: Putnam to Freud
April 9, 1912: Putnam to Ferenczi
April 29, 1912: Ferenczi to Putnam
June 4, 1912: Putnam to Freud
June 19, 1912: Putnam to Freud
June 25, 1912: Freud to Putnam
July 18, 1912: Freud to Putnam
August 1, 1912: Putnam to Freud
August 20, 1912: Freud to Putnam
September 6, 1912: Ferenczi to Putnam
September 11, 1912: Putnam to Freud
October 17, 1912: Ferenczi to Putnam
October 24, 1912: Putnam to Jones
    [incomplete]
November 21, 1912: Putnam to Freud
November 28, 1912: Freud to Putnam
December 3, 1912: Freud to Putnam
December 19, 1912: Putnam to Freud
January 1, 1913: Freud to Putnam
January 5, 1913: Putnam to Freud
January 9, 1913: Putnam to Freud
January 16, 1913: Putnam to Freud
January 21, 1913: Freud to Putnam

[Between January 21 and February
    13, 1913]: Putnam to Freud
February 13, 1913: Putnam to Freud
February 24, 1913: Putnam to Freud
March 11, 1913: Freud to Putnam
April 14, 1913: Putnam to Freud
August 6, 1913: Putnam to Freud
September 2, 1913: Putnam to Jones
    [incomplete]
October 22, 1913: Putnam to Freud
November 13, 1913: Freud to Putnam
November 29, 1913: Putnam to Freud
December 5, 1913: Putnam to Freud
December 16, 1913: Putnam to Jones
December 21, 1913: Putnam to Freud
December 25, 1913: Putnam to Freud
March 30, 1914: Freud to Putnam
April 15, 1914: Putnam to Freud
May 17, 1914: Freud to Putnam
June 2, 1914: Putnam to Freud
June 19, 1914: Ferenczi to Putnam
June 19, 1914: Freud to Putnam
July 7, 1914: Putnam to Freud
July 17, 1914: Putnam to Jones
August 19, 1914: Putnam to Jones
November 1, 1914: Putnam to Jones
[Early 1915]: Putnam to Freud
February 22, 1915: Putnam to Freud
March 9, 1915: Freud to Putnam
April 5, 1915: Putnam to Freud
May 12, 1915: Putnam to Jones
May 14, 1915: Putnam to Jones
    [incomplete]
May 19, 1915: Putnam to Freud
    [incomplete]
June 7, 1915: Freud to Putnam
July 8, 1915: Freud to Putnam
July 21, 1915: Putnam to Jones
August 13, 1915: Putnam to Freud
    [letter not sent]
September 15, 1915: Putnam to Freud
October 1, 1915: Putnam to Jones
October 6, 1915: Putnam to Freud
January 3, 1916: Putnam to Freud
January 26, 1916: Freud to Putnam
October 1, 1916: Freud to Putnam
November 12, 1916: Putnam to Jones
    [finished November 19]
March 11, 1917: Putnam to Jones
December 8, 1917: Putnam to Jones

Selected Bibliography

(Supplement to works cited)

Allen, Gay Wilson. *William James, A Biography*. New York: The Viking Press, 1967.

The American Neurological Association, Semi-Centennial Volume. New York: American Neurological Association, 1920.

Bonner, Thomas Neville. *American Doctors and German Universities; a Chapter in International Intellectual Development 1870–1914*. Lincoln: University of Nebraska Press, 1963.

Brill, Abraham Arden. *Freud's Contribution to Psychiatry*. New York: W. W. Norton, 1944.

———— *Lectures on Psychoanalytic Psychiatry*. New York: Alfred A. Knopf, 1946.

———— "Psychotherapies I Encountered." *Psychiatric Quarterly*, 21 (October 1947), 575–591.

Brome, Vincent. *Freud and His Early Circle*. London: Heinemann, 1968.

Burnham, John Cheynoweth. *Psychoanalysis and American Medicine, 1894–1918: Medicine, Science, and Culture*. Psychological Issues, vol. 5, no. 4, Monograph 20. New York: International Universities Press, Inc., 1967.

Burrow, Trigant. *A Search for Man's Sanity: The Selected Letters of Trigant Burrow, With Biographical Notes*. Prepared by the editorial committee of the Lifwyn Foundation, William E. Galt, chairman. New York: Oxford University Press, 1958.

Coriat, Isador. "Some Reminiscences of Psychoanalysis in Boston." *Psychoanalytic Review*, 32 (January 1945), 1–8.

Cotton, James Harry. *Royce on the Human Self*. Cambridge, Mass.: Harvard University Press, 1965.

Ellenberger, Henri. *The Discovery of the Unconscious*. New York: Basic Books, 1970.

Emerson, Edward W. "James Jackson Putnam." *Boston Evening Transcript*, Thursday, November 7, 1918, p. 12.

Fuss, Peter. *The Moral Philosophy of Josiah Royce*. Cambridge, Mass.: Harvard University Press, 1965.

Gauld, Alan. *The Founders of Psychical Research*. New York: Schocken Books, 1968.

Hendricks, Ives. Editor, *The Birth of an Institute*. Freeport, Maine: The Bond Wheelwright Co., 1958.

Jones, Ernest. "James Jackson Putnam," in Putnam, *Addresses on Psycho-*

Analysis. New York, Vienna, London: The International Psycho-Analytical Press, 1921.

Jung, Carl Gustav. *Memories, Dreams, Reflections.* Recorded and edited by Aniela Jaffe. New York: Vintage Books, 1961.

Lewin, Bertrand, and Helen Ross. *Psychoanalytic Education in the United States.* New York: W. W. Norton and Co., 1960.

Matthews, Fred Hamilton. "The Americanization of Sigmund Freud: Adaptations of Psychoanalysis before 1917." *Journal of American Studies,* 1 (April 1967), 39–62.

Murray, Henry. *Harvard Psychological Clinic. 1927–1957. Its Founder, Aims, Methods, Members, Graduates, and Contributions to Knowledge.* Cambridge, Mass.: 1957.

Perry, Ralph Barton. *The Thought and Character of William James.* Boston, Toronto: Little, Brown and Co., 1935, two vols.

Roback, A. A. "Morton Prince, 1854–1929." *American Journal of Orthopsychiatry,* 10 (January 1940), 177–184.

Rosenberg, Charles. *The Trial of the Assassin Guiteau; Psychiatry and Law in the Gilded Age.* Chicago: University of Chicago Press, 1968.

Taylor, Edward Wyllys. "James Jackson Putnam." *Archives of Neurology and Psychiatry,* 3 (March 1920), 307–314.

Taylor, William Sentman. *Morton Prince and Abnormal Psychology.* New York, London: D. Appleton and Co., 1928.

Washburn, Frederic Augustus. *The Massachusetts General Hospital; Its Development, 1900–1935.* Boston: Houghton Mifflin Co., 1939.

White, William Alanson. *Autobiography of a Purpose.* Garden City, N.Y.: Doubleday, Doran and Co., Inc., 1938.

Woodworth, Robert S. "Josiah Royce." National Academy of Sciences, *Biographical Memoirs,* 33. New York: Columbia University Press, 1959, 382–396.

Unpublished

Burnham, John Cheynoweth. "Psychoanalysis in American Civilization before 1918." Dissertation, Stanford University, 1958.

Fass, Paula S. "A. A. Brill — Pioneer and Prophet." Master's thesis, Columbia University, 1969.

Matthews, Frederick Hamilton. "Freud Comes to America: The Influence of Freudian Ideas on American Thought, 1909–1917." Master's thesis, University of California, Berkeley, 1957.

Ross, Dorothy. "Granville Stanley Hall, 1844–1895: Aspects of Science and Culture in the Nineteenth Century." Dissertation, Columbia University, 1965.

Sicherman, Barbara. "The Quest for Mental Health in America, 1880–1917." Dissertation, Columbia University, 1968.

Vasile, Russell George. "James Jackson Putnam — From Neurology to Psychoanalysis: A Study of the Reception and Promulgation of Freudian Psychoanalytic Theory in America, 1895–1918." Senior Thesis, Princeton University, 1970.

Biographical Notes

ALFRED ADLER (1870–1937), Viennese psychiatrist and founder of Individual Psychology, joined Freud's Vienna circle in 1902. He developed the theory that neurosis represented a compensation for inferior physical or psychological functions and argued that the will to power was a more fundamental drive than sexuality. Increasing disagreements with Freud led him to leave the Vienna Psychoanalytic Society, of which he was president, in July 1911. His early theories influenced such eclectic American analysts as William Alanson White and Smith Ely Jelliffe. He settled in America in 1935.

HENRI BERGSON (1859–1941), Putnam wrote in 1910, was the "keenest psychologist alive." He was born in Paris, graduated from the Ecole Normale Supérieure, and became professor of philosophy at the Collège de France in 1900. He was one of the new generation of explorers of the unconscious that included Freud, Janet, and Morton Prince. Freud and Bergson early read some of each other's work and, on October 23, 1913, Bergson published an article in the *Independent* that discussed the theories of Freud and Prince on dreams. Bergson's élan vital became an important concept for several American psychoanalysts, including Putnam.

SUSAN ELIZABETH BLOW (1843–1916) helped to shape Putnam's response to Freud, notably in his Weimar address. Born in St. Louis, the daughter of a wealthy entrepreneur, she later came under the influence of W. T. Harris, Hegel's foremost American exponent. In 1873 she founded the first American public school kindergarten in St. Louis on the principles of Froebel. She gave up her work in 1884 because of exhaustion and in 1889 moved to New York City and Cazenovia, N.Y. Under Putnam's care she recovered and from 1905 to 1909 was lecturer in Kindergarten at Teacher's College, Columbia University. Her extensive correspondence with Putnam touched on their favorite subjects, Goethe, Dante, Shakespeare, and, above all, philosophical idealism. She died in New York in 1916, depressed by the horrors of the Great War.

ABRAHAM ARDEN BRILL (1874–1948), whom Putnam judged to be "honest, courageous and sound," had become the leader of orthodox psychoanalysis in the United States by 1912. He emigrated alone to the United States from Austria-Hungary at the age of 15, motivated partly by hostility to his father, a commissary officer in the Imperial Army and by Prescott's histories of the New World. He painfully worked his way through the City College of New York and the Columbia College of Physicians and Surgeons, giving language and mandolin lessons. He studied under Adolf Meyer at the Psychiatric Institute on Ward's Island and in 1907–1908 with Jung and Bleuler in Zurich. He returned to practice psychoanalysis and was the first to translate Freud's major writings into English.

LOUVILLE EUGENE EMERSON (1873–1939) attended Josiah Royce's seminar on logic and received a doctorate in psychology at Harvard in 1907. While working as a psychologist at the Psychopathic Hospital of the University of Michigan, he wrote to Putnam in February 1911 of his interest in psychoanalysis and inquired about the possibility of a position in the Boston area. He was appointed psychologist in the Neurological Department of the Massachusetts General Hospital by September 1911, where he worked until 1939. He was a member of the American Psychoanalytic Association and one of the first to explore the role of family interrelationships in the neuroses.

AUGUST HOCH (1868–1919) was one of the first to introduce the psychiatric classifications of Emil Kraepelin to the United States and to take up the psychological study of the psychoses. Son of the director of the University Hospital in Basle, Switzerland, Hoch emigrated to the United States at the age of 19. From 1893 to 1905, he was pathologist at the McLean Hospital, Belmont, Massachusetts, where he knew Putnam, who found him "genuine and sympathetic." From 1905 to 1917 he taught psychiatry at the Cornell University Medical School and in 1910 succeeded Adolf Meyer as director of the Psychiatric Institute of the New York State Hospitals on Ward's Island. He retired in 1917 because of ill health and moved to Santa Barbara, California.

PIERRE JANET (1859–1947), French neurologist and psychologist, was one of the first modern explorers of the unconscious. In 1902 he succeeded Theodor Ribot in the chair of experimental and comparative psychology at the Collège de France. Putnam regarded him as "keen and able," and he deeply influenced the Boston psychotherapists. He lectured at the Lowell Institute in 1904, in Boston, and at Putnam's invitation, in 1906 at the inauguration of the new buildings of the Harvard Medical School. He became a relatively hostile opponent of psychoanalysis, objecting especially to Freud's sexual theories.

SMITH ELY JELLIFFE (1866–1945), New York neurologist, whose industry Putnam admired, was the son of a high school principal in Brooklyn. He met William Alanson White, with whom he often collaborated, in 1896, while both were working at the Binghamton State Hospital, New York. Jelliffe became managing editor of the *Journal of Nervous and Mental Disease* in 1902, and in 1911 A. A. Brill persuaded him to take up psychoanalysis. White and Jelliffe founded the Nervous and Mental Disease Monograph series in 1908 and the *Psychoanalytic Review* in 1913. He was influenced by early studies of paleontology, by Jung, Adler, and Bergson, and was one of the first workers in what became the field of psychosomatic medicine.

CARL GUSTAV JUNG (1875–1961), Swiss psychiatrist, founder of Analytical Psychology, whose "masterful ways" alienated Putnam, left the psychoanalytic movement in 1914 after two years of dispute, chiefly over Freud's theories of libido and infantile sexuality. The son of a pastor, he became lecturer in psychiatry at the University of Zurich from 1905 to 1913, and assistant to Eugen Bleuler, director of the Burghölzli Hospital and clinic. In 1907 he published *The Psychology of Dementia Praecox*, a pioneering application of Freud's theories to the psychoses; between 1904 and 1911 he developed word association tests to detect unconscious complexes. One of the greatest of the early psychoanalysts, he became increasingly preoccupied with studies of mythology, mysticism, and alchemy and with modes of achieving integration through the satisfaction of religious needs, which he regarded as inherent in the psyche.

ADOLF MEYER (1866–1950). Putnam and William James both consulted Meyer about psychiatry while he was clinical director at Worcester Insane Hospital. In Putnam's view, Meyer avoided "diagnoses" and "strict classifications" and studied each case as if it stood "wholly by itself." Perhaps the greatest American pioneer of functional psychiatry, Meyer was born in Switzerland and trained in neurology under August Forel. Hoping for greater independence, he emigrated to the United States and from 1893 to 1896 was pathologist at the Illinois Eastern Hospital for the Insane at Kankakee, and then worked at Worcester from 1895 to 1902. He directed the New York State Psychiatric Institute from 1902 to 1910 when he became professor of psychiatry at The Johns Hopkins University. He was one of the first to see the significance of Freud and Jung for psychiatry. Although never a "Freudian," he remained a member of the American Psychoanalytic Association, and trained a number of physicians who became prominent psychoanalysts.

HUGO MÜNSTERBERG (1863–1916) was born in Danzig, studied with Wilhelm Wundt, and was brought to Harvard by William James, where he became professor of psychology in 1897 and director of the Harvard Psychological Laboratory. He was a prolific scholarly and popular writer on psychotherapy, education, and criminology. He was a member of the Boston group of psychopathologists and an editor of the *Journal of Abnormal Psychology*.

OTTO RANK (1885–1939) worked as Freud's secretary and almost single-handedly directed the psychoanalytic publishing enterprises. He made important contributions to psychoanalytic studies of mythology, family interrelationships, and narcissism. After publication of his *Trauma of Birth* in 1924 he became estranged from Freud. In the 1920's he analyzed a number of Americans and, through Jessie Taft, became a significant influence in the Philadelphia School for Social Work.

THEODOR REIK (1888–1970), the son of a Viennese civil servant, met Freud in 1910, and in 1911 received a doctorate in psychology from the University of Vienna for a psychoanalytic study of Flaubert's *Temptation of St. Anthony*. He practiced lay analysis in Vienna, Berlin, and The Hague and settled in the United States in 1938. He was immensely prolific, his subjects ranging from anthropology and psychoanalytic technique to autobiography.

JOSIAH ROYCE (1855–1916), a "grateful patient," occasionally discussed philosophy with Putnam, who largely accepted his views. Royce was born in Grass Valley, California, was educated in the San Francisco public schools, and the universities of California, Leipzig, Göttingen, and The Johns Hopkins. His early writing came to the attention of William James, who brought him to Harvard in 1882. Royce taught philosophy there until 1916, and his seminar on logic became a clearing house for new conceptions in scientific method, attracting psychologists, philosophers, scientists, and physicians. Shy and awkward, Royce was profoundly interested in the meaning of community. He read deeply in the new literature of psychiatry and sexuality of the 1890's and early 1900's. With James, Putnam, Prince, Meyer, and others he was one of the circle of physicians and psychologists in Boston and Cambridge that explored hypnotism and psychotherapy.

HANNS SACHS (1881–1947), a lawyer in Vienna, joined Freud's Vienna Psychoanalytic Society in 1910 and with Otto Rank founded *Imago* in 1912. Sachs became a training analyst at the Berlin Institute in the early 1920's and in Boston, where he settled in 1932. He made psychoanalytic studies of literary and historical figures, including Caligula and Strindberg and wrote the valuable memoir, *Freud: Master and Friend.*

BORIS SIDIS (1867–1923), a political refugee, emigrated from Russia in 1887 and earned a doctorate in psychology under William James at Harvard ten years later. Temperamental and ambitious, he was one of the pioneer American psychopathologists arguing that fear was the most important cause of the neuroses. From 1896 to 1901 he was associate psychologist at the Pathological Institute of the New York State Hospitals; he practiced in Brookline, Massachusetts, from 1904 to 1909, when he established the Sidis Institute for nervous and mental disorders at Portsmouth, New Hampshire. He was a vehement opponent of psychoanalysis.

WILHELM STEKEL (1868–1940), Viennese neurologist, had been a patient of Freud and was an original member of the Vienna circle. He became an editor of the *Zentralblatt* in 1910, resigned from the Vienna Psychoanalytic Society in November 1912, but continued to edit it as his own journal. His major work was the *Sprache des Traumes,* published in 1911. Putnam considered him imaginative but "frivolous."

WILLIAM ALANSON WHITE (1870–1937) at the age of thirty-three was appointed superintendent of the Government Hospital for the Insane in Washington, D.C., in 1903 by Theodore Roosevelt. Earlier White had worked with Boris Sidis on research in psychopathology at the Pathological Institute of the New York State Hospitals and about 1909 became interested in psychoanalysis. In 1913, with Smith Ely Jelliffe, he founded the *Psychoanalytic Review.* He was a prolific writer and translator and a pioneer in psychoanalytic psychiatry.

German Texts of the Freud Letters

5 Dez 09
Wien, IX. Berggasse 19.

Dear Dr Putnam

Gestatten Sie mir, Deutsch fortzusetzen. Der Aufenthalt in Ihrem Hause war vielleicht das Inter-essante, was wir von dem grossen Amerika gesehen haben, und der Gedankenaustausch mit Ihnen trotz seiner Kürze dasjenige, was meine Hoffnung auf eine Zukunft der Psychoanalyse in Ihrem Lande am meisten bestärkt hat. Ich habe bei Ihnen ein Mass von ehrlicher Bereit-willigkeit und vorurteilsfreiem Verständnis gefunden, an das ich in Europa nicht gewöhnt worden bin, und wenn ich in Betracht ziehe, dass Sie der wahrscheinlich um ein Dezennium älter sind, kann ich mir den Respekt vor Ihrer Person zur Grundlage unserer Beziehungen nehmen. Es handelt sich gar nicht darum, ob Sie mir in allen Einzelheiten beistimmen können; meine Arbeiten wollen nichts anderes, als den Leser veranlassen, sich selbst die Erfahrungen zu holen, von denen ich spreche, und bis jetzt hat mich die Hoffnung nicht getäuscht, dass, wer dies thut, in den wichtigen Punkten zu den gleichen Ergebnissen kommen wird wie ich. Ich verlange und erwarte gar nicht, dass mir ein Leser vollkommen Glauben schenke, ohne und ehe er selbst zu den Quellen der Beobachtung herabgestiegen ist. Die meisten Menschen beweisen treulich, dass sie überhaupt nicht die Absicht haben, etwas Neues anzunehmen und billigen oder verwerfen, was ich vorbringe je nach dem jeweiligen Stand ihrer früheren Anschauungen. Von diesem Denkfehler weiss ich Sie frei, u darum erwarte ich, dass Sie sich allmälig auch von dem überzeugen werden, was Ihnen derzeit noch unglaubwürdig erscheint.

Sie finden ganz richtig heraus, dass die Dar-stellungen unsystematisch und lückenhaft sind. Dafür sind auch unsere Erkenntnisse noch sehr unvollständig, das Ganze ist erst im Werden und es ist sehr viel Raum für die Beiträge anderer Arbeiter übrig.

Unter Geldkomplex ist die Stellung der Individuen zum Geld verstanden, der selb-ständige Wert den sie darauf legen, ihre Fähigkeit mit diesem Stoff ungehindert durch unbewusste Komplexe umzugehen. Das Geldverhalten der Individuen müsste gerade in Amerika, wo die Analerotik sehr interessante Umwandlungen erfahren hat, sehr lehrreich sein. Übrigens ist die Beziehung des Geldkomplexes zur Anal-erotik ein sehr später Fund gewesen. Bei uns hier sind die Menschen in Bezug auf das Geld genau so unaufrichtig und gehemmt wie in sexuellen Dingen, und rechtfertigen so die Zurechnung des Geldes zur Sexualität.

Jede Verwendung, die Sie von einer meiner Arbeiten machen wollen, wird mir recht sein. Für Übersetzungen hat Dr. Brill das aus-schliessliche Vorrecht erhalten; er wird gewiss nichts dagegen haben, es Ihnen im betreffenden Falle abzutreten, wenn Sie es von ihm wünschen.

Dass seine Übersetzung eher gewissenhaft als schön zu nennen ist vermutete ich selbst. Er ist übrigens nicht als Ausländer zu bezeichnen; ich glaube, dass er in so früher Kindheit über das grosse Wasser gekommen ist, dass man Englisch als seine Muttersprache gelten lassen muss. Ich glaube, Ihre Klage über unsere Unfähigkeit neurotische Patienten für das Aufgeben ihrer Krankeit zu entschädigen, ist voll berecht-igt, aber die Schuld scheint mir nicht an der Therapie sondern an den sozialen Institut-ionen zu liegen. Was wollen Sie, das wir thun, wenn eine Frau über ihr verlorenes Leben klagt, wenn sie nach dem Schwinden ihrer Jugend merkt, dass sie sich um das Glück der Liebe aus konventionellen Gründen hat betrügen lassen? Sie hat Recht und wir stehen ohnmächtig vor ihr, denn wir können sie nicht mehr jung machen. Aber die Einsicht in unsere therapeut-ische Beschränkung mag unseren Entschluss bestärken, an anderer Stelle, im sozialen Leben, dahin zu wirken, dass die Menschen nicht in so hoffnungslose Positionen gedrängt werden. Aus der therapeutischen Ohnmacht muss Prophylaxe der Neurosen hervorgehen. Je energischer man übrigens in solchen Fällen das sexuelle Problem angreift, desto eher kann man wenigstens lindern. Wo es nicht so trostlos aussieht, da ergeben sich durch Sublimirung neue Lebensziele von selbst, sobald die Verdräng-ungen gelöst sind.

Die 3 Abhandlungen zur Sexualtheorie sind vergriffen. Die zweite Auflage kann nicht vor Februar auf den Markt kommen.

Ich freue mich auf die in Aussicht gestellten Photographien aus den Adirondacks und bin so unbescheiden, mir auch Ihren kürzlich veröffentlichten Aufsatz über Psychoanalyse zu erbitten, von dem Sie beim Abschied sprachen, u dessen Erscheinen mir von anderer Seite berichtet worden ist. Ferner bitte ich um *eine Zeile* Nachricht, wenn die Sammlung von "Schriften z. angewandten Seelenkunde" (6 Hefte) Sie erreicht hat. Sie ist längst bestellt worden, aber der Verleger behauptet, solche Sendungen nach Amerika gingen oft verloren. (die gleiche Sendung an Stanley Hall ist angekommen).

Mit der Bitte mich Ihrem Bruder und den liebenswürdigen Damen der Familie zu empfehlen begrüsse ich Sie

Ihr herzlich und hochachtungsvoll
ergebener Freud

28 1. 1910
Wien, IX. Berggasse 19.

Dear Dr. Putnam

Sie werden verständlich finden, wenn ich gestehe, dass ich schon lange keinen Artikel in so grosser Spannung zu lesen begonnen habe, wie Ihren ersten Aufsatz im J. of abnorm. Psychology, der an so ehrenvoller Stelle meinen Name zeigt. Was ich dann gelesen habe, konntc mich dank unserer Korrespondenz nicht mehr überraschen, aber es hat mir Freude u. Genugthuung bereitet. Ich hoffe, Ihre Äusser-rung wird einen mächtigen Eindruck in Amerika hervorrufen u der Psychoanalyse die Auf-merksamkeit Ihrer Landsleute endgiltig sichern. Besonders schön finde ich Ihre Worte auf p. 307 von: All this is wrong an. So etwas ehrt den Mann, der es geschrieben hat, nicht nur den Arzt und Forscher. Ich stehe wahrscheinlich religiös auf einem von dem Ihrigen sehr verschiedenen Standpunkt aber ich sehe, soweit sind alle ehrlichen Männer von derselben Religion. Besonderen Dank schulde ich Ihnen dann noch für die Ernsthaftigkeit mit der Sie mir in Sachen der Sex-ualität beistehen; auch das sollte selbstverständlich sein, ist es aber leider auch unter Ärzten nicht.

In einem einzigen Punkt verstehe ich Sie nicht; wie Sie Morton Prince in der Auffassung des Unbewussten Recht geben können. Ist da nicht auch das Vorurteil handgreiflich, dass die suppressed mental states hysterischer Personen "bewusst" genannt werden müssen, obwol die oberflächlichste Untersuchung zeigt, dass sie nichts von ihnen wissen (und das allein ist das Kennzeichen u zunächst der ganze Sinn des Unbewussten), das wird mir nie be-greiflich werden. Mit "awareness" hat diese Frage ja nichts zu thun. Bewusste seelische Vor-gänge melden sich beim Bewusstsein, sobald sie aktiv werden, die von uns studirten werden aktiv und doch nicht bewusst. Ist dieser Unter-schied nicht bedeutsam genug, um die Namen-gebung nach ihm einzurichten?

Ich bin natürlich sehr neugierig, was Ihre Fortsetzung bringen wird. Bei dieser Ge-legenheit erfahre ich endlich auch die richtigen englischen Übersetzungen für meine Termini. Von mir ist in nächster Zeit nichts zu erwarten. Ich muss das Jahr und die Ferien verdienen, was auch in Österreich schwere Arbeit kostet. Die zweite Auflage der "Sexualtheorie" wird in 3–5 Wochen bei Ihnen eintreffen.

Mit herzlichen Dank und Gruss
Ihr
Freud

10. 3. 10
Wien, IX, Berggasse 19.

Dear Dr. Putnam
Herzlichen Dank für Brief und zweiten Artikel. You gave us a very good character and we will take pains to deserve it.

Ihre Bemerkungen über das Wortmissver-ständnis im Streit um das Unbewusste haben mich sehr erleichtert. Es ist ja wirklich kaum möglich, dass man anders urtheilt, wenn man dieselben Phänomene studiert. Bei der Philosophie ist es etwas anderes; sie reden vom Ubw u kennen es nicht; sie haben also ein Recht es zu bestreiten. Aber wie will man *eine* Traumanalyse machen u es doch verleugnen!

Ich darf die Bemerkung wagen, dass ich von Anfang an auf dem konsequenten Stand-punkt von Bergson in dieser Sache stehe. Er ist auch der meinige, u ich sehe die Verwirrung nicht so arg, wenn man nun von dem alten Sinn von "Bw" absehen will, sich an die Thatsache hält, das für bw erklärt, was man weiss und "Ubw" das, was man, obwol es aktiv ist, nicht weiss. Dass der Name Ubw blos negativ ist, thut doch nichts zur Sache; Namen brauchen nicht passend zu sein, u uns bleibt im Fortschritt der Wissenschaft nichts übrig, als den neuen Wein in die alten Schläuche einzufüllen.

Über das Thema der Religion mit Ihnen zu sprechen, wäre mir bei Ihrer Toleranz u Aufgeklärtheit ein hoher Genuss. Vielleicht findet sich die Gelegenheit beim nächsten Kongress, da wir Sie alle zu diesem nicht erwarten dürfen. Ich fürchte, es wird doch nur wider eine fromme Wunscherfüllung. Der "gerechte Gott" und die "gütige Natur" sind doch wider nur die höchsten Sublimirungen unseres Elternkomplexes, und unsere infantile Hilflosigkeit die letzte Wurzel der Religion.
Was man im Leben sieht, macht nicht den Eindruck als gäbe es auch eine sittliche Weltordnung. Aber das ist von der Psychoanalyse unabhängig, man kann diese Religion auf sie propfen oder nicht; ich möchte sie nicht prinzipiell in den Dienst einer positiven Lehre stellen.

Die zweite Auflage der Sexualtheorie (un-verändert) geht in den nächsten Tagen an Sie ab. Ich grüsse Sie herzlich u danke Ihnen für alle Förderung unserer Sache.

Ihr
Freud

16. 6. 10
Wien IX. Berggasse 19.

Dear Dr. Putnam

Endlich bin ich wieder in der Lage, Ihnen meinen Dank für Ihre Briefe, Berichte und Zusendungen durch eine kleine Gabe von meiner Seite zu bezeugen. Meine Schrift über "Eine Kindheitserinnerung des Leonardo da Vinci" wird bereits in Ihren Händen sein. Sie enthält vieles von den Dingen, über die wir nicht gleichartig denken, und die den Inhalt der mir zugesagten Unterhaltung, hoffentlich auf europäischem Boden, bilden sollen. Ich wäre sehr geehrt, wenn ich Ihnen eine Meinungsäusserung über dieses kleine Werk entlocken könnte.

Es ist mir ferner in den Sinn gekommen, — und ich schreibe inoffiziell darüber, denn offiziell habe ich kein Recht dazu — dass nur Ihre Person und nur Boston der Ausgangs-punkt für die Bildung einer psychoanalytischen Gruppe sein können, zu welcher sich unsere Freunde in Amerika zusammen schliessen sollen, um in den in Nürnberg beschlossenen Internationalen Verein einzutreten. Ich habe gehört, dass alle grossen geistigen Bewegungen drüben in Boston geboren worden sind, und ich weiss, dass kein Anderer der allge-meinen Hochachtung so sicher ist wie Sie, und durch das Ansehen seiner unantastbaren Persönlichkeit die hart befehdete Sache der Psychoanalyse in der öffentlichen Mein-ung schützen kann. Jung, der Obmann der Internat Vereinigung ist, wird Ihnen gewiss gerne alle gewünschten Aus-künfte geben. Ich für meinen Teil bin ganz bereit, Ihnen auch für diesen Schritt danken zu müssen.

Ihr herzlich ergebener
Freud

Noordwijk aan Zee
Wien, IX. Berggasse 19
18 Aug 10

Dear Dr. Putnam

Ich habe für zwei Briefe u die versprochenen Zusendungen zu danken. In Ihrem ersten Brief hat mich Ihre Anerkennung des Leonardo u

Ihr Versprechen, die amerik. Ortsgruppe zu gründen, sehr erfreut, dagegen gekränkt, dass Sie meinen ich könnte Ihre abweichenden ideal-istischen Einsichten für "nonsense" er-klären. Ich bin nicht so eng-herzig, einen Mangel meiner Begabung zum Gesetz erheben zu wollen. Ich habe kein Bedürfnis nach einer höheren moralischen Ausgleichung, sowie ich kein musikalisches Gehör habe, u bin weit davon entfernt, mir darum die feinere Organisation zuzu-schreiben. Ich tröste mich damit, dass die Sicher-heit für die idealistischen Wahrheiten, auf die Sie nicht verzichten wollen, keine grosse sein kann, wenn schon die Grundlagen der Wissenschaft, bei denen wir uns einmütig treffen, so schwierig festzustellen sind. Aber ich respektire Sie u Ihre Art zu denken u wenn ich schon hinnehmen muss, dass ich ein gottverlassener "incredulous jew" bin, so bin ich doch nicht stolz darauf u nicht über-hebend gegen andere. Ich denke nur mit Faust: Es muss auch solche Käuze geben.

Dr. Jones, der einige Tage hier in Holland mein Gast war, erzälte, dass er Ihnen den Leonardo zu lesen gegeben. Ich hoffe, er ist seitdem vom Verleger aus in Ihre Hand gekommen, denn ich hatte Auftrag erteilt, dass alle folgenden Bände der "angewandten Schriften" an Sie gesandt werden sollten.

Ich erinnere mich daran, dass sich jetzt bald die Zeit jährt, in der ich für die Entwicklung der Ψ A in Amerika so bedeutsame Bekannt-schaft gemacht u Ihre Gastfreundschaft genossen habe, u bitte Sie den Herren und Damen Ihrer Familie meine ergebenen Grüsse zu über-mitteln.

Herzlich der Ihrige
Freud

29. Sept 10
Wien, IX. Berggasse 19.

Dearest Dr Putnam

Ich bitte Sie um Verzeihung, wenn mein Brief heute einen mir nicht gewohnten Enthusiasmus nicht verläugnen kann. Ich war selten stolzer oder züfriedener mit mir als nach der Lektüre Ihres Aufsatzes On the Etiology and Treatment of the Psychoneuroses vom 21 Juli, den ich erst heute nach meiner Rückkehr von Italien gelesen habe. Nach Ihrem Zeugnis habe ich also nicht umsonst gelebt u gearbeitet, u Männer wie Sie werden dafür sorgen, dass die Gedanken, die ich schmerzhaft genug erkannt habe, nicht für die Menschheit verloren gehen. Was will ein Einzelner mehr?

Von Ihrer Seite aber welch eine Meisterschaft der Darstellung der schwierigsten Zusammenhänge, welche Klarheit und Wahrheitsliebe, u wie erziehlich muss eine solche Darlegung auf eine Hörerschaft wirken, die noch freien Raum zur Aufnahme von Neuem in sich hat.

Ich habe in Ihren Sätzen alles, woran ich glaube, wiedergefunden, aber klarer, in breitem Zusammenhang, mitten in die kulturelle Stellung gerückt, in dies gehört, wie ver-klärt durch die grossen sozialen Gesichts-punkte des Menschenfreundes.

Ich bitte Sie jetzt um die Erlaubnis, diesen Aufsatz für unser Zentralblatt zu übersetzen. Ich kann mir keine würdigere u. kräftigere Apologie gegen die Angriffe vorstellen, gegen die wir uns hier zu wehren haben. Nur gestatten Sie, dass ich an jener Stelle, wo Sie mir persönlich ein so hohes Lob spenden, eine Auslassung mache, es würde sich für mich als den Übersetzer nicht anders schicken, besonders da ich selbst Herausgeber des Zentralblattes bin.

Von Ihrem Brief von 1 Sept. will ich nicht viel sagen. Er macht Ihnen die grösste Ehre; ich kann nur bedauern, dass meine Gedanken nicht in diese Höhen reichen.

Die Nachlässigkeit des Buchhändlers in der Zusendung des Leonardo habe ich mich bemüht zu korrigiren.

Ihr herzlich ergebener
Freud

29 Dez 10
Wien, IX. Berggasse 19.

Verehrter Herr Kollege

Ich will dieses ereignisreiche u mühselige Jahr nicht zu Ende gehen lassen, ehe ich Ihnen für Vieles gedankt habe, für die wertvollen Zusendungen Ihrer Arbeiten, für die unschätzbare Unterstützung, die Sie unserer Sache geliehen haben, für das Einsetzen Ihres Namens in Amerika gegen Missverständnisse u Verleumdungen, die mich sonst getroffen hätten. Ich wünsche Ihnen von-selbstsüchtigem Herzen-ungestörte Fortdauer Ihrer Gesundheit u Arbeitslust im Jahre 1911.

Ihr Toronto-Vortrag ist bereits im Druck und wird die *vierte* Nummer des Zentralblattes zieren. (Die dritte ist bereits erschienen). Der zweite (Washington) Vortrag, den Sie mir gleichfalls zur Verfügung gestellt haben, wird in einer späteren Nummer von Otto *Rank* übersetzt erscheinen. Sie werden gebeten, der Form zuliebe das bescheidene Honorar mit dem Übersetzer zu theilen, der im Falle des ersten Vortrags mit meiner Person identisch ist, obwol ich mich auf dem Titel nicht nenne.

Zwei kleine Sonderdrucke von mir (aus Jahrbuch u Zentralblatt) werden Sie in nächster Zeit erreichen.

Unsere Sache geht hier sehr gut. Die Oppo-sition ist auf der Höhe. Ich bin zwar schon etwas müde, aber vielleicht geht das vorüber und die nachkommenden, speziell mein prächtiger Jung, sind sehr hoffnungsvoll.

Ich habe Bleuler u Jung jetzt in München gesehen. Wir haben vor den Kongress auf Ende Sept 1911 zu verlegen und Lugano in Aussicht genommen. Bestim-mend für diese Zeitwal war die Hoffnung, unsere amerikanischen Freunde bei uns zu sehen.

Mit herzlichem Gruss
Ihr treu ergebener
Freud

22 Jan 1911
Wien, IX. Berggasse, 19.

Verehrter Herr Kollege

Unsere Neujahrswünche haben sich gekreuzt; mögen sie beiderseits in Er-füllung gehen.

Ihr Vortrag in Toronto liegt imprimirt vor mir und wird in der Januar-nummer des Zentralblattes erscheinen. Es war als ich Ihren Brief erhält zu spät, um auf Zusätze zu warten. Er bringt auch so dem Leser unerhört viel Gutes und Neues. Jung theilt mein Urtheil über ihn. Wir haben uns Ihre Erlaubnis zu Nutze gemacht, um auch Ihren Vortrag in Washington übersetzen zu lassen, der einige Monate später publizirt werden soll. Sie werden unterdess vielleicht die schöne Apologie gelesen haben die Bleuler der Psychoanalyse im neuen Heft des Jahrbuches gewidmet hat. Wir wollen abwarten, ob sie auf die erregten Gemüter in Deutschland einen besänftigenden Einfluss üben wird. Unsere nächste freudige Erwartung ist, Sie und andere Ihrer Landsleute als Mitglieder des Ψ A. Vereins auf unserem September Kongress zu begrüssen. Er wird vielleicht in Lugano stattfinden. Jung wird Ihnen alles Nähere mittheilen.

Mit vielen herzlichen Empfehlungen
Ihr getreuer
Freud

19 Febr 1911
Wien, IX. Berggasse 19.

Verehrter Herr Kollege

Ich bin sehr froh darüber, dass sie Ihr Erscheinen zum Kongress in sichere Aussicht genommen haben. Es wird also eine eindrucksvolle und nachhaltig wirkende Zusammenkunft werden.

Vielleicht sehen u sprechen wir uns schon vorher in Zürich, da wir vorhaben Jungs Gastfreundschaft im Laufe des Monats Sept und bis zum Datum des Kongresses anzunehmen. Denken Sie, welche Freude das für uns sein wird.

Ihr Toronto Vortrag ist in No 4 des Zentralblattes eben erschienen. Die 400 Sonderabzüge habe ich nach Erhalt Ihrer Arbeit telegraphisch bei Bergmann bestellt, aber noch nicht erhalten. Ich werde bei ihm anfragen, ob er sie Ihnen direkt geschickt hat. [? Ihre?] für uns nicht minder wertvolle Arbeit der Vortrag in Washington ist bereits von Herrn Rank übersetzt u wartet seinen Termin ab; wir haben bereits Raummangel im Zentralblatt.

Ich arbeite an der dritten Auflage der Traumdeutung u frage bei Ihnen an, ob Sie den-1910 gehaltenen Vortrag über Sex Symbolism in Dreams bereits veröffentlicht haben, so dass ich ihn für die neue Auflage verwerten kann.

Der nächste Halbband des Jahrbuches wird mehreres über Paranoia von Ferenczi und von mir bringen. Für den Sommer [?] ballt sich etwas wie eine grössere Synthese zusammen, für die ich vielleicht während der Kur in Karlsbad Zeit finden werde. Gegenwärtig hindern mich die Anforderungen des Erwerbs u der täglichen Praxis, mehr zu leisten. Ich freue mich aber zu sehen, dass sowohl bei Ihnen in Amerika als auch hier die Arbeiten und das Interesse für den Gegenstand Fortschritte machen. Jones ist ganz besonders thätig und unermüdlich.

Mit herzlichem Gruss Wünschen für Ihr
Wolbefinden
Ihr getreuer
Freud

27.2.11
Wien, IX. Berggasse 19.

Verehrtester Kollege

Hiemit bin ich in der Lage, mein erstes Geldgeschäft mit Ihnen abzuwickeln, indem ich Ihnen anzeige, wie Bergmann Ihre un-schätzbare im Zent. f. Ps.A. veröffentliche Arbeit honorirt hat. Die Hälfte der

hier ausgewiesenen Summe habe ich als Übersetzer in Anspruch genommen, die andere Hälfte lasse ich Ihnen durch Ver-mittlung meiner
Bank zugehen.

Von den 400 Sonderabzügen habe ich 40 zur Verteilung hier u in
den Sektionen Zürich u Berlin zurückgehalten, hoffentlich mit Ihrem
Einverständnis.

Ich will nichts Wissenschaft-liches unter diese geschäft-lichen Mitt-
heilungen mengen bleibe mit

herzlichen Grüssen
Ihr ergebener
Freud

lBeilage.

14.5.11
Wien, IX. Berggasse 19.

Verehrter Dr Putnam

Ich bitte Sie ernsthaft um Entschuldigung in zwei Punkten. Erstens
dass ich Ihnen in der Note zur Übersetzung Ihres Vortrags einen
"Charakter" gegeben. Ich wusste damals noch nicht dass Sie den
deutschen Aufsatz in Amerika versenden würden; dort muss es sich ja
höchst sonderbar ausnehmen, wenn ich, der Unbekannte, Zeugnis für
Sie ablegen will. Anders natürlich wenn Sie mich dem amerikanischen
Publikum vorgestellt haben.

Zweitens, wenn ich auf Ihren ausführlichen Brief in Sachen der
Sublimierung antworte als ob nicht der Nachtrag mit Ablehnung
einer solchen Reaktion mitgekommen wäre. Das Problem interessiert
mich zu sehr und ich meine auch Ihre Vermutung dass wir hier nicht
auf demselben Boden stehen kann Ihr Interesse für die Ψ A ab-
schwächen. Sie sagen also die Ψ A Erfahrung zeigt mir dass ich bei
meinen Patienten die Sublimierung anstreben muss wenn ich Sie wirklich herstellen will. Die Ψ A Theorie sagt mir aber nicht, warum ich so
vorgehen muss. Hier, meine ich, darf man widersprechen. Die Ψ A
Theorie erklärt es wol. Sie behauptet dass ein Trieb nicht sublimiert
werden kann, solange er verdrängt ist. Das gilt natürlich auch für jeden
Teilbetrag des Triebes. Es ist also notwendig die Verdrängung durch
die Überwindung der Widerstände aufzuheben ehe man eine Sublimierung oder eine vollständige Sublimierung erreichen kann. Das will
nun die Ψ A Therapie leisten und damit stellt sie sich in den Dienst
jeder höheren Entwicklung.

Wenn wir uns nicht begnügen zu sagen be moral and philosophical,
so geschieht es weil dies zu billig ist und bereits so oft gesagt wurde,

ohne zu helfen. Die Kunst ist den Mensch-zu *ermöglichen* moralisch zu sein und ihre Wunschtendenzen philosophisch zu beherrschen. Die Sublimierung, das Aufsuchen höherer Ziele ist natürlich einer der besten Wege um das Drängen unserer Triebe zu bewältigen. Aber das kann erst in Betracht kommen nachdem die Ψ A Arbeit der Aufhebung der Verdrängungen geleistet ist.

Wenn die Sublimierung in unseren Diskussionen wenig vorkommt so hat dies zwei Gründe, erstens weil sie nicht in Frage kommt, zweitens weil so viele unserer Patienten denen wir doch helfen wollen ungeeignet für sie sind. Es sind zum grossen Teil minderwertige Konstitutionen mit unmässig starken Trieben die besser sein wollen als sie es sein können, ohne dass sie selbst und die Gesellschaft etwas von diesem krampfhaften Wollen hätten. Es ist also humaner den Grundsatz aufzustellen: Sei so moralisch als Du ehrlicher Weise sein kannst und strebe nicht eine ethische Vollkommenheit an für die Du nicht bestimmt bist.

Wer der Sublimierung fähig ist, der wendet sich ihr regelmässig zu, sobald er von der Neurose befreit ist. Andere die es nicht können, sind wenigstens natürlicher und wahrhaftiger.

Sie können nach diesen Bemerkungen schliessen wie sehr wir uns alle freuen würden wenn wir auf dem Kongress in Weimar wirklich etwas von Ihren Ansichten uber das Verhältnis der Ψ A sur Ethik hören könnten.

In Betreff Ihrer weitergehenden Forderungen an die Ψ A möchte ich bemerken dass sie ja nur ein Instrument ist, dessen sich der Arbeiter nach den Intentionen seiner Hand bedienen kann. Ich kann mich persönlich wol in Ihre Bedürfnisse einfühlen wenn ich Ihnen auch nicht in die Versuche folge, sie zu befriedigen. Die Genügsamkeit, das Bedürfnis nach Sicherheit scheint mir das nächste Wertvolle zu sein. Es hat niemals an den erhebendsten Weltanschauungen gefehlt, aber sie waren Kinder des frommen Wunsches, der Illusion gerade wie die stolzen naturwissenschaftlichen Systeme die wir verlassen haben als wir aufs Anthropozentrische verzichten mussten. Wir kennen die menschliche Seele noch zu wenig erst wenn diese Kenntnis sich gehoben haben, werden wir wissen, was auf ethischem Gebiet möglich ist, und was man auf dem Gebiet der Erziehung — ohne Schaden thun kann um es zu erreichen.

Ich bin mit herzlichem Dank für die mich intensiv beschäftigende Zuschrift und in der Erwartung Sie im Herbst wiederzusehen,

Ihr treu ergebener
Freud

5 Okt 11
Wien, IX. Berggasse 19.

Verehrter Kollege

Sie machen sich einen schlechten Charakter zurecht. Doch weiss ich, dass ein viel schlechterer Mensch zum Vorschein käme, wenn z.B. ich mich in einer Analyse so entblössen würde, und Sie übersehen, welche Seelengrösse sich in Ihrer Aufrichtigkeit kund giebt. Es kränkt mich nur, dass Sie mir zum letzten Mal in persönlichen Angelegenheiten geschrieben haben wollen. Ich hoffe, es wird nicht so sein.

Es eilt mich nun, Ihre Fragen einzeln, soweit ich es kann, zu beantworten.

1) In Betreff Ihrer Tochter bin ich der Ansicht, dass eine Wahrscheinlichkeit von 9:1 für die Diagnose Hy. und gegen die Epilepsie spricht. Ich meine Sie brauchen es nicht eilig zu nehmen u können die Symptome vernachlässigen, wenn sich der Anfall nicht wiederholt und nichts anderes auf-tritt. Zeigt es sich aber, dass etwas progressives vorliegt, so ist eine Analyse gewiss ange-zeigt von der ich hoffe, dass sie Ihnen den Vorteil dieser Therapie in corpore pretioso zeigen wird. Ich bewahre natürlich das Geheimnis.

2. Zu Ihrem Traum kann ich bemerken, dass ich Ihre Deutung völlig korrekt finde, nur eine Überdeutung vorschlagen möchte. Die sichere Strasse, die Sie bisher vorfolgt haben, kann auch die Ihrer bisherigen Therapie sein, die neue, die sich bald so unangenehm erweist, dagegen, die der Psychoanalyse, vor welcher Sie grosse Angst zu haben scheinen. Sie fürchten sich wirklich zu sehr vor Ihren Phantasien u scheinen nicht glauben zu wollen, dass eine Übersetzung derselben in Realität völlig ausgechlossen ist. Wenn Sie diese Angst aufgeben, werden Sie auch mehr von den Phantasien erfahren, sie interessant finden u sich erleichtert fühlen. Es frappirt mich auch, dass Sie in Ihrer Zeichnung die Buchstaben ABDEFG verwenden und das C (Charles) auslassen. Leider habe ich versäumt nach dem Namen Ihrer Frau zu fragen.

3. Am wenigsten kann ich Ihrer Phantasie vom glücklichen Familienleben sagen, weil Sie sich im Motivenbericht zu ihr so sehr überstürzt und alles Mögliche, was unangenehm ist, zusammengetragen haben. Ich möchte Sie nur bitten, nicht zuviel Wert auf die Adler'schen Gedanken von Organminderwertigkeit, Protest, sich zur Geltung bringen usw zu legen, weil diese Momente oberflächlich u sekundär, auch ja meist bewusst, sind u den wirklichen Mechanismus nicht treffen. Ich sehe Sie im wesentlichen an zu früh u stark verdrängtem Sadismus — an Übergüte — leiden, der sich nun zum grösserem Teil als Selbst-

quälerei Ausgang verschafft. Hinter der Phantasie vom glücklichen Familienleben würden Sie die normalen verdrängten Phantasien von reichem Ausleben der Sexualität finden, auf deren Einfluss auch die körperliche Unbefriedigung durch die Ehefrau zurückzuführen ist. Symptome des Alterns, die ich jetzt auch kennen lerne wie ich Ihnen in Zürich erzält habe.

Immer bereit, mit Ihnen brieflich zu plaudern, wenn die Entfern-ung mündlichen Verkehr ver-hindert, zäle ich die Annäherung zwischen uns zu den Gewinnen der schönen Zeit um den Kongress.

Ich hätte bald Ihre vierte Anfrage vergessen. Ja ich meine, das Ver-kehren mit Todten wie in Ihrem Traum mit James — wenn nicht die Klausel dabei ist: Ich weiss aber, dass *er* todt ist — bedeute den eigenen Tod. Interessant, dass Sie gerade das vergessen haben.

Herzlich u ergebenst
Ihr getreuer
Freud

5. Nov 11
Wien, IX. Berggasse 19.

Verehrter Herr Kollege

Meinen schönsten Dank für das heute eingetroffene Buch über Ihren Grossvater das ich mit grossem Interesse lesen werde. Es ist gewiss nicht nur eine Pflichterfüllung sondern auch eine hohe Befriedigung wenn man von den Thaten seiner Ahnen berichten und so das Geschwätz der Wissenschaftler über die notwendige Entartung der zivilisierten Menschheit an den eigenen Namen widerlegen kann. In der That bietet gerade Ihre, die englische Rasse zahlreiche Beispiele von der Erhaltung kultureller Leistungsfähigkeit durch mehrere Jahrhunderte und viele Generationen.

Über den Zustand Ihrer Tochter lässt sich wie ich merke aus der Ferne ein Urteil absolut nicht gewinnen. Die Diagnose schwankt also noch und daher gewiss die therapeutische Ratlosigkeit. Die Anknüp-fung an eine Poliomyelitis von der Sie (ein früheres Mal) geschrieben haben, erschiene mir besonders zweifelhaft.

Ich freue mich zu hören dass unsere so spärlichen Versuche einer Analyse Ihnen keinen üblen Nachgeschmack hinterlassen haben. Die Arbeit an sich selbst ist eine unbegrenzbar fortzusetzende. Ich merke an mir wie sehr man sich jedes neue Mal in Erstaunen versetzen kann.

Die "äussere Politik" der Ψ A ruht jetzt einigermassen. Es geht nichts Neues vor. Es wird Sie interessieren zu hören, dass Ihr Vortrag in Weimar auf mich bedeutend gewirkt hat. Freilich ist meine Reaktion darauf eine ganz eigentümliche. Ich arbeite daran die Psychogenese der Religion analytisch zu verstehen und das mir persönlich fehlende religiöse Bedürfnis nach unserer Art aufzuklären. Ich studiere zu diesem Zweck Frazer, Andrew Lang, Tylor etc. und werde mich auch bald mit Ihrem verstorbenen Freund W. James beschäftigen müssen. Wenn ich zu einem Abschluss und zu Ergebnissen komme werde ich hoffentlich die wirklich Frommen nicht beleidigen müssen.

In der Hoffnung bald und Gutes von Ihnen zu hören,

Ihr

herzlich ergebener

Freud

Wien, IX. Berggasse 19.

Weihnacht 1911

Verehrter Dr. Putnam

Ich benütze den ersten Tag der Weihnachtszeit um Ihnen für Ihre letzten Zeitschriften und Sendungen zu danken. Ich werde von den Büchern gewiss sorgfältig Notiz nehmen. Dass es Ihrer Tochter gut geht, stützt wol die Diagnose auf eine harmlose Hysterie.

Meine Studien zur Psychogenese der religiösen Gefüle rücken sehr langsam vor; ich habe sehr wenig Zeit und muss vieles andere daneben thun, doch denke ich nicht daran sie aufzugeben, bedarf nur eines langen Lebens um in ihnen etwas zu erreichen.

Im Ganzen ist mir dabei zu Mute wie einem älterem Herrn, der in späten Jahren eine zweite Ehe geschlossen hat. L'amour côute cher aux vieillards. Die Arbeiten im Verein gehen gut vor sich. Wir hoffen im Frühjahr die erste Nummer der neuen nicht medizinischen Zeitschrift herauszubringen.

Mit herzlichen Wünschen zum neuen Jahre 1912.

Ihr aufrichtig ergebener

Freud

28.3.12.

Wien, IX. Berggasse 19.

Verehrter Herr Kollege

Jedesmal wenn ich von der Ψ A in Ihrer Darstellung lese gefällt mir die Sache von Neuem besser. Sie ist dann wie veredelt und verschönt und ich erkenne im Feiertagsgewand kaum die Magd wieder, die mir

die häuslichen Geschäfte besorgt. Für solche Wirkung bin ich auch
Ihrer letzter Zusendung dankbar.

Imago ist heute erschienen und rechnet auf Beiträge von Ihrer Seite.
Ich bin neugierig ob der Erfolg der neuen Unternehmung ein anderer
sein wird als nun auch die Vertreter der anderen Wissenschaften gegen
uns aufzubringen. Der nächste Erfolg wahrscheinlich, hoffentlich nicht
der endgültige.

Es tut mir leid dass Sie noch Grund zur Sorge um Ihre kleine Tochter
haben. Die Differentialdiagnose ist so unsicher wie sie ja besser wissen
als ich. Die Einzelheiten sprechen ja nur für Hysterie aber man kann
doch nie wissen.

Unser heuriger Kongress ist durch die Berufung Jungs nach New
York in Frage gestellt. Sie werden ihn gewiss dort sehen. Es ist vielleicht
besser, wenn wir in längeren Zeiträumen zusammentreffen. Wir haben
einander dann mehr zu sagen. In meinen Arbeiten über Religionspsychologie bin ich unterwegs bei der Psychologie der Primitiven aufge-
halten worden. Imago wird in diesem Jahrgang noch zwei Beiträge von
mir bringen. Das Tabu und die Ambivalenz und die Magie und die
Allmacht der Gedanken. Ein Aufsatz über die Infantile Wiederkehr
des Totemismus wird wahrscheinlich diese Arbeit abschliessen.

Ich grüsse Sie herzlich und empfehle mich Ihrer freundlichen Erinnerung

Ihr
Freud

25. 6. 12
Wien, IX. Berggasse 19.

Verehrter Herr Kollege

Es thut mir leid dass Sie sich durch Dr. Allen Starr's Äusserungen
stören liessen. Ich konnte kühl bleiben, denn ich wusste dass mir St.
persönlich ganz unbekannt ist, und das Problem, woher es auch so
genau stammen mag erschien mir nicht interessant genug. Seine Aus-
künfte über meine jungen Jahre haben mich sehr amüsiert. Ich wollte
er hätte Recht damit gehabt.

Ihr Anerbieten einige meiner kürzeren Aufsätze aus dem Zentralblatt
übersetzen zu lassen hat mich sehr gefreut obwohl ich kaum glaube
dass jene solche Auszeichnung verdienen. Ich habe schon in voriger
Woche Dr. Brill geschrieben und ihn gebeten Ihnen direkte Antwort
zu geben denn er besitzt mein förmliches Versprechen dass Über-

setzungen ins Englische durch seine Hand gehen sollen. Ich erwarte dass er ohne weiteres einwilligen wird.

Ihr Artikel in der Imago hat viel Beifall gefunden und wird vielleicht Dr. Ferenczi Anlass zu einer Entgegnung geben in welcher unser bescheidener Standpunkt vertreten werden soll. Ich war sehr erfreut von Jones zu hören dass das Interesse für die Ψ A in Amerika nicht nachlässt. Ihr Name muss uns noch viele Anhänger werben.

   Mit herzlichen Grüssen

Ihr freundschaftlich ergebener
Freud

Karlsbad
18.7.12

Verehrter Herr Kollege

Ich habe heute Brief von Dr. Brill in Sachen der Übersetzung bekommen und kann deutlich merken, dass er Einwendungen hat, mit dem Verleger nicht einverstanden ist udgl. [und dergleichen] Da er sich um die Übersetzung meiner Bücher so sehr verdient gemacht hat und ich mich vor Ihnen nicht zu schämen brauche wenn ich der Treue Opfer bringe, bitte ich Sie, auf Ihre Absicht zu verzichten. Ich will gerne jedem einzelnen meiner Freunde den Eindruck lassen dass ich ihm etwas zu Gefallen thue. Diesmal scheint Dr. Brill in diesem Falle zu sein. Ich bin hier in Kur und zur Unthätigkeit genötigt. Hoffe auch Sie in Ihrer Erholung im Camp oder anderswo und grüsse Sie mit den Ihrigen herzlich.

Ihr treu ergebener
Freud

Karersee 20. Aug. 12
Wien, IX. Berggasse 19.

Verehrter Dr. Putnam

Da es gestern genau drei Jahre waren dass ich die Reise nach Amerika antrat, die mir unter anderem Gewinn Ihre Bekanntschaft — ich darf vielleicht sagen: Ihre Freundschaft eintrug, darf ich die Beantwortung Ihres mir hierher nachgeschickten Briefes nicht länger aufschieben.

   Ich danke Ihnen herzlich dafür, dass Sie das Aufgeben der von Ihnen geplanten Übersetzungen so ohne Empfindlichkeit hingenommen haben. Ich weiss Ihr Ideal ist ein ethisches und Sie richten auch Ihr Leben danach. Von Jones habe ich gehört, dass Sie am liebsten die Analytiker als ganz vollkommene Menschen sehen möchten. Aber wie weit sind wir alle davon entfernt. Ich habe beständig persönliche Empfindlichkeiten zu beschwichtigen und mich selbst gegen solche zu wehren. Nach dem schmählichen Abfall von Adler, der ein begabter Denker aber ein bösartiger Paranoiker ist, habe ich jetzt Schwierigkeiten selbst mit unserem Freunde Jung der offenbar seine eigene Entwicklung aus der Neurose noch nicht beendet hat. Doch darf ich hoffen dass Jung der Sache im vollen Umfange treu bleiben wird und meine Sympathien für ihn haben keine grossen Einschränkungen erfahren. Nur die persönliche Intimität hat etwas gelitten.

Das spricht, meine ich, nicht gegen die Macht der Analyse sondern zeigt nur dass sie bei uns die Richtung nicht auf die eigene Person, sondern auf den andern hat und dass wir schliesslich wie ganz natürlich, auch nur mit Motoren von bestimmter nicht unbegrenzter Energie arbeiten.

Selbst gegenwärtig auf dem herrlichsten Punkt unserer Dolomiten wünsche ich Ihnen und den Ihren die schönste Sommererholung im Camp oder abroad.

Ihr treu ergebener
Freud

28. XI. 12
Wien, IX. Berggasse 19.

Verehrter Herr Kollege
Die Arbeit die Sie ankündigen (12 Nov.) ist noch nicht eingetroffen doch brauche ich sie nicht abzuwarten um zu wissen, dass sie uns aufs höchste interessieren und unserer Zeitschrift zur Zierde gereichen wird. Der Einspruch unseres Freundes Ferenczi hat die Bedeutsamkeit Ihrer Gedankengänge nicht übersehen.

Ich hoffe Sie haben nichts dagegen dass der Aufsatz in der neuen "Internat. Zeitsch. f. ärztliche Psychoanalyse" erscheint. Sie wissen dass ich durch eine Verräterei von Stekel genötigt worden bin ihm das Zentralblatt zu überlassen und mit fast allen unseren Mitarbeitern in ein neues Heim zu übersiedeln. Ihre Zustimmung zu diesem neuen Organ um die ich in einem Zirkular gebeten habe, ist hoffentlich unterwegs.

Vorigen Sonntag fand eine Zusammenkunft in München statt (Jung, Riklin, Seif, Abraham, Jones, ich und der Sekretär von Zürich in Vertretung Maeders) die einen höchst befriedigenden Verlauf nahm. Es wurde beschlossen das neue Blatt an Stelle des Zentralblatts zum offiziellen Organ zu erheben. Die Kollegen benahmen sich charmant gegen mich, Jung nicht am wenigsten. Eine persönliche Aussprache zwischen uns hat eine Menge überflüssiger Empfindlichkeiten weggeräumt. Ich hoffe auf weiteres erfolgreiches Zusammenwirken. Theoretische Differenzen brauchen es nicht zu trüben, ich werde in der Libidofrage kaum seine Modifikation akzeptieren können, da alle meine Erfahrungen gegen diese Auffassung sprechen.

Indem ich Sie herzlich grüsse und von Ihrem Wohlbefinden zu hören hoffe,

Ihr aufrichtig ergebener
Freud

3. XII. 12.
Wien, IX. Berggasse 19.

Verehrter Herr Kollege

Vielen Dank für Ihre schöne Bereitwilligkeit zur Teilnahme an unserem neuen Organ! Es ist aber gar kein neues Organ sondern unser altes Zentralblatt welches in Folge des Verrats des Redakteurs in ein neues Kleid gesteckt werden musste. Sie werden alle vertrauten Mitarbeiter in der Internat. Zeitsch. für ärztliche Ψ A wiederfinden und hoffentlich treten Sie dort häufig als Autor hervor. Ihr angekündigter Beitrag ist noch nicht eingetroffen.

Es ist natürlich dass ich viel Mühe mit meinen — Mitarbeitern habe, oft soviel wie mit der Arbeit selbst. Stekels Verlust wird allgemein als grosser Gewinn eingeschätzt.

Ich grüsse Sie herzlich

Ihr aufrichtig ergebener
Freud

1.1.1913
Wien, IX. Berggasse 19.

Verehrter Herr Kollege

Es freut mich die Thätigkeit dieses neuen Jahres mit einem Schreiben an Sie zu beginnen.

Ich danke Ihnen herzlich für Ihre Absicht unsere Zeitschrift werkätig zu unterstützen. Ebensosehr aber weil ich aus Ihren Worten zu entnehmen glaube dass Sie nicht an mir irre geworden sind trotz der vielen persönlichen Angriffe, denen ich jetzt und gewiss noch eine Zeitlang später ausgesetzt sein werde. Sie glauben mir auch, dass ich dadurch nicht sehr erschüttert bin, weil ich die psychologische Notwendigkeit solcher Vorgänge zu gut verstehe. Ich habe dabei nicht gerade Stekel im Auge, den zu verlieren eigentlich ein Gewinn war sondern wesentlich Jung den ich stark überschätzt und auf den ich viel persönliche Neigung abgelagert hatte. Wissenschaftliche Differenzen sind ja in der Entwicklung einer Wissenschaft unvermeidlich und selbst Irrtümer haben, wie ich es ja an mir selbst erfahren konnte, vieles, was fördert. Aber dass solche Abweichungen und Neuerungen theoretischer Natur mit so viel Verletzung berechtigter persönlichen Gefühle auftreten müssen, macht der menschlichen Natur allerdings wenig Ehre.

Dass ich Jung's neue Ansichten für "regressive" Irrtümer halte, ist ja selbstverständlich und hat für andere wenig Beweiskraft. Es soll da ein jeder lieber seine eigenen Erfahrungen und den Eindruck der angehörten Argumente befragen. Ich stehe dabei wie unter dem Eindruck eines Déjà vu. Ich habe all das am Widerstand der Nichtanalytiker schon erlebt was sich jetzt beim Widerstand der Halbanalytiker wiederholt.

Ihren angekündigten Arbeiten sehen wir mit grossem Interesse entgegen. Lassen Sie sich durch unser philosophisches Unverständnis nicht in der Produktion oder Mitteilung stören. Wir sind Leute, die hierfür nicht kompetent sind, weil wir auf anderen Gebieten arbeiten, aber wir hören ihnen doch andächtig zu, und nach uns werden andere, freiere Analytiker kommen, für die Ihre Anregungen fruchtbar werden können.

Mit herzlichen wünschen für ihr und der Ihriger Wohlergehen im beginnenden Jahre

Ihr getreuer
Freud

21. 1. 13.
Wien, IX, Berggasse 19.

Verehrter Herr Kollege

Ich habe Ihren Aufsatz heute erhalten, durchgelesen und werde ihn natürlich unverkürzt der internationalen Zeitschrift zuwenden, deren erste Nummer in diesen Tagen erwartet wird. Jetzt, wo sich ein Bedürfnis nach theoretischer Fortbildung der Ψ A Grundannahmen herausstellt wird es ein besonderes Interesse haben, an Ihre Postulate gemahnt zu werden.

Der zweite angekündigte Aufsatz, die Reaktion auf Dr. Reik's Bemerkung ist in der Sendung *nicht* enthalten gewesen. Betreffs seiner Verwendung erlaube ich mir folgende Bemerkung: Die Internat. Zeitschrift hält sich für die legitime Nachfolgerin des Zentralblattes, da sie den Herausgeber und 9/10 der Mitarbeiter von ihm übernommen, ihm nur Namen und Redakteur gelassen hat. Sie hat sich das Recht zugeschrieben Artikelserien Anfragen etc. die dort begonnen wurden, fortzuführen, wovon die in wenigen Lagen vorliegende erste Nummer Sie überzeugen wird. Wir bitten Sie unseren Standpunkt anzunehmen und uns die Entgegnung auf das Referat von Reik so als ob es bei uns an seinem richtigen Platze wäre, zu überlassen. Eine Beziehung zum Privatorgan von Dr. Stekel können wir nicht pflegen. Mit ergebenem Dank für Ihre Zusendung

und herzlichen Gruss
Ihr Freud

11. 3. 13.
Wien, IX. Berggasse 19.

Verehrter Dr. Putnam

Ich danke Ihnen herzlich für die versprochenen Beiträge und zuletzt für die Mitteilung Ihres Schreibens an Dr. Stekel welches über Ihre Stellung keine Zweifel bestehen lässt. Der äussere Aspekt unserer Bewegung mag sich durch den Abfall oder die Abfallsneigungen mancher Personen etwas geändert haben seit unserem letzten Zusammentreffen. Im Grunde ist nichts Schädliches geschehen und Fortschritt und Ausbreitung gehen in befriedigender Weise weiter. Es ist selbstverständlich, dass Einigkeit in der Ψ A, wo der persönliche Fehler eine so grosse Rolle spielt noch schwieriger zu erzielen ist als auf anderen Forschungsgebieten. Ich weiss nicht ob Sie uns das Vergnügen bereiten werden diesen Sept. in Europa zu verbringen und an dem für den 7/8 d.M. festgesetzen Kongress theilzunehmen. Wir würden es alle als sehr wünschenswert betrachten. Vom Befinden Ihrer Tochter schrieben Sie lange nichts, darum darf ich annehmen, dass sich eine bescheidene Neurose anstatt der gefürchteten Erkrankung bei ihr herausgestellt hat.

Was ich bei meiner schweren ärztlichen Arbeit produzieren kann findet ja regelmässig seinen Weg zu Ihnen. Meine nächste Publikation in einem Sommerheft der Imago — die vierte der Reihe — möchte Ihr besonderes Interesse erbitten, erwartet allerdings auch bei Ihnen ein Kopfschütteln zu provozieren.

Mit herzlichen Grüssen
Ihr sehr ergebener
Freud

13. XI. 13
Wien IX. Berggasse 19

Verehrter Herr Kollege

Ich danke für Ihre wiederholten Zusendungen u versuche mit meinem neuen Buch "Totem u Tabu" zu revanchiren.

Dass Sie nicht auf dem Kongress in München zugegen waren, hat auch mir sehr leid gethan. Ich weiss zwar, dass manches Ihrer theoretischen Neigungen auf der andern Seite stehen, aber es wäre gut gewesen, wenn Sie sich von der Natur der schwebenden Differenzen selbst hätten überzeugen können. Vielleicht hätte auch Ihre Gegenwart manche der Formen gemildert, in denen sich die Spaltung geäussert hat. Dass die Ψ A die Analytiker selbst nicht besser, nicht vornehmer und charaktervoller gemacht hat, bleibt für mich eine Enttäuschung. Wahrscheinlich hatte ich Unrecht, es zu erwarten.

Mit herzlichem Gruss
Ihr ergebener
Freud

30. 3. 14
Wien, IX, Berggasse 19

Verehrter Herr Kollege

Heute Ihre Arbeit aus dem Am. J. of Med. Sciences March 1914 erhalten und gelesen. Sie hat mir ausserordentlich gefallen, vielleicht am besten unter den ausgezeichneten, beredten und inhaltsreichen Schriften die Sie mir zugeschickt haben; vielleicht aber nur darum, weil sie die letzte ist. Möge sie nun nicht lange die letzte bleiben.

Ich weiss keine Stelle zu nennen, an welcher ich mich nicht voll mit Ihnen identifiziren könnte, soweit die Ψ A in Betracht kommt. Von der Philosophie verstehe ich bekanntlich nichts, mit der Erkenntniskritik (mit, nicht vor) hört da mein Interesse auf. Ich bin auch ganz mit Ihnen einverstanden, dass die Ψ A Behandlung einen Platz aufzusuchen und einzunehmen habe unter den Methoden, wie die ethische und intellektuelle Entwicklung des Einzelnen möglichst hoch zu bringen sei. Unsere Differenz ist z. Th. rein praktischer Natur u beschränkt sich darauf, dass ich die weitere Erziehung nicht in die Hände des Psychoanalytikers legen möchte. Ich glaube ja auch nicht, dass die Ψ A jede andere körperliche Behandlung überflüssig macht; doch habe ich immer gefunden dass es unmöglich ist, die Ψ A mit einer noch so berechtigten somatischen Therapie zu kombiniren, weil dann diese letztere sofort die Ψ A in den Hintergrund drängt. Ich glaube der

Grund hiefür liegt an dem ganz besonders hohen Widerstandsdruck, unter dem die Ψ A Arbeit steht, dieser kommt aber auch für den Arzt selbst in Betracht. (Die Analytiker sind ja selbst weit entfernt von dem Ideal, das Sie mit Recht fordern.) Sowie man ihnen die Aufgabe zugesteht, an der Sublimirung zu arbeiten, hasten sie von der aufopferungsvollen Ψ A Arbeit möglichst rasch weg, um zur bequemeren, erfreulicheren Thätigkeit als Lehrer und Vorbilder aller Tugenden zu kommen wie wir es jetzt in Zürich erleben. Dabei ist die Ψ A noch nicht halb fertig in der Wissenschaft geschweige denn, dass sie am Einzelnen weit genug geführt würde.

The great ethical element in the Ψ A work is truth and again truth and this should suffice for most people. Courage and truth are of what they are mostly deficient.

Yours sincerely\
Freud

17. 5. 14\
Wien IX. Berggasse 19

Verehrter Herr Kollege

Nach der Lektüre Ihres letzten Aufsatzes über Traumdeutung im J. of abn. psych. fühle ich mich gedrängt Ihnen wieder zu danken. Ich frage mich aber auch, warum andere diese einfachen Fragen nicht ebenso zu lösen wissen? Es kann doch nur an den Motiven gelegen sein, die Sie ja auch andeuten.

Ich theile gewiss den grossen Respekt nicht, den Sie den Theorien Adlers bezeugen. Sie scheinen mir den Verlust der Traumdeutung und der Lehre vom Unbewussten nicht wert zu sein. Was sie verläugnen, ist für sie charakteristischer, als was sie behaupten; mit einem grossen Teil des Letzteren sind wir ja alle einverstanden, nur kommt es für die *Auflösung der Neurosen* usw, nicht in Betracht.

Ich bin gleichzeitig so frei, Ihnen einen Aufsatz zususchicken den Sie bereits gelesen haben dürften, dessen Autor sich nicht öffentlich zu ihm bekannt hat weil er — ausnahmsweise nichts von Sexualität enthält.

In der Hoffnung dass Sie sich eines ungestörten Wolseins erfreuen

Ihr herzlich ergebener\
Freud

19.6.14
Wien, IX. Berggasse 19.

Verehrter Freund und Kollege

Ich habe mit grossen Bedauern die Nachricht von dem Hinscheiden Ihres Bruders vernommen und danke Ihnen sehr für die Zusendung des Nachrufes, mittels dessen ich gewisse Züge meiner Erinnerung von ihm, z. B. seine liebenswürdige Hilfeleistungen besser verstehe.

Ich danke Ihnen auch für die Selbstkritik in Betreff Adler's und ergreife die Gelegenheit, Sie auf eine Schrift vorzubereiten, welche Ihnen demnächst in mehreren Exemplaren — zur gütigen Verteilung unter den Mitgliedern der neuen Bostoner Gruppe von der wir noch keine Adresse haben — zugehen wird. Mir fällt wiederum wie gewöhnlich die schwerste Aufgabe zu, diesmal mich gegen Leute zu wehren, sie anzuklagen und von mir zu weisen die sich durch viele Jahre meine Schüler genannt haben und alles meiner Anregung verdanken. Ich bin keine streitbare Natur, ja ich teile nicht die so häufige Meinung, das wissenschaftlicher Streit Klärung und Förderung bringt. Aber ich mag auch die faulen Kompromisse nicht und würde nichts für eine unfruchtbare Versöhnung opfern.

Ich hoffe dass die Schweizer und ihr Anhang nach der Lektüre meiner Streitschrift im neuen Jahrbuch den Verein verlassen werden, so dass wir wieder im Wesen einig und mit freundlichen Gefühlen gegeneinander unsere Kongresse abhalten können. Möglich dass sich die Spaltung dann nach Amerika fortsetzt, wo ja Jeliffe Parteigänger Jungs ist.

Mit grossem Bedauern höre ich dass Sie auch heuer nicht nach Europa kommen werden. Ich komme auch nicht sobald nach Amerika; lassen Sie mich hoffen, dass der dünne, zwischen uns ausgespannte Faden von Korrespondenz nicht so bald reissen wird.

Ihr in Hochachtung ergebener
Freud

9 3. 15
Wien, IX, Berggasse 19.

Verehrter Freund

Ihr Händedruck über den weiten Ozean hat mich sehr erfreut. Seien Sie nur ver-sichert, dass auch die Kastaiungen dieses Krieges keine Entfremdung zwischen uns hervorrufen werden. Ich könnte mir Vorwürfe machen, dass ich Ihre Zuschriften nicht schon früher ausführlich beantwortet. Allein die Idee des Zensors lähmt die Mitteilsamkeit.

Dass Sie ein Buch schreiben, weiss ich durch Jones, von dem gelegentlich ein Brief durchdringt. Es thut mir leid zu hören dass ich es erst in einigen Monaten werde lesen können.

Die Zeit ist natürlich der Produktion nicht günstig. Zu Beginn des Krieges habe ich in einer gewaltsamen Aufraffung eine grosse Krankengeschichte geschrieben, die jetzt auf die Publikation im Jahrbuch wartet. Dann kam die Lähmung und seither arbeite ich mühselig und spärlich. Wir führen unsere beiden Zeitschriften fort. Die erste Nummer des neuen Jahrganges der Inter. Zeitsch. bringt einen technischen Beitrag von mir (Übertragungsliebe) über den ich gerne Ihre Meinung hörte. Für die nächste erste Nummer der Imago muss ich einen zeitgemässen Aufsatz über die Enttäuschung dieses Krieges schreiben, der mir gar kein Vergnügen macht, wol auch anderen nicht gefallen wird. Meine ärztliche Thätigkeit ist auf ein schlechtes Dritteil herabgesunken an der so gewonnent freien Zeit hat man keine Freude.

Zwei meiner Söhne sind bei der Armee, der eine kämpft bereits seit Wochen in Galizien und lobt bis jetzt sein Befinden sehr, der andere wird wol in einigen Wochen aus der Ausbildung an die Front kommen. Ein dritter Sohn und meine beiden Schwieger-söhne sind vorläufig noch frei. Die Frauen beschäftigen sich, soviel sie können, mit den Aufgaben die ihnen in dieser Zeit gestellt sind.

Mr [X] und Mr [Y] erinnere ich beide sehr gut. Ich danke Ihnen für alle Nachrichten über das Interesse an unserer Wissenschaft in Ihrer Nähe u konstatire mit Befriedigung, dass unser Postverkehr mit Amerika noch aufrecht erhalten ist.

Herzlich grüssend
Ihr Freud

7. 6. 15.
Wien, IX. Berggasse 19.

Verehrter Freund

Höchst angenehm überrascht! Ich meinte, dass ein Brief von hier keine Aussicht hat über den Ozean zu kommen und hatte darum auch Ihr letztes liebenswürdiges Schreiben in dumpfer Resignation nicht beantwortet. Nun erfahre ich wie un-logisch die Hoffnung macht! Dass Briefe von Amerika nach Wien kommen, ist doch noch kein Beweis dafür dass der umgekehrte Weg frei ist.

Geben Sie mir auf einer Karte einen Beweis, dass Sie diesen Brief erhalten haben. Ich habe dann den Mut, Ihnen nach Erhalt Ihres angekündigten Buches ausführlich zu schreiben, ein Mut der mir heute noch fehlt.

Mein Haupteindruck ist jedoch, dass ich weit primitiver, bescheidener, unsublimirter bin als mein lieber Freund in Boston. Ich sehe seinen edlen Ehrgeiz, seine hohe Wissbegierde und vergleiche damit meine Beschränkung auf das Nächste, Greifbarste und doch eigentlich Kleinliche, und meine Neig-ung, sich mit dem zu begnügen, was sich erreichen lässt. Ich glaube nicht dass mir die *Wertschätzung* für das von Ihnen Angestrebte fehlt, sondern mich schreckt die grosse Unsicherheit, ich bin eher ängstlich als kühn und opfere gern sovieles für die Empfindung auf festem Boden zu stehen.

Die Nichtswürdigkeit der Menschen, auch der Analytiker hat mir immer grossen Eindruck gemacht. Aber warum sollten die Analysirten durchaus die besseren sein? Die Analyse macht einheitlich aber nicht an und für sich gut. Ich glaube nicht wie Sokrates und Putnam, dass alle Untugenden in einer Art von Un-klarheit und Unwissenheit begründet sind. Ich meine dass man der Analyse zu viel aufbürdet, wenn man von ihr verlangt dass sie die jedem theuersten Ideale realisiren soll.

Also beruhigen Sie mich über das Schicksal dieses Briefes. Ich werde in meiner gegenwärtigen Isolierung doppelt froh sein antworten zu können.

> Ihr in herzlicher Freundschaft
> ergebener
> Freud

8. 7. 15
Wien IX, Berggasse 19

Verehrter Freund

Ihr Buch On Human Motives ist endlich, lange nach seiner Ankündigung, angekom-men. Ich habe seine Lektüre noch nicht vollendet, aber doch die für mich bedeutungsvollsten Abschnitte über Religion und über Ψ A schon gelesen und gebe dem Drang nach, Ihnen etwas darüber zu schreiben.

Lob und Anerkennung verlangen Sie von mir gewiss nicht. Es ist mir angenehm zu denken, dass es bei Ihren Landsleuten Eindruck machen und bei vielen die tief gewurzelten Widerstände erschüttern wird.

Auf Seite 20 fand ich die Stelle, die ich als mass-gebend für meine eigene Person gelten lassen muss. To accustom ourselves to the study of immaturity and childhood before . . . undesirable limitation of our vision . . . etc.

Ich anerkenne, das ist mein Fall. Ich bin sicherlich inkompetent, über die andere Seite zu urteilen. Ich muss wol diese Einseitigkeit gebraucht haben, um das Verborgene sehen zu können, das sich den anderen zu entziehen weiss. Dies ist also die Recht-fertigung meiner Abwehraktion. Die Einseitigkeit war auch einmal etwas Brauchbares.

Dagegen bedeutet es weniger, wenn die Argumente für die Realität unserer Ideale mir keinen starken Eindruck machen konnten. Ich kann den Übergang von der Ψ Realität unserer Vollkommenheiten zur faktischen Existenz derselben nicht finden. Sie werden sich nicht wundern. Sie wissen ja, wie wenig man von Argumenten erwarten darf. Ich will hinzufügen, ich habe gar keine Angst vor dem lieben Gott. Wenn wir einander einmal begegneten, hätte ich ihm mehr Vorwürfe zu machen, als er an mir aussetzen könnte. Ich würde ihn fragen, warum er mich nicht intellektuell besser ausgestattet hat, und er könnte mir nicht vorhalten, dass ich von meiner angeblichen Freiheit nicht den besten Gebrauch gemacht habe. (Nebenbei bemerkt, ich weiss, dass jeder einzelne ein Stück Lebensenergie re-praesentirt sehe aber nicht ein was Energie mit Freiheit (Unbedingtheit) zu thun hat. Sie müssen nämlich von mir wissen, dass ich mit meiner Begabung immer unzufrieden war und vor mir genau zu begründen weiss, in welchen Punkten dass ich mich aber für einen sehr moralischen Menschen halte, der den guten Ausspruch von Th. Vischer unterschreiben kann: Das Moralische versteht sich von selbst. Ich glaube, an Rechtssinn und Rücksicht für den Nebenmenschen, an Missvergnügen, andere leiden zu machen oder zu übervorteilen kann ich es mit den Besten, die ich kennengelernt habe, aufnehmen. Ich habe eigentlich nie etwas Gemeines und Boshaftes gethan und spüre auch keine Versuchung dazu, bin also gar nicht stolz darauf. Ich verstehe die Sittlichkeit, von der wir hier sprechen nämlich im sozialen Sinne, nicht im sexuellen. Die sexuelle Moralität, wie die Gesellschaft, am extremsten die amerikanische, sie definiert, scheint mir sehr verächtlich. Ich vertrete ein ungleich freieres Sexualleben, wenngleich ich selbst sehr wenig von solcher Freiheit geübt habe. Gerade nur soweit, dass ich mir selbst bei der Begrenzung des auf diesem Gebiet Erlaubten geglaubt habe.

Die Betonung der sittlichen Anforderungen in der Öffentlichkeit macht mir oft einen peinlichen Eindruck. Was ich von religiös-ethischer Bekehrung gesehen habe, war nicht einladend. Da war z. B. Jung, ein mir sympathischer Mensch, so lange er blind dahinlebte wie ich. Dann kam bei ihm die religiös-ethische "Crisis", mit höherer Sittlichkeit, Wiedergeburt u Bergson und gleichzeitig Lüge, Brutalität und antisemitische Überhebung gegen mich. Es war nicht das erste, nur das letzte Erlebnis, das meine Ab-neigung gegen die heiligen Bekehrten bestärkt hat.

Einen Punkt sehe ich aber, an dem ich mit Ihnen gehen kann. Wenn ich mich frage, warum ich immer gestrebt habe, ehrlich, für den Anderen schonungsvoll und wo möglich gütig zu sein, und warum ich es nicht aufgegeben, als ich merkte, dass man dadurch zu Schaden kommt, zum Amboss wird, weil die Anderen brutal und unverlässlich sind, dann weiss ich allerdings keine Antwort. Vernünftig war es natürlich nicht. Einen besonderen ethischen Ansporn habe ich in der Jugend auch nicht empfunden; es fehlt mir auch eine deutliche Befriedigung dabei, wenn ich urteile, dass ich besser bin als die Anderen! Sie sind vielleicht der erste, vor dem ich mich dessen rühme. Man könnte gerade meinen Fall also als Beweis für Ihre Behauptung anführen, dass ein solcher Idealdrang ein wesentliches Stück unserer Anlage bildet. Wenn nur bei den anderen mehr von dieser wertvollen Anlage zu bemerken wäre! Ich glaube im Geheimen, wenn man die Mittel besässe, die Triebsublimir-ungen ebenso gründlich zu studiren wie ihre Verdrängungen, könnte man auf recht natürliche psychologische Auf-klärungen stossen, und sich Ihre menschen-freundliche Annahme ersparen. Aber wie gesagt, ich weiss nichts darüber. Warum ich — übrigens meine 6 erwachsenen Kinder ebenso — ein durchaus anständiger Mensch sein muss, ist mir ganz unverständlich. Dazu noch folgende Überlegung; wenn die Kenntnis der menschlichen Seele noch so unvollkommen ist, dass es meinen armseligen Fähigkeiten gelingen konnte, so wichtige Funde zu machen, so ist es offen-bar zu früh, sich für oder gegen Annahmen wie die Ihrigen zu erklären.

Gestatten Sie mir noch einen kleinen Irrtum richtig zu stellen, der ohne Be-deutung für die Weltgeschichte ist. Ich war nämlich niemals Breuers Assistent, habe seinen berühmten ersten Fall nie gesehen, kenne ihn nur aus B's Mitteil-ungen Jahre nachher. Diese historische Unrich-tigkeit ist wohl die einzige, die Ihnen unterlaufen ist. Alles was Sie sonst über die Ψ A sagen, kann ich ohne Opfer unter-schreiben. Vorläufig verträgt sich die Ψ A wirklich mit verschiedenen Welt-anschauungen. Ob sie aber ihr letztes Wort schon gesprochen hat? Mir ist es bisher nie um die umfassende Synthese zu thun gewesen, sondern, stets nur um die Sicherheit. Diese verdient, dass man ihr alles andere opfert.

Ich grüsse Sie herzlich u wünsche Ihnen fortdauernde Gesundheit und Arbeits-lust. Selbst benütze ich die Arbeitspause dieser Zeit zur Fertigstellung eines Buches, das zwölf psychologische Abhand-lungen zusammenfassen soll.

Ihr treu ergebener
Freud

26 Jan 16
Wien. IX. Berggasse 19.

Verehrter Freund

Verkehr ist wirklich schwer in dieser Zeit. Nach dem Beispiel von Prof. Holt's Buch zu urteilen, das nicht angekommen ist, mag ich manche Zuschrift von Ihnen die mich erfreut hätte, eingebüsst haben. Um so froher bin ich, Ihre Versicherung zu haben, dass Sie meiner noch in Freundschaft gedenken und Ihr Interesse für unsere Wissenschaft fortwährend betätigen. Ihren Aufsatz über Adler werde ich gewiss eines Tages lesen können. Ich leide hier ziemlich unter der Vereinsam-ung. Meine besten Helfer, Rank, Abraham, Ferenczi sind ferne und so beschäftigt, dass wir nur selten von einander hören. Alle Entfernungen sind ja durch den Krieg ungemein vergrössert worden. Mit dem Reste der hier anwesenden und der Hilfe der noch erreichbaren Mitarbeiter halte ich die beiden Zeitschriften aufrecht. Von der Internat. Zeitsch sind 1915 6 Hefte erschienen, von der Imago 3. Ich weiss nicht ob Sie etwas davon bekommen haben. Auch meine Separata habe ich in den letzten Monaten nicht [?mehr?] verschickt.

Für grosses körperliches Wolbefinden ist es nicht die richtige Zeit; es liegt auch zu wenig daran. Zwei meiner Söhne sind im Krieg, beide bis jetzt wol und beide haben sich ausgezeichnet. Sie sind Offiziere, während mein Hamburger Schwiegersohn als Kanonier in Flandern dient. Wir sind mit Geduld gewappnet, da die Hoffnungen auf nahe Beendigung des Krieges uns getäuscht haben.

Ich schreibe die Vorlesungen die ich eben halte als "Einführung in die Ψ A" für den Druck nieder; sie sollen im Laufe dieses Jahres bei H. Heller in Wien erscheinen, können dem bereits Eingeführten nichts Neues bringen. Sie kennen meine Wünsche für ein langes otium cum dignitate et studio für Sie und Wolbefinden für die Ihrigen. Gedenken Sie wieder einmal

Ihres
herzlich ergebener
Freud

P. S.

Ich habe die Buchstaben einer mir ungewohnten Schrift hinge-malt, damit Sie der Beihilfe von E. Jones (oder besser Loo J.) entbehren können.

IX Bergg 19

Prof. J. J. Putnam
106 Marlborough Street
Boston, Mass.
U.S.A.

Wien 1 Okt. 16

Dear Friend

Bedaure sehr, so lange nichts von Ihnen gehört zu haben. Wollte Ihnen das erste Heft meiner "Vorlesungen" zuschicken, erfuhr aber, dass die Post es derzeit nicht annimmt. Also auf bessere Zeiten! Seien Sie herzlich gegrüsst.

von Ihrem
Freud

Index